# Psychiatry P.R.N.

*Cure sometimes, relieve often, comfort*

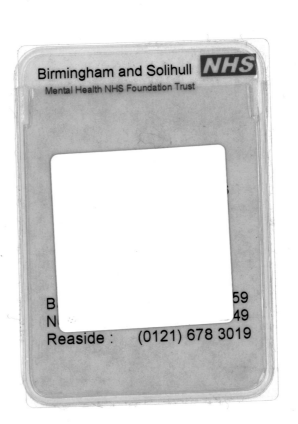

Birmingham and Solihull **NHS**
Mental Health NHS Foundation Trust

B. 59
N 49
Reaside :   (0121) 678 3019

1. From the 15th century French proverb, *Guérir quelquefois, soulager souvent, consoler toujours*. This phrase became the guiding principle of the American physician, Dr Edward Livingston Trudeau. He qualified from medical school in 1871 and was diagnosed with tuberculosis only two years later. Despite this, he dedicated his life to researching tuberculosis and built America's first sanatorium at Saranac Lake. Trudeau treated thousands of people with comfort, fresh air, rest, and good nutrition—a prescription that proved life-saving for many of his patients. In 1905, he co-founded the organization now known as The American Thoracic Society.

# Psychiatry P.R.N.

## Principles, Reality, Next Steps

*Edited by*

*Sarah Stringer*
*Laurence Church*
*Susan Davison*
*Maurice Lipsedge*

*With Illustrations by*
*Darcy Muenchrath*
*Helen Potschisvili*
*Ayesha Lodhia*

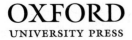
OXFORD
UNIVERSITY PRESS

# OXFORD
### UNIVERSITY PRESS

Great Clarendon Street, Oxford OX2 6DP

Oxford University Press is a department of the University of Oxford.
It furthers the University's objective of excellence in research, scholarship,
and education by publishing worldwide in

Oxford New York

Auckland Cape Town Dar es Salaam Hong Kong Karachi
Kuala Lumpur Madrid Melbourne Mexico City Nairobi
New Delhi Shanghai Taipei Toronto

With offices in

Argentina Austria Brazil Chile Czech Republic France Greece
Guatemala Hungary Italy Japan Poland Portugal Singapore
South Korea Switzerland Thailand Turkey Ukraine Vietnam

Oxford is a registered trade mark of Oxford University Press
in the UK and in certain other countries

Published in the United States
by Oxford University Press Inc., New York

© Oxford University Press 2009

British Library Cataloguing in Publication Data

Data available

Library of Congress Cataloging in Publication Data

Data available

Typeset by Graphicraft Limited, Hong Kong
Printed in Italy by L.E.G.O. S.p.A — Lavis TN

ISBN: 978-0-19-956198-8

1 3 5 7 9 10 8 6 4 2

# FOREWORD

I am delighted to write a foreword to what I believe is a ground-breaking, accessible and compassionate undergraduate textbook. When I was at medical school I quickly came to realise that there were very few books that were real 'page turners' and which could influence students in their choice of career. These included Shelia Sherlock's *Diseases of the Liver and Billary Systems*, Paul Wood's *Cardiology* and, particularly for me, Lehninger's *Medical Biochemistry*. The last influenced the whole of my career in Endocrinology. I found *Psychiatry PRN* to be similarly inspirational.

*Psychiatry PRN* is unique in that it is equally concerned with the effects of mental illness on students and doctors. It recognises that patients with psychiatric illness can sometimes be very intimidating and scary to students and that the consultation process can be extremely stressful. The approach of the authors is humane and sympathetic to all involved. It is not a patronising text in anyway, but appraises the scope and limitations of the student, doctor, patient relationships and all the therapeutic interventions.

It draws extensively from the lives of famous people in literature, fiction and non-fiction, as well as media portrayal in film and television. It also recognises that the 'celebs' can confess cathartically in public, an experience not available to ordinary people. Paradoxically this helped psychiatry to come out of the closet, if not completely— at least its head is peeping round the door. They have undoubtedly had an influence by discussing openly their own experience of suicide, physical and psychological abuse, and have made 'rehab' fashionable.

Mental illness alienates us from one another often with devastating consequences. As a former manager under the Mental Heath Act in Hackney in East London I had first hand experience of this and saw the havoc wreaked not only on the patients themselves but on their families, friends and communities.

My sister developed schizophrenia whilst a student and after many years committed suicide. Living through that I learned of her terrible anguish and my own stress, as well as my own limitations in trying to understand what was happening to her. It was relatively recently that I read a remarkable book *Night Falls Fast, Understanding Suicide*\*, that I came to terms with what had happened.

The 20th Century was seminal in unravelling some of the mysteries of the biochemistry and neuropharmacology of the brain. As well, it explored the limitations of cognitive behavioural therapy and pharmacological interventions. This is well illustrated in the publication in May 2008 by the Academy of Medical Science's report, *Brian Science, Addiction and Drugs*, which, whilst primarily about addiction, draws attention to how the 21st Century will undoubtedly bring even greater insights. It says the challenge will be to exploit the power of the multi-disciplinary approach, combining brain imaging, neuroscience, biochemistry, pharmacology and genetics with traditional psychiatric and psychological therapies.

Hopefully when you read this book you will be part of that great adventure. Those of you who take up the challenge of Psychiatry either as clinicians or as researchers for the future, your aims will be to make the future brighter for patients, their families and ultimately society itself.

Professor Dame Lesley Rees.

\*K. R. Jamison, 2001, Picador

# ACKNOWLEDGEMENTS

A huge thank you to all of our patients and students for making us think and challenging us to write *Psychiatry PRN*. Please continue to keep us on our toes.

SS: thanks to Claire for both regular and PRN TLC (yes, I owe you shoes); Martin for being the world's most patient guitarist; my brilliant family for the *can do* core beliefs.

LC: thanks to my family, especially my wife Monica and children Benjamin and Amelia for their unconditional support and love.

SD: thanks to my husband Christopher Rance for his patient technical support.

ML: thanks to Catherine Lipsedge for input on CBT and her patience and encouragement.

**Editorial Assistants**
Miss Hazel Claydon
Mrs Jennifer Haworth

**Art Team**
Ms Roxanna Chung
Dr Richard Lin
Ms Chandni Ondhia

**Culture Team**
Miss Charley Baker
Ms Anshul Deshraj
Ms Pri Lakhani
Dr Michelle Lee

**Photographs**
Mr Oli Butterworth
Dr Andrew King
Dr Richard Lin
Dr Mona Sriharan

**Advice & Feedback**
The Alzheimer's Society
Miss Charley Baker
Dr Vishal Bhavsar
Dr Zara Bolam

Dr Jessica Brock
Dr Stephen W Burton
Ms Katy Isabelle Campbell
Ms Caroline Connelly
Dr Amy Copping
Ms Rachel Crews
Mr Peter Cross
Ms Claire Davis
Dr Teif Davies
Mr Darren Felgate
Dr Fiona Gaughran
Mrs Penny Henderson
Dr Geraldine Holt
Ms Jenny Liddiard
Dr Laura Jones
Mr Jim Kelly (aged 9)
Dr Patricia Kenny
Dr Andrew King
Mr Bob Lepper
Ms Gemma McCulloch
Mencap
Dr Saman Saidi
Dr Mona Sriharan
Mr Larry Stringer
Users of www.something-fishy.org
Dr Colin Waine
Dr Deborah Woodman

**Typing, Tea, & Empathy**
Mrs Ginnie Adamson
Ms Roxanna Chung
Mrs Marion Denmark
Mrs Samantha Durrell
Dr Una Freeston
Dr Louise Gent
Mr Les Irvin
Mr Matthew J Longsborough
Mrs Julie Kitson
Mr Richard Nibbles
Ms Tracey McCord
The Quakers
Dr Saman Saidi

# BRIEF CONTENTS

# DETAILED CONTENTS

# CONTRIBUTORS

**Dr Martin Baggaley**
Consultant Psychiatrist, Medical Director, South London and Maudsley NHS Foundation Trust

**Miss Charley Baker (Literary Advisor)**
Research Associate, The University of Nottingham Conducting a study of the representation of madness in post-1945 British and American fiction, funded by The Leverhulme Trust

**Dr Ajay Bhatnagar**
Consultant Psychiatrist, North Greenwich Community Mental Health Team, Oxleas NHS Foundation Trust

**Dr Michelle Butterworth**
Consultant Addictions Psychiatrist, Kent and Medway NHS Partnership Trust; Visiting Research Associate, Institute of Psychiatry, London

**Dr Sarah Cader**
Neurology Specialist Registrar, London Rotation

**Dr Laurence Church (all 'Next steps' sections)**
Consultant Psychiatrist, Surrey and Borders Partnership NHS Foundation Trust

**Miss Hazel Claydon**
Clinical Medical Student
King's College London

**Dr Phillip Collins**
Consultant Child & Adolescent Forensic Psychiatrist, South London and Maudsley NHS Foundation Trust

**Dr Mazen Daher**
Staff Grade Psychiatrist in Addictions Psychiatry, South London and Maudsley NHS Foundation Trust

**Dr Susan Davison**
Consultant Psychiatrist in Psychotherapy, Maudsley Psychotherapy Service, South London and Maudsley NHS Foundation Trust

**Dr Mark N Haddad**
Clinical Research Fellow, Institute of Psychiatry, King's College London

**Dr Matthew Hagger**
Specialist Registrar, St Mary's Rotation, London

**Mrs Jennifer Haworth**
Clinical Medical Student, King's College London

**Dr Juliet D Hurn**
Consultant Psychiatrist, Speedwell Community Mental Health Team, South London and Maudsley NHS Foundation Trust

**Mrs Noreen Jakeman**
Principal Pharmacist for Mental Health, The Lewisham Hospital NHS Trust

**Dr Laura Jones**
Foundation Year 1 Doctor (Accident & Emergency), Cheltenham General Hospital, Gloucestershire NHS Foundation Trust

**Dr Alex Liakos**
Foundation Year 2 Doctor (Medicine & Surgery), Queen Mary's Sidcup NHS Trust

**Dr Maurice Lipsedge**
Emeritus Consultant Psychiatrist, South London and Maudsley NHS Foundation Trust; Honorary Senior Lecturer, Medical School, King's College, London

**Dr Greg Lydall**
Speciality Registrar in General Adult Psychiatry, University College London Rotation, Camden & Islington Foundation Trust, London

**Dr Amy E Manley**
Foundation Year 2 Doctor, Royal Oldham Hospital, Pennine Acute Trust

**Mr Jack Nathan**
Consultant Adult Psychotherapist, Maudsley Hospital, Institute of Psychiatry, Kings' College, London

**Dr Dimitrios Paschos**
Consultant Psychiatrist in Learning Disabilities, South London and Maudsley NHS Foundation Trust

**Dr Thomas Pollak**
Foundation Year 1 Doctor, Basildon and Thurrock University Hospitals; Honorary Research Associate at the Institute of Psychiatry

**Dr Alice M.Roberts**
Consultant Older Adult Psychiatrist, South London and Maudsley NHS Foundation Trust

**Dr Saman Saidi**
Foundation Year 1 Doctor, Centre for Clinical Research, Uppsala Universitet, Central Hospital, Sweden

**Dr Naveen Sharma**
Specialist Registrar in General Adult Psychiatry, South London and Maudsley NHS Foundation Trust

**Dr Anna Streeruwitz**
Specialist Registrar in General Adult Psychiatry, South London and Maudsley NHS Foundation Trust

**Dr Sarah Stringer (all 'Reality' sections)**
Staff Grade Older Adult Liaison Psychiatrist,
South London and Maudsley NHS Foundation
Trust; Honorary Clinical Tutor at the Institute
of Psychiatry

**Professor Janet Treasure**
Director of the Eating Disorders Unit, South London
and Maudsley NHS Foundation Trust; Professor,
King's College London

**Ms Deborah A Walker**
Consultant Psychotherapist in CBT, South London
and Maudsley NHS Foundation Trust

**Dr Sheena Webb**
Chartered Clinical Psychologist, Child & Adolescent
Mental Health, Oxleas NHS Foundation Trust

## Artists

Risk factor drawings by Ayesha Lodhia, Student,
King's College, London, United Kingdom

Clinical signs drawings by Darcy Muenchrath,
Toronto, Canada

Chapter opening drawings by Helen Potschisvili,
Student, Central Saint Martins College of Art and
Design, London, United Kingdom

# WALK THROUGH PREFACE

## Part 1 – Overview in Psychiatry

In just under 30 pages, this succinct section of the book frames the subsequent 14 chapters, which are dedicated to clinical conditions. Readers may come back to this section many times, but we suggest students read it *at least* once, and in particular, before going on placement (paying special attention to brief chapters on Safety and Essential Interview Skills).

We hope readers will find that psychiatric assessment and formulation (Chapter 1) become more familiar ground with the introduction of Vincent van Gogh as their first patient.

> ### Your first patient
>
> **History**
> *Name*
> Vincent Willem van Gogh
>
> *Date of birth*
> 30 March 1853
>
> *Background information*

## Part 2 – Clinical Conditions: Principles, Reality, Next Steps

*Psychiatry PRN* contains core content for psychiatry education, but gives prominence to clinical and practical skills, as well as exam preparation. We've taken the medical shorthand of PRN (*Pro Re Nata*) to inform the structure of this part of the book, dividing it into the following areas: Principles, Reality, and Next Steps.

Each chapter opens with *Principles*, which cover the key characteristics of a psychiatric condition. This is the typical ground of textbooks, and this book covers those same learning outcomes for medical students, but is arguably more succinct than standard texts.

The *Reality* section offers a practical articulation of clinical skills for the novice. This involves sample dialogue (highlighted with a blue tint) that might form part of the psychiatric interview, which reflects common presentations and the difficulties often encountered by medical students. The content in this section includes a general approach (Tips, Tricks and Cautionary Tales), leading to a sample interview, moving on to indicative stations for Objective Structured Clinical Examinations (OSCEs). This section has been designed to help students and lecturers get the most out of their contact time in the classroom, and to optimize preparation for placements, for the benefit of students and patients alike.

> **Suicidal ideation** (see Suicide Reality for more, p.63)
>
> • Things have been awful recently. Is it ever so bad that you want to die?

> ### 1. Alcohol misuse history (15 minutes)
>
> **Candidate's instructions**
> John Darwin is a 40-year-old builder who has been told to see the GP by his manager. You are a medical student attached to the GP surgery.
>   Please take a history of alcohol use.

The *Next Steps* section provides patient management problems in order to illustrate early working life as a doctor. Importantly, these sections highlight where psychiatric considerations overlap with medical and surgical management.

Some chapters are smaller than others as we've made coverage proportionate with typical curricula. For this reason, not all chapters include OSCE stations, to help students focus on the most clinically relevant areas.

> ### Poor rehabilitation following a heart attack
>
> You are the junior doctor on a cardiology team. Mr Jacobs is a 74-year-old man who was admitted to your ward in a dishevelled state two weeks ago, following a myocardial infarction. He has a history of congestive cardiac failure and stroke. The team are frustrated because he is not making the expected progress in his rehabil-

Discussion of medication is covered as part of management on a chapter by chapter basis, where relevant, as opposed to having a dedicated chapter on psychopharmocology. Generic names are used and readers are specifically referred to current formularies and manufacturers' instructions.

> **Antipsychotics**
>
> Antipsychotics are dopamine antagonists; they block post-synaptic D2 receptors. In general, the greater the affinity, the more effective they are in treating positive symptoms, caused by dopamine excess. Extrapyramidal side effects (EPSEs), due to generalized dopamine blockade, are

Similarly, we haven't included a dedicated chapter on forensic psychiatry, but risk considerations are brought to your attention throughout the book wherever you see this icon.

The following icons are interspersed throughout the book to denote:

 TIPS 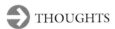 THOUGHTS  FACTS

Lecturers may have alternatives to share with their students in order to help unlock understanding, particularly of difficult or subtle areas.

> **References / Further reading**
>
> Each chapter contains references to scholarly journal and book sources. Additionally, cultural references are provided in 'film strips', which suggest further resources in the form of films, books, and quotations.

## Illustrative Content

It's a bold endeavour to include illustrations in a psychiatry textbook, but student reviewers have encouraged us to do so. The illustrations in the book will have fans and critics, but we hope the material is memorable and thought-provoking—for both camps. As with all of the content in the book, the illustrative material is designed to aid students in their understanding of psychiatric illness. At no stage has it been our intention to take a reductionist approach, nor to stereotype any particular group. Some of the drawings may be a little disturbing, but then the *lived experience* of psychiatric illness often falls into the same category.

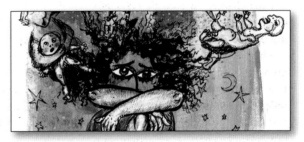

All of the chapters dedicated to clinical conditions open with an impressionistic drawing. We hope these add to the visual appeal of the book. In addition there are ten line drawings in the book, that are designed as a sort of visual mnemonic—to encourage students to think and remember. Some drawings depict clinical signs, and/or are designed to be suggestive of the experience of a particular condition, e.g. withdrawal from opiates. A small selection of black & white drawings are dedicated to risk factors and offer more in the way of visual mnemonics. All of these drawings are available online to facilitate use in the classroom or for personal study.

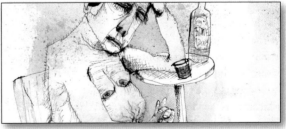
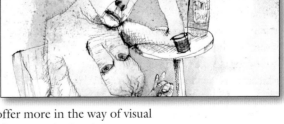

Photographs are included and are mostly found in the chapters on Substance Misuse and Organic Psychiatry. Photographs have been carefully selected to illustrate things students may not have seen before, such as particular 'street' drugs, or brain images where lesions are clearly evident.

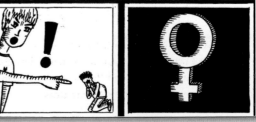

www.oxfordtextbooks.co.uk/orc/stringer/

Four scenarios have been professionally filmed in order to allow students to *preview* certain psychiatric interviews and rehearse their own clinical skills. We hope that lecturers and students will find the clips form useful preparation for seminars and, in particular, that they help to allay any apprehension ahead of placements. The interviews depicted are designed to be realistic, not perfect, so should provoke some useful tutorial discussion.

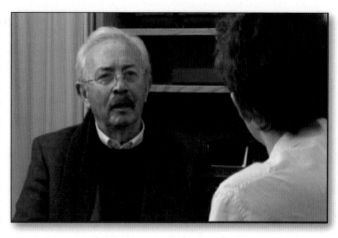

Clips are dedicated to a Mini-Mental State Examination (MMSE), depression, post-traumatic stress disorder, and assessing risk of self-harm. Lecturer and student preferences guided the choice of topics for these clips.

Also online is the *Take Me With You Guide to Assessment*, which can be downloaded, along with instructions on how to perform and mark the MMSE.

## OSCE mark sheets

Indicative mark sheets are hosted online for all of the sample OSCE stations in the book. Students can use/download these to test themselves on the OSCE stations in the book. Assessment criteria may vary depending on the year of study and institution, so these sheets are provided for general reference only—check local guidelines.

In addition to the indicative mark sheets, we've included an extra OSCE station and accompanying mark sheet for chapter 9.

**1. History of psychosis (15 minutes)**

Mark sheet for 'History of psychosis' (Rita Olsworth)

| | Satisfactory | Poor/omitted |
|---|---|---|
| **Introduction (1)** | | |
| • Gives full name and role | | |
| • Explains purpose of interview and gains consent | | |
| **History (2)** | | |
| • Duration of symptoms | | |
| • Possible triggers/stressors/life events | | |
| **Current symptoms (max 7)\*** | | |
| • Delusions | | |
|   • General content (persecutory, reference) | | |
|   • Tests conviction | | |

## Podcast

 If you like the editors' style in this book, you can hear them talk about one of their specialist topics, so go online to see which of the four Editors is speaking.

## Self assessment resources

Each chapter in Part 2 of the printed book opens with some questions, by way of a challenge to existing learning and to shape what is covered in the chapter. We've provided the answers online, along with additional self-assessment resources, in the form of Q&A items and interactive cases, which have marking functionality.

## Links

Further references to psychiatry organizations are provided as active web links. More information on some of the cultural frames of reference which are used in the book have been included as well.

## Illustrations

Finally, all of the drawings which were commissioned for the book are available online. As a lecturer, you can download these for discussion in teaching sessions. Students may wish to download the pictures in order to annotate them for revision.

# 1 PSYCHIATRIC ASSESSMENT

*Thomas Pollak, with Sarah Stringer and Maurice Lipsedge*

Starry, starry night.

Paint your palette blue and grey,

Look out on a summer's day,

With eyes that know the darkness in my soul.

*Vincent (Starry, Starry Night)*—Don McLean[1]

The information contained in the following assessment is drawn from a number of sources, particularly *The Illness of Vincent van Gogh* (Blumer 2002) and *The Yellow House* (Gayford 2006). Vincent's views on his alcohol consumption have been elaborated to show symptoms of alcohol dependence.

## Your first patient

### History
*Name*

Vincent Willem van Gogh

*Date of birth*

30 March 1853

*Background information*

Vincent van Gogh was brought to Hotel Dieu Hospital, Arles, by police on the morning of 24 December 1888. The police were contacted following an incident the previous night when Vincent threatened his friend, Paul Gauguin, with an open straight razor. He fled the scene and later reappeared at a brothel on Rue du Bout d'Arles, asking to see a prostitute named Rachel. He gave her his severed earlobe, saying, 'Guard this object very carefully'. He then left. Police discovered blood-soaked towels near the bottom of the stairs in his house, and found Vincent unconscious in his bedroom, bleeding from his left ear.

*Presenting complaint*

'I am having frightful ideas . . . I fear that God has abandoned me.'

*History of presenting complaint*

Vincent reports that for the past 4 weeks he has been aware of God punishing him. Although he denies hearing God

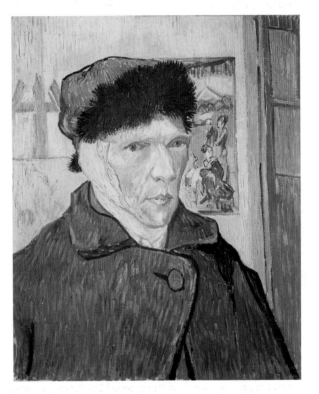

FIGURE 1.1 Self Portrait with Bandaged Ear, 1889 (oil on canvas) by Vincent van Gogh (1853–1890). © Samuel Courtauld Trust, Courtauld Institute of Art Gallery/The Bridgeman Art Library

speak to him, he says he receives divine 'communications' that only he can understand. He would not elaborate as to their nature.

He says that his thoughts have become more confused over the previous 3–4 weeks, their speed increasing to the point that 'the noise inside has become unbearable'. He reports losing the need for food, sleeping only 2 or 3 hours a night, and having to work constantly 'to regain God's favour' through his art.

Vincent does not report elevated mood but says that his mood changes as quickly as his thoughts and has been doing so for a month.

Vincent is unable to say what has caused the change in him, but referred to the 'impending treachery' of Mr Gauguin. He gave no explanation for cutting off his ear, stating that his reasons were 'quite personal'.

## Past psychiatric history

Vincent reports two previous episodes of depression, each lasting a few months. The first followed rejection by a girl in London during his early twenties. The second followed dismissal from his post as an evangelist in Belgium when he was 25. He never saw a doctor for these. Subsequent to both episodes, Vincent reports periods of immense energy and productivity where he pursued his goals of religion and art with great intensity and needed less for sleep.

## Past medical history

Vincent has suffered from gastrointestinal irritability for most of his adult life; no cause has been identified. He claims to suffer from 'seizures' but did not elaborate on these. At 29 he was treated for gonorrhoea as an inpatient in The Hague.

## Drug history

No prescribed medications.
No known drug allergies.

## Family history

Vincent's mother, Anna Cornelia, is still alive; his father was a preacher and died 3 years ago. Vincent is the eldest of six surviving siblings (Figure 1.2). Exactly one year before Vincent was born, his mother gave birth to a still-born boy, also named Vincent Willem. Vincent believes that his name is cursed. There is no family history of mental illness.

## Personal history

### Birth and early development

Vincent was born in Groot-Zundert, in The Netherlands. His mother's pregnancy and labour are believed to have been unremarkable. Developmental milestones were reached normally, although doctors had some concerns over apparent craniofacial asymmetries. Vincent's parents told him that he was a clumsy boy.

### Family background and early childhood

Vincent described himself as a moody child, often disobedient and with few friends. His early interests were

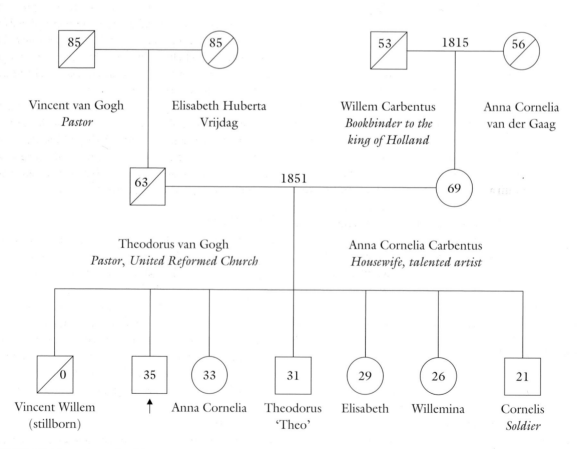

**FIGURE 1.2** Vincent van Gogh's genogram

flowers, birds, and insects, but he preferred to play alone. His younger brother Theo was always his closest friend, although Vincent described himself as being distant from his parents and other siblings.

## Education

Until the age of 12, Vincent was taught at home by a governess. He then went to boarding school until starting middle school in Tilburg, where he learnt to draw. His attendance and marks were satisfactory, although he neither worked particularly hard nor excelled in any subject; notably, he showed no special aptitude for art. At 25, Vincent began a theology degree, but dropped out within the first year.

## Occupation

Vincent worked as an apprentice for an art dealer in his uncle's company from the age of 16, travelling to Brixton, London, as part of his job. He returned to Britain at 23 to work as a supply teacher in Ramsgate. Two years later, having cut short his theology degree, Vincent became a preacher in Belgium. This was also short-lived, as he was dismissed by the church for failing to maintain a sufficiently tidy appearance. Aged 27, he took up art in Brussels.

For the past 8 years he has lived and worked as an artist in Antwerp, Neunen, Paris, and The Hague. He has had little financial success and is largely funded by his brother Theo.

## Psychosexual/relationships

Vincent's romantic life has been characterized by unrequited love and rejection. In particular, there were two unreciprocated infatuations during his twenties, one in London and the other in Etten. The second of these rejections led Vincent to deliberately harm himself, burning his hand with a lamp.

While living in The Hague, at 28, Vincent began a relationship with a prostitute named Sien, a single mother with a drinking problem. Vincent's family disapproved and placed considerable pressure on him to end the relationship, which he eventually did.

In Arles, Vincent has made frequent use of prostitutes, whom he describes as his 'sisters of mercy', although he has recently reduced contact with them because of a loss of libido. Nevertheless, he enjoys a particularly close relationship with a prostitute named Rachel.

## Substance misuse

### Alcohol

Vincent admits to drinking alcohol daily to 'stun' himself when 'the storm inside gets too loud'. He notes that without alcohol he becomes shaky and sweaty, and desperately craves a drink. Vincent reports that he needs increasing amounts of alcohol, and is currently drinking eight glasses of absinthe and 1.5 bottles of red wine a day. He has been drinking beer and wine in moderation since his late teens and started drinking absinthe 8 years ago. In the past 2 months Vincent has drunk in the mornings, causing Mr Gauguin to criticise his drinking and make Vincent feel both guilty and angry. He has never tried to give up drinking completely, but has thought about cutting down. Vincent recognizes a loss of control upon drinking and frequent blackouts when intoxicated. He has had fights with Mr Gauguin that he has not remembered subsequently, and has been barred from numerous inns in Arles for aggressive behaviour while drunk.

### Smoking

Vincent has smoked a pipe since his teens, now using 15g of tobacco per day.

### Other substances

Vincent also admits to occasionally chewing his lead-based paints, and sipping the turpentine that he uses to thin his paints. He did not offer reasons for this.

### Forensic history

Nil formal, but note aggression when drunk.

### Premorbid personality

Vincent reports that as an adolescent he was prone to lengthy periods of low mood but was 'not quite miserable'. He describes himself as hard-working and a loner. He often feels overwhelmed by setbacks, struggling to get back on track afterwards. Vincent enjoys travel and frequently moves between cities.

Vincent has strong religious convictions. Politically and morally, he believes passionately in social justice, particularly for the poor. This has shaped his life to the extent that he gave up most of his possessions to work among the poor as an evangelist in Belgium. As an artist, he claims to be producing art 'for the people'.

### Social history

Vincent's brother, Theo, is always on hand with emotional and financial support. Despite offering practical help, Vincent's mother often makes disparaging remarks about his behaviour, which she regards as odd.

Vincent moved to Arles in February 1888, with the intention of establishing a 'southern school' of artists in the South of France. For the past 9 weeks he has lived with Paul Gauguin, an artist from Paris, in a shared house he refers to as 'The Yellow House'. The citizens of Arles have not welcomed Vincent, viewing him as an eccentric.

### Collateral history

Mr Gauguin reports that over the past 9 weeks, Vincent has become increasingly irritable, flying into unpredictable rages and talking to himself. He has also been obsessed with religious issues, and speaks of profound meanings in his paintings, which are not obvious to others. He has been sleeping little, eating poorly, drinking heavily, and painting continuously. In the past month alone, Vincent has produced over 25 paintings, describing them as the best he has ever done. On one occasion Mr Gauguin noticed Vincent staring into space, his hand shaking. He dropped his paintbrush and seemed confused afterwards, unable to recall this event. Mr Gauguin believes that he may have triggered Vincent's deterioration by expressing his intention to leave Arles; he suggests that the prospect of living alone terrifies Vincent.

Mr Gauguin thinks that Vincent may have cut off his ear and given it to Rachel in emulation of a common practice in the bullfighting arenas around Arles, where a victorious bullfighter cuts off a bull's ear and presents it to his beloved.

## Mental state examination

### Appearance and behaviour

A gaunt 35-year-old white man with red hair and beard, his head bandaged, with blood seeping through on the left-hand side.[2] He was appropriately dressed in a blue cap with a furry trim and matching winter coat. He appeared unwashed, with sallow skin and coal marks on his face. He smelled of alcohol and smoked his pipe nervously throughout the interview. He had difficulty maintaining eye contact and was frequently distracted by objects in the room, particularly the yellow sunflowers arranged in a vase. Vincent whispered to himself throughout the interview, apparently responding to someone or something. He looked tense, and at one point paced the room in an agitated manner for 10 minutes. Although he was not keen to engage, there was no evidence of aggression.

### Speech

Pressure of speech: volume varied from a whisper to a shout when agitated. Tone switched between irritable, gloomy, and excited. Vincent complained that he 'could not keep up' with his thoughts and found the speed of them distressing. He showed flight of ideas, with rapid changes in topic.

### Mood

Subjectively: 'Black, black as the night!'
Objectively: Labile: switching rapidly between euphoria, tearfulness, and irritability.

### Thought

Religious themes predominated, although it was difficult to establish specific beliefs. He stated on a number of occasions that God had forsaken him and had been communicating to him through everyday objects. At one point he said, 'I am in the Garden of Gethsemane'.

He expressed persecutory delusions regarding Mr Gauguin, whom he accused of conspiring against him with other artists from Paris. Vincent would not elaborate on their alleged plans but could not be convinced of their innocence.

Vincent reported no thoughts of self-harm. When asked about his ear, he replied, 'That affair is over now'. He denied thoughts of harm to others, including Mr Gauguin.

### Perception

Vincent denied illusions or hallucinations in all modalities. However, it seems likely that he was experiencing auditory hallucinations as he whispered to himself as though talking to someone. He was also probably experiencing visual hallucinations since his eyes repeatedly tracked something unseen as if it moved around the room.

### Cognition

Vincent scored 29 out of 30 on the Mini Mental State Examination. He lost one point for not knowing which floor of the building he was on.

### Insight

Vincent showed partial insight into his condition. Although he admitted that he was ill, he insisted that the illness was a 'malady of the soul' inflicted upon him by God. He agreed to admission and to taking medication, but suggested that medicines were unlikely to work as 'they could not undo God's doing'.

## Psychiatric assessment

Psychiatric assessments can seem overwhelming; they are longer, more detailed, and have more subsections than in other medical specialties. Vincent's assessment should give you a vivid example of how to structure a history and mental state examination (MSE), demonstrating where to place the information you gather during an assessment. This section will now take you through the principles of the history and MSE, explaining relevant terms and ending with Vincent's formulation.

Before starting, be aware that the exact division of information in the history and MSE is controversial, reflecting the difficulty of summarizing a whole life into neat categories. The most important thing is that you listen to your patient's story and present it in a way that helps others understand why *this* person is suffering *this* problem at *this* time. Your assessment should lead people through the information so that your preferred diagnosis doesn't ambush them. To do this, include all the information needed to make a confident diagnosis and exclude competing diagnoses—as well as the details that bring your patient to life.

## Psychiatric history

### Background information

Set the scene with the patient's name, age, sex, and ethnicity. Explain how they came to present to the hospital or clinic and whether admission was informal (voluntary) or under a section of the Mental Health Act.

### Presenting complaint

'Always use the patient's own words'—this keeps their story fresh and stops you from misinterpreting their problem from the start. Useful starting questions might be:

- What led up to you coming into hospital?
- Have you been having any problems recently? Can you tell me about them?

### History of presenting complaint

Describing the period leading up to admission, assess the presenting complaint as you would in any history. Use NOTEPAD to ensure that you include:

- **N**ature of problem
- **O**nset
- **T**riggers
- **E**xacerbating/relieving factors
- **P**rogression (improving, worsening or staying the same; intermittent or continuous)
- **A**ssociated symptoms
- **D**isability (effect on life)

The nature of the presenting complaint is the form the problem takes, e.g. a worry, mood, delusion, hallucination, physical ailment, social problem.

Before finishing, summarize the patient's problem and ask them:

- Is there anything else you think I should know?

> Associated symptoms are guided by *your* knowledge. Patients may not know that depression is associated with insomnia and hopelessness, so ask specific questions.

### Past psychiatric history

Ask about previous contact with psychiatric services, problems treated by the GP, and times of severe stress or depression which the patient handled alone.

- Has anything like this ever happened before?
- Have you had any stress-related or mental health problems before?

Find out when past episodes occurred, how long they lasted, and whether they required admission to hospital or use of the Mental Health Act. Note past diagnoses and treatments, highlighting treatments that helped. Always check for previous risky behaviour while unwell (self-harm, suicide attempts, or violence).

### Past medical history

List past and present physical problems; not only can physical problems relate to the presentation (e.g. multiple sclerosis can cause depression), but awareness of them is vital in arranging treatment.

### Drug history

List the patient's current medications, both prescribed and over-the-counter. Always note drug allergies and side effects.

### Family history

Drawing a genogram with the patient is the clearest way to present their family. For each relative, include:

- Name, age, occupation
- Mental illness
  - Has anyone in your family suffered from stress or had to see a doctor for mental health problems?
- Physical illness
- Age and cause of death, if applicable.

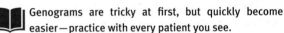 Genograms are tricky at first, but quickly become easier—practice with every patient you see.

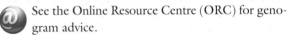 See the Online Resource Centre (ORC) for genogram advice.

### Personal history

This is the patient's life story. At first, include as much detail as possible in each section, learning how to ask questions and order information. With experience, you can act more like a film-maker or biographer, focusing on the headline events that created this person or relate in some way to their problem.

**Birth and early development**

Unless you are assessing a child or someone with a learning disability or neurological problems, it is usually enough to ask two questions:

- Do you know if there were any problems with your mother's pregnancy and your birth?
- As far as you know, did you walk and talk at the normal ages?

As a general rule of thumb, if someone doesn't know much about these things, they were probably 'normal' (i.e. a full-term spontaneous vaginal delivery with normal milestones). If there *were* any problems, find out details, including:

- Prematurity
- Labour complications/birth trauma/interventions, e.g. Caesarean section
- Time in special care/being unable to go home immediately
- Need for paediatric follow-up

## Family background and early childhood

Record periods of serious or lengthy illness, separation from parents, and neglect or abuse.

- What was it like growing up in your family?
- What were your parents and siblings like? How did you get on with them?
- Was early childhood a happy or a difficult time?

## Education

This section gives a lot of information about personality and social abilities, and some idea about intelligence. Note age and level of achievement on leaving education, e.g. three A-levels (grades BBD).

- What was school like for you?
- Did you have any problems at school?

Also explore more specific issues:

- What were your friendships like?
- Were you shy or outgoing?
- Were you bullied or did anything traumatic happen?
- Were you ever in trouble for things like bullying or truanting?
- Did you get on with teachers?
- Were you near the top, middle, or bottom of the class?

## Occupation

Chronologically list your patient's jobs, including durations and reasons for leaving jobs (e.g. promotion/resignation/dismissal). Did they enjoy working? Look for trends, e.g. numerous brief jobs that ended due to arguments with employers. This may say something important about their interpersonal relationships or response to authority.

## Psychosexual/relationships

List relationships chronologically, using common sense to decide how detailed this should be. Which was the longest relationship and what happened? What were the characteristics and can your patient see any recurring patterns?

- Age of first intercourse and number of sexual partners
- Long-term/brief

- Monogamous/not
- Heterosexual/homosexual/bisexual
- Quality of relationships (e.g. abusive, supportive)
- Marriages or civil partnerships

If currently in a relationship, ask about duration, partner's name and occupation, and whether they are content. Ask if there are any sexual problems.

### Substance misuse

This should cover past and present use of drugs, alcohol, and cigarettes. The easiest method is to take each drug individually and ask when it was first used, tracking forward from that point. Look specifically for route and amount used, including changes over time (increased amounts suggest tolerance). Note attempts at abstinence and formal detoxifications. Also note specific problems due to drug misuse (e.g. hepatitis, withdrawal fits).

### Forensic history

This covers criminal behaviour.

- Have you ever been in trouble with the police?

List offences, noting seriousness, convictions, and sentences. Clearly record details of any violent or sexual offences in the notes. Find out whether offences were committed while unwell, and think about symptoms that might increase risk, e.g. paranoia may cause someone to lash out for perceived self-protection. Consider possible forensic issues relating to your patient's disorder, e.g. theft to afford a drug habit.

 **It's often worth asking people if they ever broke the law without being caught.**

### Premorbid personality

This tries to understand *what the person was like* before they became unwell. A lot of information is reflected in the rest of the personal history, e.g. someone who bullied others at school, physically abused their partner, and lost multiple jobs after arguing with managers might be reasonably viewed as somewhat volatile.

- Before all this happened, what kind of person were you?
- How would your friends describe you?
- How do you cope under pressure?
- Do you have any strong religious or moral views?

### Social history

The social history is the patient's *current* day-to-day situation. It should cover:

- Housing (type, rented/owned, flatmates)
- Finances, including benefits

- Current employment/training
- Activities or interests
- Carer's duties
- Social network

 **Always check for final points:**

- You've told me a lot today. Is there anything we've not covered that you think I should know?

### Collateral history

A history from someone who knows the patient well is useful—especially if the patient can't or won't talk to you. Other people may be better placed than the patient to say whether behaviour or personality have changed. You need your patient's consent to actively contact their family or friends, since the act itself indicates that there is something medically or psychiatrically wrong with them. If a relative approaches *you* (e.g. while on the ward), there is no breach of confidentiality in listening to them, although you must explain that you cannot reveal your patient's information without permission. If collateral historians do not want the patient to know what they have said, document this and write the information on a separate (removable) page in the notes—consider the potential impact upon interpersonal relationships if the patient chooses to access their notes.

Don't *assume* that collateral historians are good witnesses. People may give misleading or deliberately *false* information!

## Mental state examination

*Past* psychopathology belongs in the history; if it is *present* it goes in the mental state examination (MSE). The MSE, like any other medical examination, describes your findings when you examine the patient. In a physical examination you would not report jaundice if the patient was not yellow—even if you knew that they had liver disease, or *were* jaundiced yesterday. Likewise, don't mention hallucinations in a patient's MSE unless they are hallucinating *when you see them*. Patients often present 'normally' and reporting this is as crucial as reporting pathology in accurately depicting their mental health, and monitoring deterioration or recovery. If your MSE does not show the psychopathology of the recent history, note this clearly to draw attention back to the history and ensure that it isn't overlooked (e.g. 'no hallucinations elicited in any modality, in contrast to the history obtained').

The MSE comprises:

- Appearance and behaviour
- Speech
- Mood

- Thought
- Perception
- Cognition
- Insight

Most of the MSE is covered during the history; if your patient has spent the last hour emphatically explaining the conspiracy against them, don't repeat this simply because you are 'now doing' the MSE.

### Appearance and behaviour

Imagine watching a film with the sound off. Everything you could describe would be included in appearance and behaviour (although you may want to add smells). A good description should highlight diagnostic clues and enable *anyone* to walk onto the ward and easily identify your patient.

#### General appearance

Start with age, sex, build, and ethnicity. Then note:

- Hair, make-up, clothing
- Physical problems (e.g. hemiparesis, hearing aid, dehydration)
- Scars, piercings, tattoos
- Self-care: well-kempt or self-neglecting (e.g. dishevelled, stained clothing, malodorous)

Clothing deserves a special mention if inappropriate (e.g. a bikini in the winter) or striking in some way. Sometimes it reflects the underlying mood (e.g. dark clothes in depression; bright garish clothes in mania). Very loose or tight clothing may indicate recent weight loss or gain.

#### Body language

- Facial expression, e.g. smiling, scowling, fearful
- Eye contact, e.g. responsive and appropriate/staring/downcast/avoidant/distracted
- Posture, e.g. hunched shoulders in depression
- Activity level: overactive or underactive?
- Describe *what* they are doing, e.g. 'Pacing restlessly around the room'
- Movements may seem slowed (motor retardation) in depression, or speeded up in mania

#### Other movements

- Extrapyramidal side effects are caused by antipsychotics (see p.80 for more), e.g.
  - Akathisia: unpleasant restlessness causing agitation
  - Parkinsonism: shuffling gait, 'pill rolling' tremor, slowed movements, and rigidity
  - Tardive dyskinesia: rhythmic involuntary movements of the face, limbs, and trunk, e.g. grimacing, chewing

- Repeated movements
  - Mannerisms: appear goal-directed (e.g. sweeping hair from face)
  - Stereotypies: not goal-directed (e.g. flicking fingers at air)
  - Tics: purposeless, involuntary movements involving a group of muscles (e.g. blinking)
  - Compulsions: rituals the patient feels compelled to undertake (e.g. hand-washing)
- Catatonic symptoms: these are rare, e.g. waxy flexibility (see p.78 for more)

## Rapport

Are they withdrawn and cold; polite and friendly; rude or *guarded* (suspicious or deliberately with-holding information); disinhibited (e.g. removing their clothing)?

## Other

- Responding to hallucinations, e.g. watching 'nothing', talking to an unseen companion
- Smells, e.g. body odour, urine, alcohol

### Speech

Because of the overlap between them, speech and thought are difficult to separate: speech is our window to the patient's thoughts. Think of speech as a train, and the patient's thoughts as the passengers.

- *Speed* is the rate of speech.
- The number of passengers is the abundance of thoughts.
- *The route* is the way that thoughts progress, linking from one idea (*station*) to the next.

Therefore normal speech and thought would be a train travelling at normal speed, while reasonably full of passengers. The train would travel a logical route from Station A to Station B.

The train can obviously drive too quickly or too slowly (increased or decreased rate of speech and under-lying thoughts). It can also:

- Drive too quickly, whilst overcrowded with passengers. This is *pressure of speech*, reflecting underlying *pressure of thought*. It feels like machine-gun fire and is hard to interrupt. It is usually seen in mania.
- Drive slowly with few passengers. This is *poverty of speech*, reflecting underlying *poverty of thought*, and is usually seen in depression.
- Stop without warning and throw all the passengers off. This is *thought block*: the complete emptying of the mind of thoughts, shown in speech by a sudden halt. It is sometimes seen in schizophrenia.

With normal speed and passengers, the train can make an unnecessary lengthy detour via lots of minor peripheral stations, finally reaching Station B. This is *circumstantial speech*, reflecting underlying *over-inclusive thinking* which adds excessive details and subclauses to every sentence.

While overcrowded and speeding, the train can make a series of sudden detours, quickly passing through a number of unexpected stations. This is *flight of ideas*. The route is understandable, because there is always a reason for each detour. Ideas may be linked normally, or through rhymes or puns; sometimes new ideas arise from distractions in the room. Although the original plan was to reach station B, this was lost along the way and the destination changed; this keeps happening, and so the goal of thinking is never maintained for long.

*Derailment* may occur. The train can leave the tracks, ending up at a new destination completely unrelated to the original route. This may happen in schizophrenia and is very difficult to follow, since the patient's speech is muddled and illogical, with no understandable con-nections between thoughts. This is also called *loosening of associations* or *knight's move thinking*—the latter because of the indirect movement of the knight in chess.

Although the train would usually progress from Station B to Station C, in *perseveration* it becomes stuck at Station B. Answers to questions are repeated inappropriately, e.g.

**You:** What's your name?

**Elvis:** Elvis.

**Y:** How old are you?

**E:** Elvis.

This usually occurs in organic states (e.g. dementia).

The above terms will not always be relevant, but every patient's speech can be described in terms of:

- **Rate:** fast, slow, or normal.
- **Volume**: loud, soft, or normal, e.g. shouting, whispering.
- **Tone**: the emotional quality of speech, e.g. sarcastic, angry, glum, calm, neutral. Loss of the natural lilt and stresses in sentences produces monotonous speech.
- **Flow**: speech may be spontaneous, or only when prompted; hesitant, or with long pauses before answers; garrulous and uninterruptible.

Also note:

- Dysarthria—impaired articulation
- Dysphasia—impaired ability to comprehend or gener-ate speech

- Clang associations (rhyming connections, e.g. bang, sang)
- Punning (playing on words with the same sounds but different meanings, e.g. tire, tyre)
- Neologisms (made-up words)

### Mood

Mood and affect are sometimes used synonymously, although they are a little different. Overall, *mood* is like a lake, into which you throw a stone—the ripples you then see are the *affect*. In other words, mood is the pervasive experience of the patient; affect is the momentary changing state we observe from the outside. Mood divides into:

- **Subjective:** how the *patient* says they are feeling, recorded in their own words.
- **Objective:** what *you think* about the patient's emotional state, e.g. low, elated, irritable, anxious, perplexed, etc. As well as naming the mood, you can comment on its variability:
  - Labile—very changeable mood, e.g. flitting quickly between anger, tears, and laughter (like getting unexpected *waves* rather than ripples from the lake analogy).
  - Flat/blunted—lack of normal variability (as if the stone has no effect on the surface of the lake).

Mood is *incongruent* if your patient's report of their mood does not match their presentation, e.g. they giggle as they say they feel deeply depressed.

If the patient's mood shifts appropriately with the conversation and is neither particularly 'up' nor 'down' you can write, 'Reactive and neither elated nor depressed'.

 Don't list symptoms of depression (e.g. appetite, sleep) under Mood in the MSE; save them for the history.

### Thought

The content of thought is the patient's *beliefs* and *ideas*. Simply writing *persecutory delusions* gives very little information, so give verbatim examples or fully describe content.

 Even if there is nothing 'abnormal' you need to record something! What is your patient thinking about?

#### Preoccupations and worries

Preoccupations are recurrent thoughts that can be put aside by the patient. *Worries* are similar, but cause a feeling of anxiety or tension.

- What kinds of things do you worry about?
- What's on your mind?

### Delusions

A delusion is a fixed belief, held despite rational argument or evidence to the contrary. It cannot be fully explained by the patient's cultural, religious, or educational background. Occasionally the belief is true, but this is coincidental, since the reasoning behind it is illogical and faulty, e.g. a patient might rightly believe that his wife is cheating on him, but the belief began only because she burned his dinner.

Delusions feel as real as any other thought. If you were *deluded* that you were a medical student, this belief would feel as real as the belief you currently have that you are a medical student. No-one could convince you otherwise because you would *know* it was true and other people's disbelief would annoy you. This can make it difficult to ask about delusions! Fortunately, delusions generally relate to things that are important to the patient, and so are often referred to while talking. Your job is to listen sensitively and explore anything unusual.

 Be alert to the evasive replies of the guarded patient.

>> See Schizophrenia Reality (p.83) for tips on asking about delusions.

True *primary delusions* are rare. These arise completely 'out of the blue' in someone without prior mental health problems. You are *much* more likely to discover *secondary delusions*, which follow another abnormal experience, such as an abnormal mood or a hallucination (e.g. on hearing a disembodied voice, a patient then believes they are being stalked). *Systematized delusions* occur when delusions grow and build on each other, connecting into a delusional system. Delusions can be categorized by theme.

- **Grandiose delusions:** exaggerated beliefs of being special or important
  - e.g. being rich and famous.
- **Persecutory (paranoid[3]) delusions:** beliefs that others are trying to persecute or cause harm
  - e.g. people are spying on the patient.
- **Nihilistic delusions:** beliefs regarding the *absence* of something vitally important
  - e.g. the patient is dead, homeless, or their organs are rotting.
- **Delusions of reference:** beliefs that ordinary objects, events, or other people's actions have a special meaning or significance for the patient
  - e.g. news reports relate to them, objects are arranged as 'signs'.
- **Delusions of control:** beliefs that outside forces control the patient in some way.

- **Passivity**: the belief that movement, sensation, emotion, or impulse are controlled by an outside force, e.g. as if someone has a remote control for the patient's actions.
- **Delusions of thought interference**: these occur against the person's will and feel like an invasion of privacy.
  - Thought withdrawal: the belief that someone/ something is removing thoughts from the patient's head.
  - Thought insertion: the belief that thoughts are being placed into the patient's mind, so that they are thinking someone else's thoughts.
  - Thought broadcasting: the belief that thoughts are broadcast to others. This is different from people guessing someone's thoughts by reading body language.

- **Delusions of jealousy**: despite the name, these are actually delusions of *infidelity*. The patient believes their partner is cheating; it usually affects men.
- **Amorous (erotomanic) delusions**: the belief that someone is in love with the patient. This is more common in women.
- **Delusions of guilt**: the belief of having committed an awful sin or crime.
- **Hypochondriacal delusions**: the patient believes that they have an illness.

*Partial delusions* are like delusions but not held quite as firmly—there is a little doubt (partial conviction). These include beliefs that are 'nearly' delusional on the way into a psychotic episode and delusions that are weakening with recovery. Under close questioning, someone with a partial delusion would agree that it was possible their belief *could* be wrong, e.g. due to their imagination playing tricks on them.

### Overvalued ideas

These are reasonable ideas pursued beyond the bounds of reason. The patient's life revolves around the idea to the point that it causes distress to them or others. For example, a man might become reasonably annoyed when his neighbour fills her front garden with unsightly garden gnomes, believing that they 'make the neighbourhood look cheap'. It is *not* reasonable to be preoccupied to the point of giving up work to take the neighbour to court and finally destroying the gnomes with a hammer! The overvalued idea here is that the gnomes make the neighbourhood look cheap.

### Obsessions

These are recurrent, unwanted, intrusive thoughts, images, or impulses which enter the patient's mind, despite attempts to resist them. Deep down, the patient knows that the thought is irrational, unlike a delusion where the patient absolutely believes it to be true. They also recognize the thought as their own—it isn't placed into their head by some outside force, unlike thought insertion.

Obsessions are unpleasant and make the patient feel acutely uncomfortable or anxious, with themes such as contamination, aggression, sex, religion, or infection, e.g. 'I've got AIDS'. This discomfort is often 'undone' by a compulsion. *Compulsions* are repeated, stereotyped, and seemingly purposeful rituals that the patient feels compelled to carry out. They may also be resisted, since the patient again feels that they are senseless. Compulsions can be actions (e.g. hand-washing) or thoughts (e.g. counting), but are included under Thought because of their close association with obsessions. If they are observed during the interview, they belong under Appearance and Behaviour.

- Do you have thoughts that keep coming into your head even though you try to block them out?
- Some people have rituals that they feel they need to do in a very exact way. Do you do anything like that?

### Thoughts of harm

Everyone must be assessed for thoughts of harm to self or others. Document all thoughts with full details of any plans, e.g. any preparations, intended method and timing, victim's details, etc. (See p.57 for more information on self-harm and suicide, and p.82 for harm to others.)

### Perception

Perception relates to the patient's sensory world. All five modalities should be explored; if they are normal, you can simply state 'No illusions or hallucinations in any modality'.

### Illusions

An illusion is the *misperception* of a stimulus. People are more likely to make perceptual mistakes when they are drowsy, unable to attend to the stimulus, extremely emotional, or can't see or hear clearly (e.g. someone who is scared of spiders mistakes a patch of dirt for a spider while cleaning a poorly lit shed).

Illusions are common in healthy people but also occur in mental illness, particularly delirium (where consciousness is clouded).

### Hallucinations

A hallucination is a perception in the *absence* of a stimulus, e.g. hearing a voice when no-one has spoken. Hallucinations feel as real as any other perception, so you can't ask 'Do you have hallucinations?'

>> *See Schizophrenia Reality (p.85) for tips on asking about hallucinations.*

Check all modalities.

- **Auditory**, e.g. music, voices.
- **Visual**, e.g. flashes, animals.
- **Touch**
  - **Tactile**: superficial feelings on or just below the skin, e.g. feeling of being scratched.
  - **Deep sensation**: internal feelings, e.g. feeling of the heart being twisted.
- **Olfactory**, e.g. smelling smoke.
- **Gustatory**, e.g. tasting 'poison' in food.

Voices may be in the second person (addressing the patient directly as 'you') or the third person (as 'he/she'). Those particularly suggesting schizophrenia discuss or argue about the patient, give a running commentary of the patient's actions, or say the patient's thoughts aloud (thought echo). Always describe what the patient is experiencing, e.g. second-person auditory hallucinations of an unfamiliar male voice shouting, 'Your mother is a prostitute!'.

Healthy people *do* experience hallucinations, although these are usually brief, e.g. on waking (hypnopompic hallucinations), on falling asleep (hypnagogic hallucinations), or following a bereavement (e.g. hearing the dead person speaking). Hallucinations can signify severe mental illness. Auditory hallucinations are the most common; visual hallucinations suggest organic illness (e.g. brain tumour).

### Depersonalization and derealization

Both experiences are an unnerving feeling of unreality and you may have experienced one or both when tired or anxious. They occur in many disorders, especially anxiety states.

- **Depersonalization:** the person feels unreal: detached, numb, or emotionally distant.
  - Do you ever feel as if you aren't quite real?
- **Derealization:** the world feels unreal, e.g. 'like a film set'.
  - Do you ever feel as if the world around you is not quite real?

Don't worry about naming all the psychopathology—straightforward description is better, e.g. rather than stating 'Lilliputian hallucinations', describe the tiny little people seen by the patient.

### Cognition

Cognition is the umbrella term covering thinking and remembering. It includes orientation, attention, concentration, and memory, all of which are affected by the patient's level of consciousness.

By the time you have taken the history, you should have a reasonable understanding of the patient's general cognition. If your patient is alert and has given a clear, detailed, and accurate history it is reasonable to note their attention, concentration, and memory as grossly normal. Orientation to time, place, and person may again be clear from the history, although to be certain you might briefly check these. Any concerns should lead to formal testing with the Mini Mental State Examination (MMSE).

 See p.16 and ORC.

### Insight

Insight is never simply *present* or *absent*; there are different levels of awareness that something is wrong.

- Awareness that behaviour or symptoms are seen as abnormal by others.
  - Do you think your friends would say that you're different to usual?
- Agreement that the behaviour or symptoms are abnormal.
  - Do you think there's anything wrong with you at the moment?
  - Is this normal for you? How are you different to usual?
- Understanding that problems are due to *mental* illness (not, e.g. physical illness).
  - What do you think is causing X? Could it be stress or mental illness?
- Agreement that this illness requires treatment.
  - Do you think that the doctor's treatment will help?
  - Would you be happy to try the treatment?

Insight can be patchy, e.g. a patient may not think that they are ill, but takes medication because they believe it satisfies the Mafia, stopping their persecution.

### Final thought

A *full* assessment includes a physical examination. Always take a chaperone when examining patients, but remember that many people don't want repeated physical examinations by students.

## Formulation

The formulation presents the most important points from the history and examination before outlining further management and prognosis.

### Case synopsis

- Background information: name, age, occupation, ethnicity, marital status.
- Brief summary of current episode.
- Relevant past history.

- Examination
  - Salient features of MSE.
  - Important physical findings, e.g. hemiparesis, jaundice.

### Differential diagnosis

Start with your *preferred diagnosis* and then list other differentials, from most to least likely. For each, add reasons for and against the diagnosis. Keep the list short and don't show off by naming rare or eponymous conditions unless certain you are right! Remember that organic states 'trump' all other conditions (see p.27 for diagnostic hierarchy).

### Risk

Risk to self and others must be mentioned, e.g. suicide, self-harm, violence, neglect. Risk is graded as low, moderate, or high.

### Aetiology

From the information gathered in the history and examination, consider the causes of your patient's illness. *Predisposing* factors make people vulnerable to a disorder; *precipitating* factors trigger it; and perpetuating factors prevent recovery. Use a grid to help you to organize this material (Table 1.1).

**TABLE 1.1** Aetiology example

|  | Biological | Psychological | Social |
|---|---|---|---|
| Predisposing | e.g. genetics | e.g. personality | e.g. childhood abuse |
| Precipitating | e.g. drug misuse | e.g. helplessness | e.g. life event |
| Perpetuating | e.g. ongoing pain | e.g. pessimism | e.g. lack of support |

Social and psychological factors are often intermingled, e.g. redundancy has an obvious psychological impact. The same factor can be mentioned more than once as its effects can both precipitate and perpetuate the illness. You don't need to fill every box.

 **Consider whether aetiological factors can be removed or reversed as part of the management.**

### Investigations

Investigations exclude physical causes of the problem (e.g. hypothyroidism in depression); check general physical health and provide baseline measures before starting medications.

- Biological, e.g. blood tests, CT scans
- Psychological, e.g. symptom rating scales, IQ testing
- Social, e.g. collateral history, contact GP

### Management

Management is *holistic*, since medication alone cures very little. Think about immediate, medium-term, and long-term care—again, a grid helps (Table 1.2).

**TABLE 1.2** Management example

|  | Biological | Psychological | Social |
|---|---|---|---|
| Immediate | e.g. alcohol detoxification | e.g. reassurance | e.g. hospital admission |
| Medium term | e.g. regular medication | e.g. cognitive behavioural therapy | e.g. assist with benefits |
| Long term | e.g. trial without medication | e.g. psychodynamic psychotherapy | e.g. retraining |

### Prognosis

Give your opinion on the patient's prognosis, both for their current episode of illness and long term. Include positive and negative prognostic factors to support your view.

## Formulation: Vincent van Gogh

### Case synopsis

Vincent van Gogh is a 35-year-old single Dutch artist. The police brought him to hospital on 24 December 1888 after he threatened a friend with a razor, and then cut off his own ear and gave it to a prostitute. He has not explained his actions but has mentioned 'frightful ideas' and being forsaken by God. Over the past 9 weeks he has become increasingly irritable, and has painted incessantly. There is a 4-week history of divine 'communications' and the feeling of being punished by God. During this time, his thoughts have been confused and fast, his mood labile, and his appetite and libido low, and he has been sleeping only 2–3 hours a night. Relationship problems with his friend, Mr Gauguin, could have triggered this episode, and substance misuse may have exacerbated his symptoms.

He suffered two episodes of depression in his twenties, neither of which was formally treated; both followed losses. Each episode gave way to a period of immense energy and creativity. He has self-harmed once before, burning his hand when he was 28. Vincent has had relationships with prostitutes since his twenties. He contracted gonorrhoea when he was 29 and has a possible history of seizures.

He drinks excessive alcohol, chews lead-based paints, and sips turpentine.

On MSE, he was unkempt, distracted, agitated, and labile, and appeared to be experiencing visual and auditory hallucinations. Speech was pressured and he showed flight of ideas. He was preoccupied with religious themes and paranoid delusions.

Physical examination was unremarkable, other than the amputation of his left earlobe, which was sutured and free from infection.

## Differential diagnosis

1. **Bipolar affective disorder** (BPAD): current episode mixed affective (see p.41).
   - *For*: A current mixture of manic and depressive symptoms, in the context of previous depressive episodes and possible hypomania. Depressive symptoms include low mood, appetite, and libido, and the conviction of being abandoned and punished by God. Manic symptoms include reduced need for sleep, increased creative energy, and flight of ideas.
   - *Against*: Organic causes are still to be excluded.
   - *Severity*: Severe, since psychotic symptoms (hallucinations and delusions) are present.

2. **Organic disorders** must be excluded.
   - **Temporal lobe epilepsy**
     - *For*: A probable history of seizures. Mood and psychotic symptoms can be associated with seizures, and absinthe is known to lower the seizure threshold.
     - *Against*: Unclear description of seizures.
   - **Neurosyphilis (general paresis of the insane)**
     - *For*: History of sexually transmitted disease and sex with prostitutes. Neurosyphilis can present with seizures and mood disturbance.
     - *Against*: No symptoms or physical signs of syphilis, e.g. Argyll–Robertson pupil, tremor, leg weakness, or memory impairment. Symptoms normally take 10–20 years from infection to be expressed.
   - **Lead encephalopathy**
     - *For*: Chewing lead-based paints. Seizures, hallucinations, abdominal pains, irritability, and mood changes.
     - *Against*: No confusion, vomiting, ataxia, or peripheral weakness.

3. **Substance misuse**
   - **Comorbid diagnosis of alcohol dependency/ harmful use of other substances**
     - *For*: Features of dependency: tolerance, withdrawal, craving, loss of control, use despite harm. Admits eating paints and drinking turpentine.
     - *Against*: No evidence of salience, reinstatement after abstinence, or narrowed repertoire. No definite harm from paints or turpentine.
   - **Delirium tremens**
     - *For*: Chronic heavy drinking, hallucinations.
     - *Against*: Neither tremulous nor disoriented.
   - **Alcoholic hallucinosis**
     - *For*: Chronic heavy drinking, hallucinations.
     - *Against*: Mood component present and *visual* hallucinations.

4. **Schizoaffective disorder**
   - *For*: Psychotic *and* affective symptoms together.
   - *Against*: Affective symptoms predated psychotic symptoms.

## Risk

Although Vincent denies thoughts of harm to self or others, he is at *high* risk for both because he has recently cut off his earlobe and threatened a friend. Ongoing substance misuse increases his impulsivity and he has a past history of aggression in the context of intoxication.

## Aetiology

**TABLE 1.3** Aetiology—Vincent van Gogh

|  | Biological | Psychological | Social |
|---|---|---|---|
| Predisposing | ?Neurodevelopmental abnormalities (suggested by craniofacial asymmetries, clumsiness) | Low self-esteem secondary to repeated rejection by partners<br>History of depression | Financial hardship and reliance on brother<br>Lack of artistic recognition |
| Precipitating | Substance misuse<br>Lack of sleep | Threatened loss (departure of Mr Gauguin) | Social rejection in Arles<br>Critical family (mother) |
| Perpetuating | Lack of sleep<br>Substance misuse | Fear of public humiliation following recent events | Isolation |

## Investigations

1. Blood tests: FBC, U&E, LFTs, γGT, TFTs, lead levels.
2. Sexually transmitted disease screen, including syphilis serology.
3. Consider CT head: recent history of 'seizures' with hallucinations.
4. Electroencephalogram (EEG).
5. Collateral histories: Theo van Gogh and Rachel (the prostitute).

## Management

**TABLE 1.4** Management—Vincent van Gogh

|  | Biological | Psychological | Social |
|---|---|---|---|
| Immediate | Alcohol detoxification<br>Medical review of ear | Reassurance<br>Carer support (Theo) | Admission<br>Prevent access to alcohol |
| Medium term | Refer to physicians if evidence of lead poisoning/syphilis/epilepsy<br>Start mood stabilizer (e.g. lithium) | Education and motivational interviewing for substance misuse<br>Cognitive behavioural therapy<br>Safe-sex education | Alcoholics Anonymous<br>Find accommodation (landlord refusing to take him back) |
| Long term | Monitor for side effects of mood stabilizer | Psychodynamic psychotherapy, e.g. explore issues relating to loss of stillborn brother | Social skills training: improve ability to relate to women<br>Assist in exhibiting art/finishing theology degree |

### Risk management

In the short term, admission to hospital will reduce access to knives and victims. He should be observed closely for evidence of ongoing related psychotic symptoms. Longer term, treatment of the underlying illness will reduce risk, though repeated assessment is needed.

### Prognosis

In the short term, Vincent's prognosis is likely to be good, since he has agreed to take medication and has a supportive brother. Longer term, he will probably experience further episodes, especially having experienced episodes already. Compliance with medication will improve his prognosis, although his comorbid substance misuse, male sex, poor employment history, and psychotic features are poor prognostic indicators. He is at high risk of self-harm and suicide.

### Follow-up information

Vincent was diagnosed with epilepsy by Dr Felix Rey, at the Hotel Dieu Hospital. He was prescribed potassium bromide (a popular anti-epileptic at the time), which seemed beneficial, short-term. Paul Gauguin returned to Paris and never saw Vincent again. After discharge, Vincent suffered numerous psychotic relapses, probably precipitated by continued absinthe drinking. In 1889 he admitted himself to an asylum in St Rémy, where he remained for a year, experiencing at least three further relapses. Here he produced around 300 works of art, including *Starry Night*. On 27 July 1890, Vincent shot himself in the chest in a field outside Auvers. He died at home, two days later, with Theo by his side, having received virtually no recognition of his art during his lifetime.

Over 30 diagnoses have been proposed for Vincent's presentation, including bipolar affective disorder, schizophrenia, neurosyphilis, lead poisoning, Ménière's disease, and acute intermittent porphyria.

Although there was no family history of mental illness at the time of Vincent's admission, members of his family became ill after his death.

- Theo died in 1891 at the Medical Institution for the Insane following a 'mental and physical collapse' possibly due to syphilis.
- Willemina (sister) may have suffered schizophrenia. She was institutionalized and died in an asylum in 1941.
- Cornelis (brother) was a soldier, officially killed in action in 1900. Unconfirmed reports claim that he killed himself.

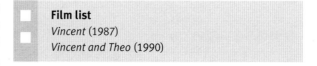

**Film list**
*Vincent* (1987)
*Vincent and Theo* (1990)

## Notes

1. Copyright Don McLean (admin: Universal Songs Inc.).
2. The painting is drawn from a mirror, hence the appearance of the *right* ear being bandaged.
3. *Paranoid* is an umbrella term, meaning that something relates to the self. In the broadest sense, all delusions are paranoid, since they in some way refer to the patient. Paranoid delusions officially include persecutory, grandiose, jealous, and erotomanic delusions. Nevertheless, paranoid has come to mean *persecutory* in common parlance.

## References/Further reading

Arnold, W.N. (2004) The illness of Vincent van Gogh. *Journal of the History of the Neurosciences*, **13**, 22–43.

Blumer, D. (2002) The illness of Vincent van Gogh. *American Journal of Psychiatry*, **159**, 519–26.

Gayford, M. (2006) *The Yellow House: Van Gogh, Gauguin and Nine Turbulent Weeks in Arles*. London: Penguin.

Loftus, L.S. and Arnold, W.N. (1991) Vincent van Gogh's illness: acute intermittent porphyria? *British Medical Journal*, **303**, 1589–91.

Sims, A. (1988) *Symptoms in the Mind: An Introduction to Descriptive Psychopathology*. London: Ballière Tindall.

Voskuil, P.H. (2005) The illness of Vincent van Gogh. *Journal of the History of the Neurosciences*, **14**, 169–75; author's reply, 176.

# THE *TAKE ME WITH YOU* GUIDE TO ASSESSMENT

## History

Background information
'Presenting complaint'
History of presenting complaint
Past psychiatric history
Past medical history
Drug history
Family history
Personal history
- Birth and early development
- Family background and early childhood
- Education
- Occupation
- Psychosexual/relationships

Substance misuse
Forensic history
Premorbid personality
Social history
Collateral history

## Mental state examination

Appearance and behaviour
Speech
- Rate
- Volume
- Tone
- Flow

Mood
- Subjective
- Objective

Thought
- Preoccupations and worries
- Delusions
- Overvalued ideas

- Obsessions
- Thoughts of harm

Perception
- Illusions
- Hallucinations
- Depersonalization and derealization

Cognition—see MMSE
Insight

## The Mini Mental State Examination

 For instructions on how to perform and mark the MMSE, go to the ORC.

1. Orientation to time (day, date, month, season, year) = **5 points**

2. Orientation to place (floor/building/town/city/country) = **5 points**

3. Registration (apple, penny, table) = **3 points**

4. Attention and concentration = **5 points**
    (a) 'World' backwards *or*
    (b) Serial sevens test

5. Delayed recall (apple, penny, table) = **3 points**

6. Naming (pen, watch) = **2 points**

7. Expressive language ( *No ifs, ands, or buts*) = **1 point**

8. Reading and comprehension (CLOSE YOUR EYES) = **1 point**

9. Write a sentence = **1 point**

10. Copy pentagons = **1 point**

11. Three-stage command = **3 points**

Take this paper in your left hand, fold it in half, and put it on the floor.

# 2 SAFETY

*Sarah Stringer*

Students often worry about being attacked by psychiatric patients. The reality is that only a minority are aggressive and *very* few are interested in attacking medical students! Aggression and violence are often preventable, so maximize your safety by reading this section *before* you enter the wards.

📖 As a student, do *not* get involved with ward Control and Restraint (C&R) incidents. Get out of the way and usher away other patients to keep them safe.

## 1. Dress code

Clothing should be practical and non-provocative—not low-cut, tight, or short. Avoid logos or labels. Anything around your neck could be grabbed and pulled, so avoid ties, scarves, necklaces, and ID badges should be on quick-release lanyards.

## 2. Stick together

Never interview alone. Mixed-gender pairings are helpful; one of you can always chaperone.

## 3. Work with the staff

Introduce yourself to the staff; they can't support you if they don't know who you are. Request a tour of the ward, noting exits and how the alarms work. Ask for help in choosing patients to interview, always check the notes and with staff for a past history of violence and current risk issues.

- Who would be good to interview *today*?
- Is there anything I should know before seeing them?

Never interview a patient without telling someone first. Ask staff to check on you intermittently (e.g. by adding you to the list of patients on 15 minute observations).

## 4. Prepare your room

Use interview rooms with windows so that staff can see you. Arrange chairs beforehand.

- Sit nearest the door and preferably within reach of an alarm.
- Ensure a clear path to the door.
- Keep 'personal space' between chairs. Sitting too close heightens tension and places you in grabbing distance.

## 5. No drink or drugs

Drugs and alcohol increase aggression: never interview intoxicated patients.

## 6. Behave yourself

*Your* conduct will help keep you safe.

- Courtesy is essential. Gain consent to interview, explaining that it is voluntary and can be terminated at any time.
- Gain permission before taking notes; stop writing if your patient appears suspicious.
- Never argue with patients, laugh at them, or dismiss their beliefs.
- Be sensitive to culture, age, and gender.
- Give the 'right' amount of eye contact (staring feels threatening; inattentive eye contact looks uninterested/scared).
- Don't intimidate: question gently, use open body language, and sit at the patient's level.

## 7. Read the signs

Most aggression can be predicted by recognizing the warnings that violence *may* follow.

- *Verbal warnings*
  - **Direct threats:** take these seriously!
  - **Abuse:** swearing or insults
  - **Tone:** angry, sarcastic, threatening, or rude
  - **Volume:** shouting or prolonged silence
- *Physical warnings:*
  - Prolonged staring/narrowed eyes/angry frown/dilated pupils
  - Fast breathing/sweating/facial reddening or blanching
  - Gritting teeth/clenching fists/trembling/agitation
  - Leaning over you
  - Pacing (don't let people walk *behind* you)
  - Violent gestures, e.g. pounding the table.

## 8. Trust your gut

Always listen to your 'gut' feeling. If you start feeling unsafe (even if you don't know *why*), end the interview and leave. No history-taking is ever important enough for you to endanger yourself.

### 9. De-escalation and escape

While exiting or resolving *mild* hostility:

DO

- Keep your tone and body language calm—no sudden movements.
- Give your patient space.
- Apologize if *you've* upset them.
- Empathize and feed back their feelings, e.g. 'It's frustrating for you'.
- Tell them that they are frightening you.
- Back out. Never turn your back on someone who threatens you.
- Tell staff immediately.

DON'T

- Say, 'Calm down'. This implies that you think they are *unreasonably* angry; it is inflammatory.
- Touch them.
- Make jokes.
- Stand to 'match' a patient who stands; stay seated or back out. *If* currently standing, don't stand face to face or put your hands on your hips. Standing to their side, shoulder-on, is less confrontational and makes you a smaller target.

### 10. If you *are* assaulted

- Get help (shout and press the alarm): staff will intervene when they know you are in danger.
- Get away.
- Have a full physical check by a doctor.
- Complete an incident form.
- Contact the consultant(s) responsible for you and your patient to debrief and gain support.
- Take the rest of the day off.
- Seek further support if needed (e.g. counselling).
- Contact the police in serious assaults.

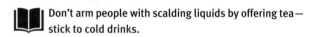 Don't arm people with scalding liquids by offering tea— stick to cold drinks.

>> *For more advice, go to Mania reality (p.50).*

## Further reading

Royal College of Psychiatrists (2006) *Safety for Psychiatrists* (Council Report CR134). London: Royal College of Psychiatrists. Available online at: http://www.rcpsych.ac.uk/files/pdfversion/cr134new.pdf

# 3 ESSENTIAL INTERVIEW SKILLS

*Sarah Stringer*

Excellent communication skills are the key to working with people, and the principles are the same whether with friends, colleagues, or patients; or in social, clinical, or exam situations. General and specific tips follow, with OSCE (Observed Structured Clinical Examination) advice in the next chapter.

## Interview skills

### Introduce yourself and settle down

#### The first moment

Smile and make eye contact as you introduce yourself, since it shows that you are confident and trustworthy. Immediately using someone's first name can be offensive; address your patient formally, and then ask what they like to be called.

- Hello, Mr Smith . . . Are you happy to be called Mr Smith, or do you prefer something else?

#### To shake or not to shake?

Shaking hands works for some people but not others. If your patient has severe arthritis, you may hurt them. If OCD, they might spend the interview looking for a sink to wash their hands. Some cultures don't sanction handshaking (e.g. Muslim women may not feel comfortable shaking hands with men). If you *do* shake hands, do it well; perfect your 'shake' on a friend, avoiding aggressive crunches or limp clammy shakes.

#### Explain yourself!

Explain why you want to talk and give them the chance to refuse. Saying 'I want to take a history' makes no sense to non-medics. Try something like:

- I'm a medical student. Stella (the nurse) said you'd be a really good person for me to talk to and learn from. Have you got time to talk?

Remember that you may be the tenth student this week to request an interview. If they refuse, ask if they'd like to talk another time, or let them know how long you are available in case they change their mind.

 **Getting involved in ward activities lets you chat with patients before requesting formal interviews.**

### Comfort and privacy

Respect your patient's confidentiality by finding somewhere private to speak. If they want to bring a friend or family member, let them. Allow time to get comfortable and move your chair into a good position to talk. Sit at roughly 90 degrees to your patient. Facing your patient head-on feels antagonistic, but sitting side by side causes neck strain. If your patient leans or shuffles backwards, you are too close. Be aware of your own personal space and how comfortable the distance feels.

### Active listening and body language

Active listening is about offering the other person your undivided attention to give them the message, 'What you're saying matters to me'. Some doctors employ *anti-listening* techniques, leaving their patients feeling unimportant and misunderstood.

 Try to *really* listen to someone today without doing anything else. How does this differ from your 'normal' listening? What happens?

---

**BOX 3.1** Anti-listening techniques with translations

Wriggling/fidgeting = My bladder's full.

Rushing = I've got more important things to do.

Glancing around the room = How do I get out?

Crossed arms/legs = I don't want to hear this. Why are you still talking?

Staring eye contact = I wonder how long I can go without blinking.

Slouching = Bored.

Interrupting = I'll take over from here. I know best.

Blank facial expression = Hmmm . . . Beans on toast for tea tonight?

Writing notes constantly = I don't have to look at you if I do this.

---

#### Silence

Silence gives your patient space to talk. It is hard to listen when two people talk at once, especially if you are one of them. You can make intermittent 'listening noises' (uh-huh/mmm) to let your patient know that you haven't fallen asleep or passed away.

Allowing a silence to last a moment or two longer than normal may help someone to mention something that is difficult to talk about.

### Body language

The general rule is to sit still, lean slightly forward, and keep your body language 'open' (not hunched with all your limbs crossed). Try to make eye contact, nod when you agree with things they say, and facially, *look interested*. Don't be disheartened if the other person doesn't give *you* eye contact; just be ready to meet their gaze if they look up.

 Tilting your head to one side *very slightly* lets the speaker know that you are listening.

Comfort is essential, since you don't want to keep wriggling into new 'listening poses' every few minutes. Although crossed legs are not advised, if you sit most comfortably with your legs crossed, fine—cross them to point your body *towards* the other person, rather than showing off the side of your thigh and buttock.

If you lean *too* far forward, nod *too* much, and make *excessive* eye contact, you will look scary.

When people get on well they unconsciously copy each other's movements (mirroring). Mirroring deliberately but subtly can help the interviewee to feel understood.

Making notes keeps your history accurate but can ruin rapport. Give your undivided attention for the first few minutes before explaining that you will take notes to ensure that you don't muddle up their story. Jot down major points and stop writing if the conversation becomes more sensitive.

## Question style: open, closed, or clarifying?

- *Closed questions* give a choice of yes or no answers, e.g. Are you 60?

- *Clarifying questions* let patients give specific one-word or short answers, e.g. How old are you?

- *Open questions* encourage the patient to talk and answer the question as they want to. They often start with *how*, *why*, or *what*, or might be ordinary sentences asked as questions, e.g. What's it like being 60?/Tell me more about that . . . ?

Start with an *open* question, but try to be relevant. Woolly questions like, 'How are you?' may result in conversations that never reach the deeper issues. This is fine in a relaxed ward environment, but needs honing when time is pressured. Relevant open questions might be:

- How were things going before you came into hospital?

- I don't know anything about why you came to hospital. Could you tell me what happened?

Now, settle back and listen.

Medical students often slip into checklists, chanting closed questions at the patient. For example:

**You:** Was your pain sharp?

**Peter:** No.

**Y:** Did it burn?

**P:** No.

**Y:** Was it crushing?

**P:** Yes.

**Y:** Did it get worse with breathing in?

**P:** No.

**Y:** Or with exercise?

**P:** Um . . . No?

**Y:** Was it in the centre of your chest?

**P:** Yes.

**Y:** Have you had it before?

**P:** Yes.

**Y:** Were you short of breath?

**P:** Yes.

**Y:** Did it improve with GTN?

**P:** With what?

**Y:** That medicine in your hand.

**P:** My spray?

**Y:** Yes. Your GTN spray. Did it get better with your GTN spray?

**P:** No.

This is a very slow and clumsy way of taking histories.

Contrast this with the *funnel*, where you
start with an open question or two,
before 'funnelling'
the answers
down with
clarifying
or closed
questions.

For example:

**Y:** What happened? *(open)*

**P:** I ran upstairs and the pain came on suddenly—crushing me, like an elephant sitting on my chest, right here [*puts clenched fist over central chest*]. I couldn't breathe. I was terrified! I could feel the pain spreading into my jaw and down my left arm. It was just like the last time I had a heart attack. I wanted to get my spray, but it was downstairs, and when I moved, the pain got worse.

**Y:** It must have been frightening. How long did it last? *(clarifying)*

**P:** Half an hour.

**Y:** Did you notice anything else? *(clarifying/closed)*

**P:** Um . . . I was really sweaty.

**Y:** Did you feel sick? *(closed)*

**P:** Yes.

Start a new funnel with each new topic. Medicine is pressurized enough without making every history a game of twenty questions.

### Combination questions

Try to avoid *double- or triple-barrelled-questions* (lots of questions squashed into one). People generally remember and answer the first or last things you asked.

> **You:** Have you had trouble sleeping or eating less or more than usual, or are you low on energy and would you say you're a bit constipated?
>
> **Ben:** I'm not constipated.

Another combination question to avoid is the *leading question*. This combines a question with the answer you expect.

> **Y:** You haven't been taking your medicine, have you?
>
> **B:** !

Unsurprisingly, it tends to annoy people.

## Get the story

Psychiatry is rich with stories. Just as you won't understand a novel by opening random pages and reading unrelated sentences, you won't understand your patient's story by firing unrelated questions at them. Gathering a story needs *curiosity*, *links*, and *detective work*.

### Curiosity

If a friend told you that someone followed them on the way home, you would be curious and full of questions, e.g.

- Who followed you? (Expand understanding of the delusional system)
- Do you know why you were followed? (Expand understanding; look for persecutory, guilty, or grandiose themes)
- Has it happened before? (Duration of episode/past psychiatric history)
- Could there possibly be an innocent explanation for the stalker? (Test conviction)
- Did anyone else see it happen? (Reality check)
- Have you told the police? What did the police say? (Reality check)

- What did you do? What do you plan to do about it? (Risk assessment)

If you can do this for a friend, you can do it for a patient.

### Links

Jumping around different parts of the history feels awkward. By linking your questions to the things your patient says, your history will feel smooth and your patient will know that you have listened to them. Examples might be:

- *Linking duration to precipitating factors:*

> **Berndt:** I've been feeling nervous for two months now.
>
> **You:** Did something happen two months ago?

- *Linking delusions to auditory hallucinations:*

> **Holly:** The police have been following me for a week.
>
> **You:** Over the past week, have you ever heard them talking?

- *Linking sleep and energy:*

> **Alfaz:** I only get about three hours' sleep a night.
>
> **You:** That's not good! Does it leave you feeling tired?

With a little creativity, you can link most things. You can also gently redirect the interview this way without being too pushy.

### Detective work

People rarely tell you everything, straight away. Although you will need to ask direct questions about symptoms, look for clues that hint at symptoms or an interesting storyline, and focus the conversation onto these hints.

A simple *reflection* is often enough, e.g.

> **Mrs Getty:** They made it impossible for me.
>
> **You:** *They . . . ?*

> **Mr Smith:** My wife was always up to no good . . .
>
> **You:** Up to no good?

If your patient has quickly moved on, don't jump in suddenly since it may make them wary of answering (e.g. 'Wait! You did *what* to his grandmother?'). Instead, log the clue and wait for the right moment to return to it calmly and redirect the conversation, e.g. 'You mentioned something about his grandmother . . . ?'

## Empathize

If you enjoy setting fire to ants with a magnifying glass, you may find empathy tricky. Empathy is sometimes described as 'walking in someone else's shoes', and is a kind of non-magical mind-reading.

### Imagine

When you watch a film or play, you switch on your imagination to understand what the characters are feeling. However, if you don't want to let the story seem too 'real', you can switch off your imagination (e.g. wondering how long the zombies in the film spent in make-up takes the fear from horror movies).

As doctors, we sometimes need to switch off to protect ourselves from the harrowing situations we encounter, *but* if we never switch on, patients and their problems make no emotional sense to us—and patients pick up on this. So try switching *on*. For example, if *you* were being stalked, how would *you* feel? Angry? Scared? Suspicious of everyone?

### Listen

As well as *imagining* how people feel, *listen* to what they're saying. Sometimes the message is really clear but often you must read between the lines for the extra clues in what is *not* said.

Vocal cues include tone, volume, and pace of speech. Body language cues include eye contact, facial expression, body posture, and gestures. If someone speaks sadly, softly, and slowly while looking tearful, they are clearly communicating sadness, even if they say they are fine.

## Showing empathy

You need to communicate that you have picked up on a feeling, either verbally or non-verbally. This tells your patient that you have not only heard them, but understand them.

### Verbally

Avoid platitudes (e.g. *Every cloud has a silver lining*) or saying, 'I know how you feel'. These expressions show that you *don't* understand how someone is feeling at all. The classic medical school phrase is '*That must be very hard for you*', but if you never say this in real life, it tends to sound forced and artificial. Instead, listen to yourself when a friend tells you about something bad that has happened. What do you say to *them*? Gather two or three of these phrases and use them with patients. As long as they are not full of expletives, they will probably be the best thing you can say.

Try not to worry about the exact words you use, since the key is *how* you say it. You can actually say almost anything (even, '*That must be very hard for you*'), if you say it and mean it. Keep a kind tone and speak softly while holding eye contact—this is no time to look uncertain or shifty.

Sometimes it helps to name the emotions that people are experiencing. Read your patient's body language—if they are clearly holding back tears you can gently state the obvious:

- It makes you feel sad.
- I can see this is really upsetting you.

This legitimizes your patient's feelings and tells them that you can cope if they want to openly feel that way. If you get it wrong, just ask how they *are* feeling.

### Body language

If you are naturally empathic, your face will probably automatically adopt an empathic expression when someone tells you something emotional. However, it is worth finding a mirror and checking the 'empathy face' you pull—you may be surprised to find that you look constipated or cross, rather than concerned and kind! You don't want to overdo it, but you *do* need to register expressions; just raising your eyebrows or frowning may be enough.

Shuffle your chair closer or lean in, if needed—it lets you speak more softly about delicate issues and also adds a hint of solidarity. If they shuffle or lean away from you, they don't want you that close.

### Touch

Touch is a difficult area. Some people dislike being touched by anyone, some only allow their closest friends and family to touch them, and some people warmly touch everybody they meet. Culture, upbringing, personality, and previous experience all build into this—both for you and your patient. Touch can be unwanted and unpleasant —or therapeutic and supportive, depending on how it is done and how it is interpreted. Never touch someone if it makes *you* feel uncomfortable. If in doubt, *don't*. Think about why you want to touch. If it is to make yourself feel better, *don't*. If you genuinely want to offer comfort, reassurance, or kindness—you should do so.

'Safer' areas include forearms, elbows, shoulders, and backs, since they are fairly non-sexual. You might place your hand on the patient's arm or back and hold it there whilst they cry. Be sensitive: if your patient flinches or shrinks back, apologize and give them space.

> If you want to touch someone, ask yourself how it would be seen if your consultant or the patient's partner walked in at that moment. If you would stop or have to explain yourself, you are probably doing something wrong.

### Tissue issues

Allow people to cry. Shoving tissues at them at the first sign of a tear gives the message, 'Stop crying—*I* don't like it!' If your patient is clearly uncomfortable—struggling to wipe their face with their sleeve, for example—offer tissues. Tissues sometimes let people cry *more*, because they know that they can mop the tears afterwards.

📖 Empathy is not just about the sad emotions; it includes laughing *with* someone and smiling when they are happy or proud of themselves.

## The four rescue skills: what to do when you get stuck

Silence is important. Being able to leave gaps and silence in an interview is a sign of confidence and shows that you are not afraid of hearing difficult things. It also gives your patient the chance to set the pace of the interview. An *awkward* silence is a different matter entirely. It can feel acutely embarrassing when you go blank ('dry up') and have nothing to say. The four rescue skills that end these silences are *reflection*, *asking for concerns*, *summarizing*, and *asking for questions*.

### Reflection ('Reflection . . . ?')

When you have nothing to say, *say what they said*. Reflection is much easier and less intrusive than making up a clever statement or question to encourage your patient to keep talking; it is a simple echo. Reflection can end short silences when your patient dries up, loses concentration, or becomes self-conscious.

**Sheila:** Well, at first I was a bit nervous . . . [*pause*]

**You:** Nervous . . . ? (*or* A bit nervous . . . ?)

It prompts your patient to talk more about the subject that you have reflected on. Say it softly, sink into the background, and let it hang in the air. Try it out on unsuspecting family and friends—if they notice it, you've got it wrong. Experiment with your timing and tone of voice, or emulate television interviewers who do it well.

### Asking for concerns

Asking for concerns is a useful trick when you dry up and may unearth important issues which change the emphasis of the whole interview if asked early enough.

- Is there anything else worrying you?
- What's your biggest worry?

### Summarize

Students tend to summarize only at the end of interviews, but summarizing is more than a full stop and can again be very helpful if you go blank. As well as buying you time and covering an embarrassing silence, it demonstrates that you *have* been listening, while letting you check that you've understood what your patient said. Do not say, 'I'd like to summarize', since it sounds

contrived and is something you would never say normally. Instead, try something like:

- *Let me check I've got this right.* You've been low since your husband left you, three months ago. You've no energy, can't enjoy anything, and have problems sleeping and eating. You feel really guilty and hopeless about ever returning to work as a teacher. Is that right? (± Was there anything else?)

Your patient can then agree, correct, or expand on the information you've summarized. Having briefly gone through your list of symptoms in the summary, you have also reminded yourself that you didn't ask about suicidal thoughts (etc.).

📖 Summarizing is not repeating *everything* your patient has just said, word for word. The skill is in mentioning the main facts to draw together the story so far.

### Asking for questions

As with *asking for concerns*, this can make good use of gaps in the flow of your interview. Patients' questions often remind you to cover important things you may have forgotten.

**You:** OK. Is there anything you'd like to ask *me*?

**Miss Munroe:** So are these tablets alright with my diabetes?

**Y:** (*I forgot to check past medical history!*) That's a good question. First, tell me about your diabetes . . .

## Closing

Interviews that either limp to a standstill or end abruptly can ruin an otherwise brilliant conversation, leaving you and your patient feeling dissatisfied. Instead:

- Summarize what you have covered during the interview. Have you missed anything?
- Ask for questions and answer them.
- Ask for concerns and address them.
- Thank your patient for their time.
- Say goodbye. Smile, make eye contact!

If you do not know the answers to their questions, say so. You may be able to find out the answers for them from the ward staff or your consultant (do not offer to do this unless you plan to follow it up and return). Never give false reassurance about a concern. Simply hearing someone's worries can be therapeutic; you don't need to 'fix' everything.

## Finally: the issue of 'gaining rapport'

Most people have a favourite doctor or nurse, and often describe them as having 'the most wonderful bedside manner'. This bedside manner is the elusive 'rapport' we aim for with our patients; it is *getting on with people.* This is partly a case of good communication skills, but also a lot to do with the kind of person you are and the kind of person your patient is. For this reason, remember to take your personality with you onto the wards. Be professional and polite at all times, but don't let 'being on your best behaviour' make you bland. Hold onto your sense of humour, individuality, and ability to react to things: people want to be looked after by people, not robots.

 You will not get on with everyone you meet or treat, but you should always *try* to.

## Further reading

Silverman, J., Kurtz, S., and Draper, J. (2005) *Skills for Communicating with Patients.* Oxford: Radcliffe Medical Press.

Von Fragstein, M., Silverman, J., Cushing, A., *et al.* (2008) UK consensus statement on the content of communication curricula in undergraduate medical education. *Medical Education*, **42**, 1100–7.

Washer, P. (ed.) (2009) *Clinical Communication Skills.* Oxford: Oxford University Press.

# 4 HOW TO SUCCEED IN PSYCHIATRY OSCEs

*Sarah Stringer*

OSCEs differ between medical schools, but the following tips should help you in psychiatry stations, wherever you are.

## Before the exam

### Get feedback before it is too late

There is little benefit in discovering during the OSCE that your 'bedside manner' is an unbearable form of torture; find out and fix problems early on.

- See as many patients as you can and *ask them* afterwards how they felt you did and how you could improve. Patients are your experts.
- In pairs, take turns to observe and give feedback on each other's bedside manner.
- *Change*, according to your feedback, especially if there are recurring themes.

### University rules

- Ensure that you know the format of the exam, timings, bells, and rules about entering and leaving stations, as well as the potential for rest stations or double stations.
- Find out how your university writes their instructions—in particular, which line is the Task Line (see below).

### Practise OSCEs

Practising OSCEs with your friends is essential. Take turns to act, interview, examine, and give feedback to fine-tune your skills. The role-plays at the end of the chapters, along with a small selection available on the online resource centre, should help you.

- Time stations accurately to set your internal clock to the OSCE length.
- Do more than one OSCE at a time to help practice pressurized entrances and exits. Learn how to block out a 'bad' performance and move on to the next station.
- The bigger the audience, the better. If you can cope with a few people watching, the actual station will be less frightening. Practising alone in front of the mirror can only help so much.
- If you worry that other candidates' noise will distract you through the thin cubical walls, try practising with the radio on in the background.
- Filming your performance will help you spot your own strengths and weaknesses.

## In the exam

### A. Read the instructions

Although it is very brave to attempt a station without the assistance of instructions, it is unhelpful. *Read* the note outside the station.

> **e.g. 'You are a third-year medical student attached to a GP surgery. Gregory Pearce is a 19-year-old student who has been having a stressful time at college. He has attended because his parents are worried about him. *The GP has asked you see him and take a history of psychosis.'*

Find out how your university writes their instructions—in particular, which line is the Task Line. This may be the first line, but can be the last line of the instructions, following a chunk of writing about this patient and their issues. If you read the Task Line *first* and then read the rest of the story, you will be in the right frame of mind to take in the relevant information, and won't be thrown by an unexpected task (especially if there is a lot of information about the patient).

In theory, as you stand there you should run over the main topics you would like to cover. Unfortunately, this is the point where most students draw a complete blank, rather than a mind-map. Don't panic. Instead:

- Learn the patient's name (*Gregory Pearce*).
- Memorize the reason for attending (*his parents are worried*).
- Pick up clues (stress at college).
- Prepare your introduction.
- Prepare your first open question.

## B. Beginnings

➜ An OSCE student once interviewed his patient from *behind*, simply because this was the position of the chairs when he entered the room. Move the chairs if you need to!

1. Walk in and *succinctly* introduce yourself.

   Introduction = greeting + their name + your name + your status.

   > **You:** Hello, Mr Pearce? I'm *[insert your name]* a third-year medical student.
   >
   > **Greg:** Hi.

📖 Ask permission to sit down, rather than standing over your patient: tell them who you are and why you're there. Getting to the same height as the other person will stop you seeming threatening or overbearing.

2. Explain why you are there.

   > **Y:** The GP's asked me to have a quick chat about how things have been recently. Is that OK with you?
   >
   > **G:** OK.
   >
   > **Y:** Thank you.

This has gained Mr Pearce's consent for the interview; there is usually no need to expand on consent (or confidentiality) unless you are asked to.

3. Ask a *relevant open* question.

   - I understand that you've come in because your parents are worried about you. *What do you think they are worried about?*
   - Your doctor told me that you've been having a stressful time at college. *What's been happening?*

4. Settle back and listen.

📖 The classic response to 'What brought you here today?' is 'An ambulance, Doctor'. This is not funny, especially in an OSCE.

## C. Main body

1. Believe that your actor is a patient and that you are doing this for real—or you will under-perform. Include things that you would do in a real situation, such as offering to find patient information leaflets or website addresses. Don't mime handing over invisible leaflets or tissues (it looks silly). Always say that you would ask a senior if you have been asked to make a decision that you feel is beyond your capabilities; this is what you would do in real life.

2. Stay calm and confident (this relaxes patients and examiners alike). If you are working within your limitations you have nothing to worry about—your university is looking for *safe* doctors, not *perfect* doctors. If you don't know the answer to a question, say so rather than making one up.

   - I don't know—but I'll check with my consultant and let you know.

3. Use your skills:

   - Active listening and body language
   - Ask questions (open, closed, clarifying)
   - Get the story (curiosity, links, detective work)
   - Empathize and show empathy
   - Rescue skills (reflection, concerns, summary, questions)

## D. Endings

Most universities give some kind of one-minute warning. This is the time to rein in the interview, if you haven't already started to draw things to a close. Cover anything critical. For example, if you are talking to a depressed patient and you have not asked about suicide, ask *now*. Quickly clarify any important points you've missed, but try to finish the consultation:

- Final summary
- Ask for questions and answer them
- Ask for concerns and address them
- Thank you and goodbye

Do not leave early. A full psychiatric history can take more than an hour, so there will always be more questions to ask (and marks to gain) in an OSCE. In some medical schools you are not *allowed* to leave until your time is up, which can leave you feeling rather awkward if you *try* to leave and can't. On the other hand, do not procrastinate once the bell goes or you may be manhandled out of the station by the examiner.

## E. Afterwards

No matter how badly things go, never dwell on the nightmare of the previous station. Unless you walk into your next station with a black eye and bloody nose, the new examiner will be unaware of your track record. Each station is a fresh challenge.

## Further reading

Michael, A. (2003) *OSCEs In Psychiatry: Prepare for the New MRCPsych.* Edinburgh: Churchill Livingstone.

# 5 CLASSIFICATION AND DIAGNOSIS

*Alex Liakos*

Diagnoses are useful shorthand for complex illness concepts: they let patients and doctors know what the problem is. This validates a patient's symptoms and offers a way forward, essentially saying, 'I believe you and know how to help you, because I've seen this problem before'. Diagnoses also allow professionals to share their experiences and accumulate an evidence base for treatment of a disorder.

There are also problems with diagnoses. They may be unreliable or culturally specific: different doctors may diagnose the same patient with different problems. Additionally, once diagnostic 'labels' have been stuck onto people, they are difficult to peel off and can lead to lifelong stigma and misunderstanding.

There are two main classification systems (Table 5.1):

- ICD (International Classification of Diseases)
- DSM (Diagnostic and Statistical Manual of Mental Disorders)

Diagnoses are usually considered hierarchically: those higher up 'the pyramid' take precedence over those below (Figure 5.1). Therefore clinicians need to exclude organic causes of symptoms (denoted O on the pyramid) before diagnosing anything else. Since some diagnoses share symptoms, patients' experiences may fit into more than one category; treatment usually first targets the diagnosis highest up the pyramid.

Although you will become very good at diagnostic 'pattern recognition', don't get carried away by it. It remains a simple label which can never convey the unique experience of each of your patients, no matter how similar their symptoms are. Diagnose thoughtfully and be prepared to be wrong sometimes. Remember that *unusual* experiences are often different from *abnormal* experiences, and that symptoms without disability need no diagnosis at all.

➜ In 1972, eight healthy volunteers were admitted to psychiatric wards after attending hospitals, complaining only of a voice saying words like *thud*. Despite behaving 'normally' and stating the voice had gone, all were treated with antipsychotics and most diagnosed with schizophrenia. On average, admission lasted nineteen days.

## References/Further reading

Rosenhan, D.L. (1973) On Being Sane in Insane Places. *Science*, **179**, 250–8.

**TABLE 5.1** ICD vs. DSM

|  | ICD | DSM |
|---|---|---|
| Current edition | ICD-10 (1992) | DSM-IV (1994) |
| Developed by | World Health Organization (WHO) | American Psychiatric Association (APA) |
| Scope | All disorders | Mental health only |
| Categorization method | Matching descriptions to broad diagnostic guidelines | Definitive inclusion and exclusion criteria |
| Categories | 10 categories | 5 axes |

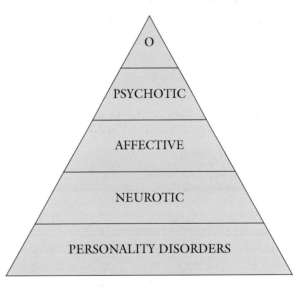

**FIGURE 5.1** The diagnostic pyramid

# 6 MENTAL HEALTH AND THE LAW

*Hazel Claydon and Jennifer Haworth*

In certain situations, it is essential to detain or treat people against their will. As in most countries, the UK has a legal framework for the detention of people suffering from mental illness so as to safeguard the rights of patients *and* protect them from themselves and others. There are two areas of mental health law that you need to know as a medical student or junior doctor:

- The compulsory admission and treatment of mental illness
  - governed by The Mental Health Act 2007.[1]
- Consent and capacity
  - governed by the Mental Capacity Act 2005.

## Mental Health Act 2007 (MHA)

The MHA is concerned with a wide range of issues from admission to discharge of people suffering from a 'mental disorder' who are considered to be a *risk to themselves or others*. 'Mental disorder' is defined very broadly by the MHA as 'any disorder or disability of the mind'. The sections of the MHA that you need to know are listed in Table 6.1.

Key points to note with regard to the MHA:

- People can only be detained if appropriate medical treatment is available.
- Sections do not apply for the treatment of physical disorders.

- Patients held under Sections 2 and 3 have the right to appeal against their detention.

Only 10–15% of all inpatients in mental health units are admitted under the MHA—most are there voluntarily.

## Mental Capacity Act 2005 (MCA)

*Capacity* is the ability to make decisions and is presumed to be intact unless proven otherwise. It relates to *specific* decisions, and should be assessed separately for each decision. *All* doctors must be able to assess capacity.

'Unwise' decisions do not mean that someone lacks capacity. Instead, according to the MCA, a person lacks capacity if, at the time in question, they are unable to make a decision for themselves because of an impairment of their mind/brain (whether permanent or temporary).

To have capacity, a person must be able to:

- understand the information relevant to the decision;
- retain that information;
- use or weigh that information as part of the process of making the decision;
- communicate their decision (whether by talking, using sign language or any other means).

Capacity is lacking if *any* of these abilities are missing.

**TABLE 6.1** Major Mental Health Act sections

| Section | Purpose | Maximum duration | Application | Recommendation |
|---------|---------|------------------|-------------|----------------|
| 2 | Admission for assessment | 28 days | AMHP | 2 doctors (at least one Section 12 approved*) |
| 3 | Admission for treatment | 6 months | AMHP | 2 doctors (at least one Section 12 approved) |
| 5(2) | Holding order for a patient already on the ward | 72 hours | – | 1 doctor |
| 136 | Police order to remove a person appearing to suffer from a 'mental disorder' from a public place to a 'place of safety' | 72 hours | – | Police officer |

*A Section 12 approved doctor is someone with proven expertise in the diagnosis and treatment of mental disorder (usually a psychiatrist). AMHP, approved mental health professional.

If it is decided that someone lacks capacity, steps may be taken in their *best interests*. These steps should be the least restrictive of their rights and freedoms, should allow them to participate as much as possible in the decision-making process, and should take into account their personal beliefs. A health professional's decision that a person lacks capacity, while an everyday implicit occurrence, is important with potentially huge ramifications, so tread carefully and respectfully!

>> *For practical guidance on capacity issues, see p.144.*

>> *For practical guidance on capacity issues, see p.144.*

## Note

1. The MHA only covers England and Wales:

   http://www.opsi.gov.uk/acts/acts2007/ukpga_20070012_en_1

   Scotland is covered by the Mental Health (Care and Treatment) (Scotland) Act 2003:

   http://www.opsi.gov.uk/legislation/scotland/acts2003/asp_20030013_en_1

   Northern Ireland is covered by the Mental Health (Northern Ireland) Order 1986:

   http://www.opsi.gov.uk/RevisedStatutes/Acts/nisi/1986/cnisi_19860595_en_1

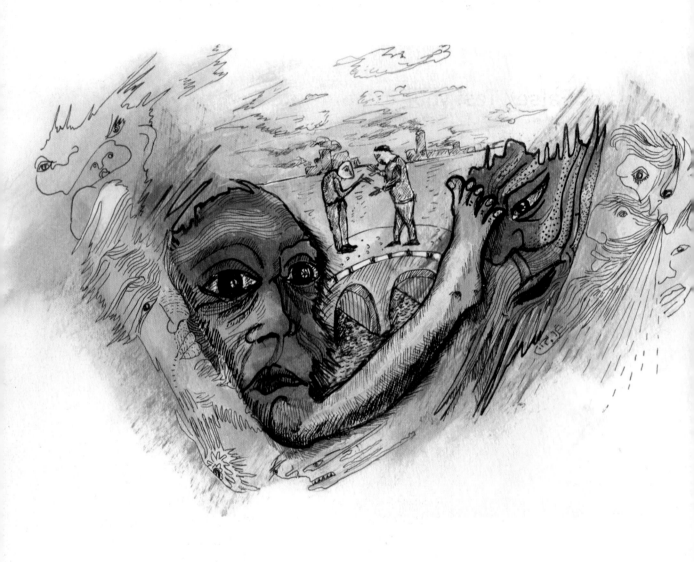

# 7 Affective disorders

*Greg Lydall, Mazen Daher, Noreen Jakeman, and Sheena Webb*

## True or False? Test your existing knowledge—answers in the chapter and online

1. Mood fluctuations are commonly pathological in humans.

2. Adverse childhood experiences are associated with depression in adulthood.

3. The S allele of the serotonin transporter gene promoter region confers greater susceptibility to depression following life events than the L allele.

4. Antidepressants decrease the overall level of central monoamines.

5. Anhedonia is the inability to feel sadness.

6. Depression in elderly patients can cause forgetfulness of a severity mimicking dementia.

7. Childhood depression should be treated with antidepressants.

8. Hypothyroidism is a side effect of lithium.

9. Mirroring should be employed when interviewing manic patients.

10. When depression following a heart attack is severe enough to prevent rehabilitation, the prognosis is so poor for patients over 70 that arrangements should be made for nursing home accommodation.

## Contents

# PRINCIPLES

## Introduction

Moods fluctuate as part of the normal human experience, but mood (or 'affective') *disorders* are illnesses where the main feature is excessively high or low mood. People often use the term *depression* to describe a transient healthy feeling of sadness. However, clinical depression is no more like feeling sad than falling in love is like having a crush. Likewise, mania is very different from the normal experience of happiness.

Although people may only experience a single affective episode, mood disorders generally run a relapsing and remitting course, referred to as either *unipolar* (recurrent episodes of *depression*) or *bipolar* (episodes of mania *and* depression). Where the term 'depression' is used in this chapter it means unipolar depression.

## Epidemiology

Depression is more common than bipolar affective disorder (BPAD), and has a female predominance. Full details are given in Table 7.1.

**TABLE 7.1** Epidemiology and twin concordance of depression and BPAD

|  | Depression | BPAD |
|---|---|---|
| Male : female | 1:2 | 1:1 |
| Lifetime risk[a] | 16.6% | 3.9% |
| 12 month prevalence[b] | 6.7% | 2.6% |
| Twin concordance rates (MZ:DZ)[c] | 44%:20% | 40%:5.4% |

[a] Kessler *et al.* 2005a
[b] Kessler *et al.* 2005b
[c] McGuffin *et al.* 2003

## Aetiology

### Genetics

Mood disorders run in families. Rather than a single 'gene for depression' (or BPAD), a combination of genes probably increases the risk of mood disorders. There is overlap between the inheritance of BPAD and depression: the relatives of depressed people are at increased risk of depression, while the relatives of those with BPAD are at higher risk of both BPAD and depression.

Adoption studies show that children of depressed parents have a higher risk of depression even when raised in 'depression-free' adoptive families. Complex models of genetic and environmental interactions have superseded the nature–nurture debate, there being a genetic contribution at the level of temperament, behaviour, and response to stress (Cadoret 1978). Only some people become depressed following stress, while others remain well. The serotonin transporter gene gives an example of genetic susceptibility to stress. Its promoter region has two versions: an S (short) allele and an L (long) allele. If someone with the S allele suffers three or more life events, their risk of depression trebles, whereas this has no effect on the depression risk for someone with the L allele (Caspi *et al.* 2003).

➡ Depression *can* come out of nowhere (especially when there is a strong family history). This can feel hard to cope with because there seems nothing to legitimize the depression: 'I've nothing to be sad about'.

### Childhood and life experiences

Adverse childhood experiences are associated with later depression, operating through their impact on confidence, trust, and self-esteem. These include early childhood abuse, relentless criticism, parental loss, and perceived lack of affection.

In adults, *vulnerability factors* increase the risk of depression by reducing resilience to adverse situations. They include unemployment, lack of a confiding relationship, lower socio-economic status, and social isolation.

---

**BOX 7.1** Brown and Harris study of women in Camberwell, London

This study (Brown and Harris 1978) showed that life events did not always precipitate depression, but were more likely to do so if other *vulnerability factors* were already present:

- three or more children under the age of 14 at home
- not working outside the home
- lack of a confidante
- loss of mother before the age of 11.

These associations seem less relevant in BPAD, perhaps because of the stronger genetic component.

---

## Life events

Life events have been classified according to their degree of stressfulness (Box 7.2). An excess of life events may occur in the 3 months before an episode of depression, and the risk of depression increases sixfold in the 6 months following life events (Paykel 1994).

BOX 7.2 The Holmes–Rahe Social Adjustment Scale (Holmes and Rahe 1967)

1. Death of spouse.
2. Divorce.
3. Marital separation.
4. Jail term.
5. Death of a close relative.

'Loss events' are particularly important in depression. The obvious example is bereavement, but *loss* comprises a wide range of events, including loss of role (e.g. following retirement) and loss of autonomy (e.g. following physical or mental ill health). If these losses cannot be mourned, depression may ensue.

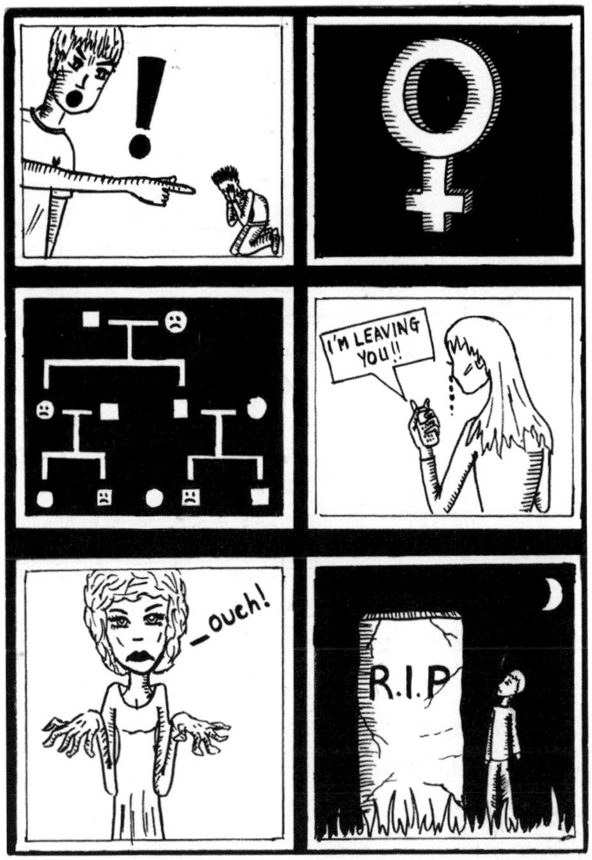

Both negative and positive life events can precipitate mania, although as BPAD evolves over time, environmental triggers become less important. The puerperium, sleep deprivation, and flying across time zones can all trigger manic episodes.

> Although depression may be 'understandable' (e.g. following an adverse life event), this does not mean that it should be left untreated.

## Physical causes

Physical illness is associated with depression. Chronic pain can precipitate depression and is linked with an increased suicide risk. Physical illnesses which directly *cause* depression include Cushing's syndrome, hypothyroidism, stroke, Parkinson's disease, multiple sclerosis, and hyperparathyroidism, although the processes are not fully understood. Some medications (e.g. beta-blockers and antihypertensives) can cause depression, as can illicit drugs such as stimulants (e.g. cocaine).

Mania can be caused by physical disorders such as Cushing's syndrome, head injury, or multiple sclerosis. Steroids, antidepressants, and stimulants can all trigger mania.

## Main theories of affective disorders

### Behavioural and cognitive theories

Seligman's studies led to the *learned helplessness* model of depression (Maier and Seligman 1976). Dogs repeatedly given unavoidable electric shocks eventually gave up trying to escape even when conditions changed and they were freed. Depressed people learn that they cannot change their situation and effectively give up trying.

Beck's model of depression informs cognitive behavioural therapy (CBT). It shows how negative thinking can depress mood, which generates negative thoughts,

FIGURE 7.1 Risk factors for depression

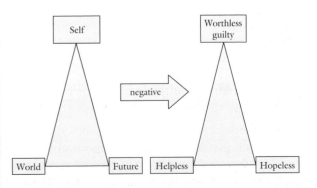

FIGURE 7.2 Beck's negative cognitive triad in depression

resulting in a downwards spiral into depression. He proposed a negative *cognitive triad* of views on the self, the world and the future, whereas in mania he defined a positive triad.

## Psychoanalytical theories

Psychoanalysts believe that early experience, particularly the quality of early relationships, determines the risk of later depression. Mental states are viewed as a kind of internal drama. Depression can be understood as a cruel relationship between a harsh critical judge and a helpless inadequate agent. In mania the agent rebels and denies vulnerability, defending against depression.

## Neurochemical theories

*The monoamine hypothesis* states that depression is the result of a deficiency in brain monoamine neurotransmitters.

- Noradrenaline (NA):
  - affects mood and energy.
- Serotonin (5-hydroxytryptamine, 5-HT):
  - affects sleep, appetite, memory, and mood.
- Dopamine (DA):
  - affects psychomotor activity.

Drugs that deplete monoamines (e.g. reserpine) can cause depression, whereas most antidepressants increase 5-HT and NA levels. Findings in depression include:

- ↓plasma tryptophan (a 5-HT precursor)
- ↓cerebrospinal fluid (CSF) levels of 5-hydroxy indoleacetic acid (5-HIAA; a 5-HT metabolite) levels in suicide victims
- ↓CSF homovanillic acid (a dopamine metabolite).

These suggest monoamine deficiency in depression. The hypothesis does not explain the 4–6 week delay in mood elevation by antidepressants, despite their more rapid chemical effects, e.g. 5-HT reuptake inhibition.

Mania may be related to dopamine overactivity. Bromocriptine (a dopamine agonist), amphetamine, and cocaine increase dopamine levels, and can induce manic symptoms, whereas antipsychotics (dopamine receptor antagonists) can treat mania.

## Endocrine abnormalities

Cortisol is the main stress hormone, and may mediate between stressful life events and the biological changes in depression, possibly by damaging hippocampal neurons. In 50% of depressed patients, dexamethasone (a synthetic glucocorticoid) fails to suppress cortisol secretion. However, non-suppression also occurs in mania, schizophrenia, and old age, and therefore is not diagnostically useful.

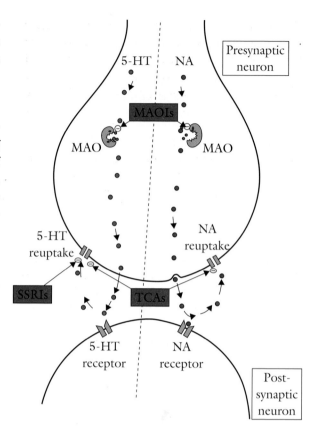

**FIGURE 7.3** Simplified diagram showing the mechanism of antidepressant action. 5-HT, serotonin; MAO, monoamine oxidase; MAOIs, monoamine oxidase inhibitors; NA, noradrenaline; SSRIs, serotonin-specific reuptake inhibitors; TCAs, tricyclic antidepressants

## Depression

### Clinical presentation

Dementors are among the foulest creatures that walk this earth. They infest the darkest, filthiest places, they glory in decay and despair, they drain peace, hope, and happiness out of the air around them. Even Muggles feel their presence, though they can't see them. Get too near a Dementor and every good feeling, every happy memory will be sucked out of you.

*Harry Potter and the Prisoner of Azkaban*—J.K. Rowling[1]

The experience of depression, as described through the metaphor of Dementors, is horrible. Although diagnosis only requires two weeks of symptoms, this can feel like an eternity for the sufferer.

### Core symptoms

The *core* symptoms of depression are:

- *low mood*
- *anergia*
- *anhedonia.*

Diagnosis requires at least two of these symptoms. As well as feeling pervasively low, people may describe irritability, anxiety, or tearfulness. Diurnal variation of mood can occur, where one part of the day feels worse (classically the mornings). *Anergia* is low energy, described by patients as feeling 'tired all the time'; they may not finish tasks because they quickly feel worn out, and this can hugely affect their ability to function. Movements may be obviously slowed down (psychomotor retardation). *Anhedonia* is the loss of enjoyment and interest in activities they previously enjoyed.

### Cognitive symptoms

The person feels worthless, useless, and unlovable. They guiltily dwell on past misdeeds. Their view of the future becomes pessimistic and they lose confidence in themselves. Things can look so bad that suicide seems the only option. Poor concentration and memory can be frustrating. Memory impairment in the elderly can be so extreme that the picture resembles dementia (i.e. pseudodementia). Thinking can also feel slowed.

### Biological symptoms

An altered sleep pattern is common, typically as *initial insomnia* (difficulty falling asleep) or *early morning wakening* (waking at least 2 hours earlier than normal). Less common is hypersomnia, which may coexist with hyperphagia and weight gain. More commonly, appetite for food and sex is suppressed, leading to weight loss and a strain on relationships. Physical symptoms, such as constipation, aches and pains, and dysmenorrhoea, may be problematic.

### Psychotic symptoms

These may emerge in very severe depression. Auditory hallucinations are often unpleasant derogatory voices. Rarely, visual hallucinations of scenes of destruction or evil spirits may be seen. Delusions are often nihilistic or persecutory. Nihilistic delusions follow the theme of 'nothingness'—e.g. the world has ended; the patient is dead; their organs are blocked or decomposing. If experiencing persecutory delusions, the patient may feel that they deserve persecution or punishment, linking in with guilt feelings. Guilt itself may progress to a delusional level, even to the extent that the patient believes they have committed some terrible crime, despite being blameless.

Depression is graded as *mild, moderate, severe*, or *severe with psychotic features*. This reflects both the number and severity of symptoms, and the effect on functioning. Biological symptoms tend to emerge as the severity increases, with psychotic symptoms only seen in the most severe cases. Suicidality, psychotic symptoms, severe self-neglect, or ceasing to eat and drink are the most worrying features.

---

**BOX 7.3** Subtypes of depression

- *Seasonal affective disorder* (SAD) presents predictably with low mood in the winter. There are usually *reversed biological* symptoms of overeating and oversleeping.
- *Atypical depression* has no seasonal variation, but again shows reversed biological symptoms and may retain mood reactivity.
- *Agitated depression* is depression with psychomotor agitation (instead of retardation), e.g. restlessness, pacing, hand-wringing.
- *Depressive stupor* is when psychomotor retardation is so profound that the person grinds to a halt. They become mute and stop eating, drinking, or moving.

## Differential diagnosis

1. **Physical causes**, e.g. hypothyroidism, head injury, cancer, 'quiet' delirium.
2. **Adjustment disorder**: unpleasant but mild affective symptoms follow a life event, but do not reach the severity needed to diagnose depression.
3. **Normal sadness**: try not to medicalize; people are allowed to be sad sometimes.
4. **Bereavement**: normal grief should not be diagnosed as depression (see Box 7.4).

---

**BOX 7.4** Bereavement

Grief is a *normal* response to loss. The normal stages of grief are:

- **Numbness**
- **Pining**
- **Depression**
- **Recovery**

Grieving people may feel that they are 'going mad' or will never recover. They may hear or see the dead person, experience immense anger, guilt, anxiety, or sadness, and feel overwhelmed by sudden 'pangs' of grief. You need to listen, explain, and normalize their experiences, rather than medicalize grief by dispensing antidepressants. Occasionally, there is an abnormal grief reaction, where the grief is:

- **Extremely intense** (reaching the level for depression; disabling the person)
- **Prolonged** (>6 months) without relief *or*
- **Delayed** (no sign of an emotional response).

These ideas are only guidelines; grief is an individual experience. Look for evidence that the person is moving *forward* (even if slowly) to a point where the loss is slightly less painful than it was at first, and don't expect this to happen quickly. Worry when grief gets 'stuck'.

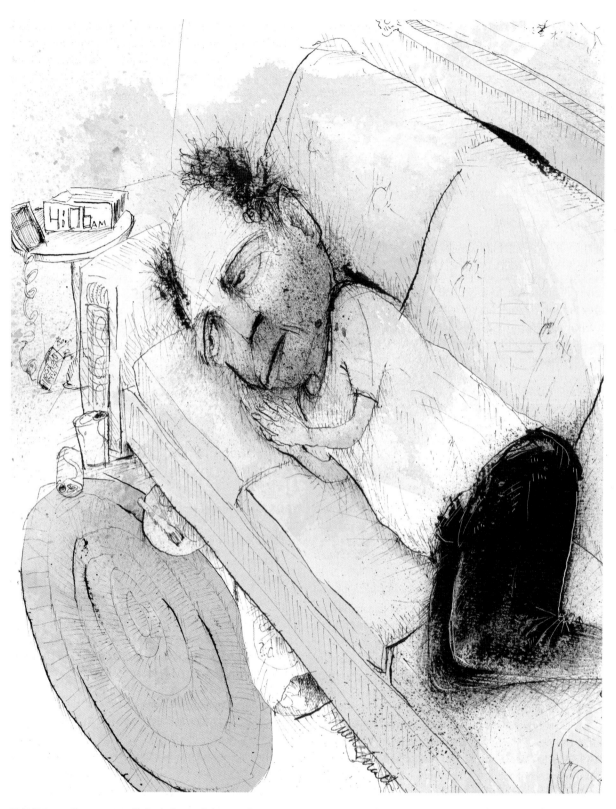

**FIGURE 7.4** How many clinical signs of depression can you identify in this artist's impression? Compare this to the experience of mania (see Figure 7.6)

5. **BPAD/schizoaffective disorder/schizophrenia**: look for previous manic or psychotic features.

6. **Substance misuse**: alcohol and drugs may cause depression or be a form of self-medication.

7. **Postnatal depression/puerperal illness** (see p.196)

8. **Dementia**: depression can affect memory so badly that the patient appears to have dementia (i.e. pseudo-dementia); dementia can begin with affective changes.

## Investigations

1. Collateral history.

2. Physical examination.

3. Blood tests (include others as suggested by history and examination):
   - TFT (to rule out hypothyroidism)
   - FBC (anaemia causes fatigue)
   - G or HbA$_{1c}$ (diabetes causes fatigue).

4. Rating scales can measure severity or monitor treatment response, e.g. Beck Depression Inventory (BDI), Hospital Anxiety and Depression Scale (HADS).

5. CT or MRI head are *never* routine, but may help to rule out *suspected* cerebral pathology.

## Management

Mild depression often resolves spontaneously and GPs commonly adopt a 'watchful waiting' approach or refer for supportive counselling or problem-solving therapy. If necessary, Community Mental Health Teams can provide support at home, e.g. through Home Treatment Teams. Consider inpatient treatment if there is a significant risk of suicide or self-harm.

Advice on sleep hygiene, exercise, and self-help, and access to CBT or counselling may be sufficient in managing mild depression. Social stressors must be addressed and interventions might include time off work, respite for carers, refuge from abusers, debt advice, or support groups.

### 1. Psychological treatment

This is the first step to treating mild depression and is ideally always involved in moderate or severe depression, with antidepressants, as necessary.

### Cognitive behavioural therapy (CBT)

CBT is a way of thinking about thinking. This brief goal-oriented therapy focuses on the *here and now* and views psychological problems as a result of the patient's distorted perceptions of themselves, the world, or the future (Hawton *et al.* 1996). The therapist helps the patient to notice negative automatic thoughts (NATs), triggered by day-to-day situations and resulting in

unhelpful moods and behaviours. Mood, thought, and behaviour are mutually reinforcing. With time, the patient learns how distorted core beliefs and dysfunctional assumptions, often set up in childhood, feed into a vicious circle. CBT targets thoughts and behaviours, with the aim of making changes that have a knock-on effect on mood.

### CBT for depression

Depressed people often believe that they are worthless and life is hopeless. A vicious circle is set up: the negative perception of events leads not only to lowered mood, but to unhelpful behaviour that withdraws the person from the world around them, further confirming their view that they are useless and unlovable (Figure 7.5).

CBT aims to challenge negative beliefs and increase the patient's daily exposure to positive stimulating activities. Activity scheduling helps the patient to engage in behaviours that will enhance energy levels, develop interests, and provide a sense of achievement. The patient is asked to practise challenging their NATs as and when they arise. They are made aware of common thinking errors, e.g.

- *Generalization*—'I *always* mess *everything* up'.
- *Minimization*—'I only passed that exam by chance. It doesn't mean I'm good enough'.

Distorted beliefs are tested through:

- *Discussion* during sessions, e.g. 'How do you know for sure that no-one cares about you?'
- *Behavioural experiments* between sessions, e.g. inviting a friend to dinner to test out the idea that nobody wants to spend time with them.

The therapist helps the patient to build an alternative set of more *realistic* beliefs about themselves, e.g. 'I'm not perfect, but I'm OK'. Towards the end of therapy, relapse prevention focuses on ensuring that old thinking and behavioural habits do not re-emerge.

### Psychodynamic psychotherapy

The developing relationship between therapist and patient is the key issue in psychodynamic psychotherapy. The patient applies their unconscious templates of relationships, derived from past experience, to the new situation with the therapist, e.g. 'I will be rejected'/'The therapist will let me down'. These distorted expectations or *transferences* are more felt than thought, and the emotional atmosphere in the room informs the therapist's interpretation, e.g. 'You're afraid I'll humiliate you'/ 'You expect me to dislike you'. Putting words to the feelings allows the patient to recognize their hidden beliefs and re-evaluate them in the light of current reality.

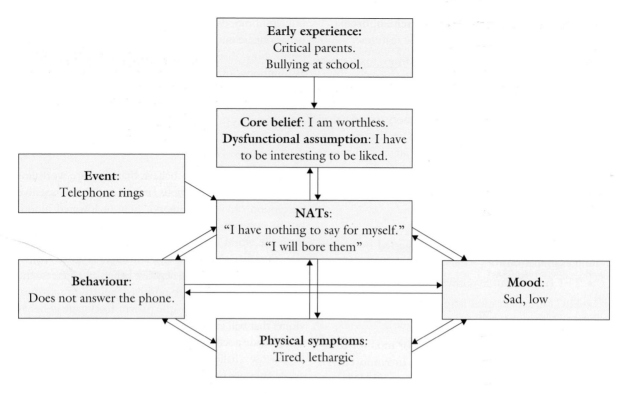

FIGURE 7.5 Example of CBT formulation for depression

**Interpersonal therapy**

This focuses on main themes of unresolved loss, psycho-social transitions, relationship conflict, and social skills deficit.

*2. Pharmacological treatment*

Antidepressants increase the overall level of monoamines at the synapse by decreasing either reuptake or break-down (Figure 7.3). Over time, the serotonin and central beta-adrenergic receptors become downregulated (decrease in number), which is thought to account for the 4–6 week delay in antidepressant effects.

Antidepressants are usually indicated for moderate to severe depression, *ideally with psychotherapy*. In psychotic depression, an antipsychotic is added. All antidepressants are effective in treating depression, but selective serotonin reuptake inhibitors (SSRIs) are usually the first choice because of their relatively mild side effects and safety in overdose *compared with older drugs*. Treatment should continue until the patient is no longer depressed and *then* for a further 6 months to prevent relapse. In recurrent depression, treatment should continue for much longer (e.g. 2 years). The maintenance dose of the antidepressant should be the same as for acute treatment, since lower doses are rarely effective.

All antidepressants can cause hyponatraemia or some degree of sexual dysfunction; most lower the seizure threshold (use with care in epilepsy). Antidepressants should be avoided in mania or hypomania. Advise patients not to drink alcohol while on antidepressants because of increased sedation, and never to drive if feeling drowsy on antidepressants. Explain that the onset of action is delayed, and outline the major side effects (Table 7.2).

**SSRIs**

SSRIs enhance serotoninergic neurotransmission by blocking the reuptake of serotonin into the pre-synaptic nerve terminal.

**Tricyclic antidepressants (TCAs)**

These inhibit the reuptake of NA and 5-HT. The use of TCAs is falling out of fashion. Due to cardiotoxicity they can be lethal in overdose so should be avoided where there is a risk of suicide.

**Monoamine oxidase inhibitors (MAOIs)**

MAOIs inhibit the metabolism of monoamines, thus increasing their synaptic levels. They are rarely used nowadays because of the dangers of a hypertensive crisis due to a build-up of noradrenaline when eating tyramine-rich foods (e.g. mature cheese, yeast extracts, and fermented soya beans). They should not be combined with other antidepressants.

Childhood depression is treated psychologically; antidepressants should only be prescribed by specialists, and are indicated for the most severely depressed children.

**TABLE 7.2** Comparison of antidepressants

| Class | Example | Common side effects |
|---|---|---|
| Selective serotonin reuptake inhibitors (SSRIs) | Fluoxetine<br>Sertraline<br>Paroxetine<br>Fluvoxamine<br>Citalopram<br>Escitalopram | Nausea, vomiting<br>Appetite/weight change<br>Blurred vision<br>Anxiety and agitation<br>Insomnia, tremor, dizziness<br>Headache<br>Sweating |
| Serotonin and noradrenaline reuptake inhibitors (SNRIs) | Venlafaxine<br>Duloxetine | As for SSRIs, but also:<br>Constipation<br>Hypertension<br>Raised cholesterol |
| Noradrenergic and specific serotonin antidepressant (NASSAs) | Mirtazapine | Sedation<br>Increased appetite/weight<br>Oedema |
| Noradrenaline reuptake inhibitor antidepressants (NARIs) | Reboxetine | Dry mouth<br>Constipation<br>Excessive sweating<br>Urinary problems<br>Insomnia<br>Tachycardia |
| Tricyclic antidepressants (TCAs) | Amitriptyline<br>Clomipramine<br>Imipramine<br>Lofepramine<br>Dosulepin | Tachycardia, arrhythmias<br>Dry mouth<br>Blurred vision<br>Constipation<br>Urinary retention<br>Postural hypotension<br>Sedation<br>Nausea, weight gain |
| Monoamine oxidase inhibitors (MAOIs) | Phenelzine<br>Tranylcypromine | Hypertensive crisis (the 'cheese reaction')<br>Postural hypotension, dizziness<br>Drowsiness, insomnia<br>Headache<br>Blurred vision<br>Nausea and vomiting<br>Constipation |
| Reversible inhibitors of monoamine oxidase A (RIMAs) | Moclobemide | Agitation/anxiety<br>Sleep disturbance<br>Nausea<br>Hypertension |
| Miscellaneous | Trazodone<br>(5-HT reuptake blockade and 5-HT$_2$ antagonist)<br><br>St John's wort<br>(herbal, unlicensed) | Sedation<br>Dizziness, postural hypotension<br>Tachycardia<br>Nausea<br>Constipation, diarrhoea<br>Tremor<br>Photosensitivity<br>Anxiety, dizziness<br>Gastrointestinal symptoms,<br>Fatigue, headache |

**Look out for patients who respond 'too well' to antidepressants: all antidepressants can switch people with BPAD from depression to mania. BPAD may be undiagnosed if your patient is yet to suffer their first manic episode.**

**St John's wort can treat mild depression, and seems to work similarly to SSRIs. It can induce metabolizing enzymes, risking drug interactions, e.g. making the oral contraceptive pill (OCP) ineffective.**

### Stopping and swapping

Although antidepressants are not addictive, if suddenly stopped, they can cause unpleasant *discontinuation symptoms*. These vary with the drug, but include 'flu-like symptoms, 'electric shock' sensations, headaches, vertigo, or irritability. Always withdraw antidepressants over a few weeks.

Antidepressants of different classes can interact dangerously: *check before changing*. Some can be cross-tapered; others need a drug-free washout period. *Serotonin syndrome* is caused by excess serotonin (e.g. from giving two antidepressants at once). It is potentially life-threatening and symptoms include restlessness and sweating, myoclonus, confusion, and fits.

### Poor response

Treatment resistance (refractory depression) is the failure to respond to two adequate trials of different classes of antidepressants at adequate doses and for a period of 6–8 weeks (Souery *et al.* 1999). Up to 30% of patients may be treatment resistant, but always re-examine the diagnosis and check that the patient is taking their medication! The dose can be increased, the drug changed, the *class* of drug changed; specialists may employ augmentation strategies, e.g. (Rush *et al.* 2006):

- *Lithium*
- *Tri-iodothyronine* ($T_3$) or *levothyroxine* ($T_4$)
- *Buspirone* is an anxiolytic drug that acts on $5HT_{1a}$ receptors. It has no antidepressant action alone, but may have a synergistic effect when combined with SSRIs.

#### *3. Non-drug options*

### Electroconvulsive therapy (ECT)

ECT can be a fast and life-saving treatment in severe or psychotic depression, e.g. if the patient has stopped eating and drinking. Past treatment *was* both frightening and painful but has been refined over the years, now using electrodes to produce a generalized tonic–clonic seizure while the patient is anaesthetized. The main concern is that some people experience a degree of memory loss after the procedure.

### Light therapy

A light box can be used to treat SAD, compensating for the fewer hours of daylight in the winter that are thought to be responsible for the disorder.

## Prognosis

Approximately 50% of patients will have at least one more episode. Each episode lasts on average 8–9 months, but treatment can reduce this to only 2–3 months. Psychotic depression has a poorer prognosis, but shows a better response to ECT. Up to 15% of people with major depression eventually take their own lives.

**In depression the most important risk is suicide (see p.60); however, do not overlook other areas, e.g. self-neglect and malnutrition secondary to poor motivation and appetite disturbance. This is particularly common in the elderly or those with psychotic symptoms.**

# Mania

**My thoughts were so fast that I couldn't remember the beginning of a sentence halfway through. Fragments of ideas, images, sentences, raced around and around in my mind like the tigers in a children's story. Finally, like those tigers, they became meaningless melted pools. Nothing once familiar to me was familiar. I wanted desperately to slow down but could not.**

**(Jamison 1995)**

## Clinical presentation

To diagnose a *manic* episode, symptoms should last for at least a week and prevent work and ordinary social activities. Less severe symptoms, not entirely disrupting the patient's ability to function, lead to a diagnosis of *hypomania*. Hypomanic periods may be quite productive, since thoughts, energy, and confidence are overflowing, but not so chaotically as not to be put to creative use.

#### *Core symptoms*

Whereas mood, energy, and enjoyment are *lowered* in depression, these are all *raised* in mania. *Elevated mood* varies from carefree cheerfulness to elation and uncontrollable excitement, though irritability and aggression can replace these. Mood may be *labile*, switching quickly between different emotions. People describe *boundless energy*, and are *overactive*, busy, restless, and talkative. *Increased enjoyment and interest* may prompt the person to indulge in many new activities, meeting lots of new 'friends'.

#### *Cognitive symptoms*

*Inflated self-esteem and confidence* lead the person to believe that they are gifted, attractive, creative, intelligent, and extremely special. Optimism makes the future look very hopeful and the world seems full of opportunity. Exciting ideas abound, thoughts race, and concentration dissolves; despite being very distractible, the patient will often feel as though they can think more clearly than ever. Speech becomes pressured and topics change rapidly (flight of ideas).

## Biological symptoms

Sleep is dramatically reduced, and people may be up all night without feeling tired. They develop voracious appetites for food and sex (although they may be so busy they forget to eat). Behaviour may become reckless, disinhibited, and inappropriate, and with raised libido, risky sexual liaisons can take place. Previously timid people may spend excessively, drive recklessly, or gamble their money away. Drugs or alcohol can become new interests and serve to make the patient even more disinhibited.

## Psychotic symptoms

In severe illness, optimism develops into grandiose delusions of, for example, an important mission, fame, or special powers. Persecutory delusions may arise if the patient believes that others are jealous of them. Auditory hallucinations may reflect the elevated mood, e.g. prime ministers or saints talking to the patient.

The *diagnosis* of BPAD can be made when a patient has suffered a manic episode and *any other* affective episode, whether depressed, hypomanic, manic, or mixed (elements of both depression and mania at once).

---

**BOX 7.5**  BPAD subtypes

- **Type I BPAD**
  - *Manic* episodes interspersed with depressive episodes.
- **Type II BPAD**
  - Mainly recurrent depressive episodes, with less prominent *hypomanic* episodes.
- **Rapid cycling BPAD**
  - Four or more affective episodes in a year.
  - More common in women.
  - May respond better to sodium valproate.

---

**TABLE 7.3**  Summary of depression and mania

| Factor | | Depression | Mania |
|---|---|---|---|
| Duration | | 2 weeks | 1 week |
| Core symptoms | Mood | Low | High (elated or irritable) |
| | Energy | Low (anergia) | High |
| | Interest/enjoyment | Low (anhedonia) | High: new activities or contacts |
| Cognitive | Self | Worthless | Grandiose, superhuman |
| | | Decreased confidence | Increased confidence |
| | | Guilty | Guilt-free |
| | World | Helpless; the world feels overwhelming | Capable; the world can be dominated |
| | Future | Hopeless, pessimistic | Hopeful, optimistic |
| | Concentration | Poor | Poor, very distractible |
| | Memory | Sometimes impaired | Sometimes forgetful secondary to poor concentration |
| Biological | Sleep | Usually decreased | Decreased |
| | Appetite/weight | Usually decreased | Increased (though may not have time to eat) |
| | Libido | Low | High |
| Psychotic | Hallucinations | Auditory (>visual): often unpleasant, derogatory | Auditory (>visual): may be pleasant, or important people |
| | Delusions | Nihilistic | Grandiose |
| | | Persecutory | Persecutory |
| Risk | Self | Suicide | Suicide |
| | | Self-harm | Spending/gambling |
| | | Neglect | Reckless driving |
| | | | Substance misuse |
| | | | Self-neglect |
| | | | Exhaustion |
| | Others | Rarely | Aggression |
| | | | Sexually inappropriate behaviour |

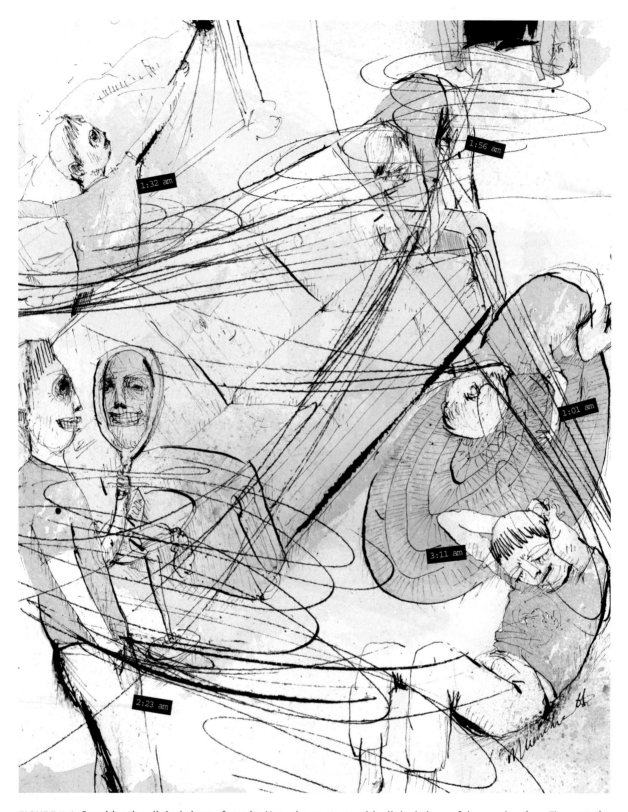

FIGURE 7.6 Consider the clinical signs of mania. Note the contrast with clinical signs of depression (see Figure 7.4)

Don't assume that racing thoughts and plenty of energy are always enjoyable—patients may find them distressing and overwhelming.

Patients may be able to exert some control over their symptoms for a short time, which can be misleading in a brief interview.

## Differential diagnosis

1. **Organic** causes must always be excluded, e.g.
   - Drug-induced states, e.g. amphetamines, cocaine
   - Dementia
   - Frontal lobe disease
   - Delirium
   - Cerebral HIV
   - 'Myxoedema madness' (paradoxically, a state of frenzied activity in extreme hypothyroidism).

2. **Schizophrenia/schizoaffective disorder**: psychotic symptoms precede and outweigh affective symptoms.

3. **Cyclothymia**
   - This is persistent mood instability with many episodes of mild low mood and mild elation. None of the episodes are sufficiently severe or prolonged to meet criteria for even mild depression or hypomania.

4. **Puerperal disorders** (see p.196) .

## Investigations

1. Collateral history.
2. Physical examination.
3. Blood tests: FBC, TFTs, CRP to exclude infection or thyroid problems; other tests as indicated.
4. Urine drug screen.
5. CT/MRI brain to exclude organic causes, if indicated.

## Management

### 1. Pharmacological treatment

#### Mood stabilizers

These drugs 'even out' the extreme highs of mania and the profound lows of depression, although they tend to be most effective against mania. The three main drugs used are lithium, sodium valproate, and carbamazepine. Their mechanism of action is currently uncertain, although the anticonvulsants may act on sodium channels or GABA (gamma aminobutyric acid), an inhibitory neurotransmitter in the nervous system.

#### *Lithium*

Various theories have been proposed to explain lithium's mechanism of action, but none have yet been proven. Lithium's therapeutic range is 0.6–1.0mmol/L, but it has a narrow therapeutic index, becoming toxic from

---

1.2mmol/L (Box 7.6). Lithium levels must be checked a week after starting or changing the dose, monitored weekly until a steady therapeutic level has been achieved, and then every 3 months. U&Es and TFTs should be monitored every 3–6 months, since lithium can cause renal impairment and hypothyroidism.

 Lithium levels are taken 12 hours post-dose.

Care is needed if switching between lithium citrate (usually liquid) and lithium carbonate (usually tablet), since they contain different amounts of lithium.

#### *Valproate*

Valproate is an anticonvulsant, but treats acute mania and provides prophylaxis in BPAD. Valproic acid is the active drug, but it is usually given as the sodium or semi-sodium salt in the hope of lessening adverse effects (valproic acid, sodium valproate, and semi-sodium valproate are all variations of the same drug). Plasma levels do not need monitoring, as there is no generally accepted therapeutic range and dose-related toxicity is not usually a problem.

#### *Carbamazepine*

Carbamazepine is another anticonvulsant, which can cause toxicity at high doses. It induces liver enzymes that metabolize many drugs, including itself, making it essential to monitor carbamazepine levels closely and to check for drug interactions before prescribing. It is less effective than lithium, but is a second-line treatment in BPAD prophylaxis.

Some people feel that mood stabilizers curb creativity or blunt their normal reactivity, and this may be a reason to discontinue medication. If you felt more confident and happy than you'd ever felt before, would *you* take a tablet to 'bring you down'?

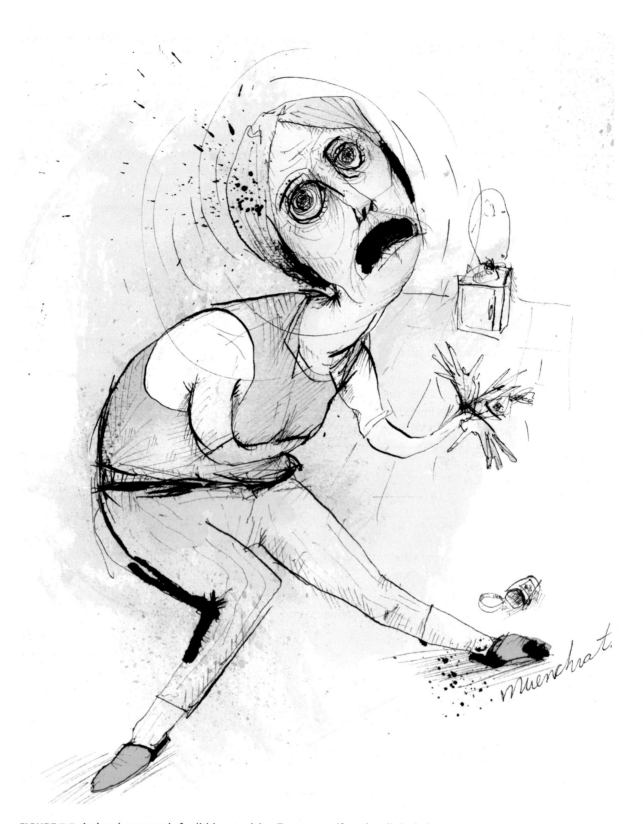

FIGURE 7.7 A visual mnemonic for lithium toxicity. Test yourself on the clinical signs

## Other drugs used for mood stabilization

*Antipsychotics* such as olanzapine are used in the manic phase and may be continued as prophylaxis after the mood has settled. Generally, atypical antipsychotics (e.g. olanzapine, risperidone, or quetiapine) are chosen over typicals because they have fewer side effects (see p.79).

*Other anticonvulsants*: lamotrigine is effective as prophylaxis, especially in bipolar II disorder. Topiramate and gabapentin are being assessed for effectiveness as mood stabilizers.

**TABLE 7.4** Side effects of mood stabilizers

| Drug | Side effects |
|---|---|
| Lithium<br>*Monitor levels!* | Mild tremor<br>GI effects, nausea, vomiting<br>Polyuria, polydipsia<br>Arrhythmia<br>Hypothyroidism<br>Weight gain |
| Valproate | GI effects, nausea, vomiting, diarrhoea<br>Liver failure<br>Thrombocytopenia<br>Hair loss<br>Weight gain |
| Carbamazepine<br>*Monitor levels!* | Rash<br>Leucopenia<br>Dizziness, ataxia<br>Drowsiness, fatigue<br>Nausea, vomiting<br>Oedema, fluid retention<br>Weight gain<br>Hyponatraemia<br>Enzyme induction may decrease levels of other drugs, making them ineffective (e.g. OCP) |
| Lamotrigine | Skin rashes which may be life-threatening<br>Headache, tiredness<br>Nausea<br>Dizziness<br>Insomnia<br>Arthralgia and back pain |

### Acute treatment of mania or hypomania

Stop all medication that may induce symptoms, including antidepressants, drugs of abuse, steroids, and dopamine agonists. Mania can lead to exhaustion if not adequately treated, so monitor food and fluid intake and prevent dehydration.

*If treatment free*, give an antipsychotic *or* a mood stabilizer. A short course of benzodiazepines is often added for sedation, since sleep deprivation can worsen mania and contribute to physical collapse. If symptoms are severe or response is poor, the antipsychotic and mood stabilizer may be combined.

*If already on treatment*, optimize the medication. Check compliance, adjust doses, and consider adding another agent (e.g. if already on optimal dose of mood stabilizer, an antipsychotic may be added). Again, short-term benzodiazepine treatment can help.

Electroconvulsive therapy may be used if patients are unresponsive to medication or risk life-threatening over-activity and physical exhaustion.

### Long-term treatment

Long-term treatment is needed after even a single manic episode, since further episodes are highly likely and potentially devastating. Mood stabilizers are used and other drugs added when symptoms arise or when facing stress that could precipitate relapse (e.g. antipsychotics or benzodiazepines). Patients can often identify relapse indicators and initiate medication themselves.

Depression in BPAD can be difficult to treat, since antidepressants can switch the mood to mania. To lessen the chance of this, antidepressants should only be given in combination with a mood stabilizer or antipsychotic as 'cover'. Monitor closely for signs of mania, and if manic symptoms re-emerge, stop the antidepressant immediately.

Medication may be cautiously and slowly withdrawn if the patient has been symptom-free for a sustained period. The patient should be made aware of the risk of relapse and fully involved in this decision.

After withdrawal of mood stabilizers, review your patient *more*—rather than *less*—frequently, to identify relapse early.

Patients should know that suddenly stopping medication (particularly lithium) can trigger a manic episode.

### 2. Psychological treatment

#### CBT

Psycho-education is essential. Therapist and patient work together to identify relapse indicators, such as insomnia or uncomfortably increased energy. By recognizing these signs, patients can establish strategies to avert relapse. Relapse prevention strategies include:

- Developing routine
- Ensuring good-quality sleep
- Promoting a healthy lifestyle
- Avoiding excessive stimulation/stress (often easier said than done)
- Addressing substance misuse
- Ensuring drug compliance

CBT also identifies the excessively positive thoughts that occur in mania, and helps patients to test them out and regain a sense of perspective. CBT can reduce relapse rates, shorten episodes of illness, and decrease the length and number of hospitalizations.

### Psychodynamic psychotherapy

This is useful in some cases, when mood is stabilized.

### 3. Social interventions

These include family support and therapy as well as aiding return to education or work.

## Prognosis

Manic episodes often begin abruptly and are normally shorter than depressive episodes, lasting between a fortnight and 5 months. Recovery is usually complete between episodes, although remissions become shorter with age and depressions become more frequent. Fifteen per cent of people with BPAD kill themselves, although long-term treatment with lithium reduces this to the same levels as for the general population.

> **Risks due to poor judgement, increased impulsivity, sexual disinhibition, and irritability should be considered. The risk of suicide is not always recognized; remember that affective lability seen in mania can involve extreme sudden distress or sadness. This carries significant risk of suicide, especially when psychotic symptoms are also present.**

# REALITY: DEPRESSION

## General approach: tips, tricks, and cautionary tales

### 1. Don't say, 'I know how you feel'

Although this *seems* empathic, it usually comes across rather badly, causing irritation or even frank anger that you could expect to *know* how awful someone else's experience feels. Paradoxically, it's often more empathic to say, 'I can't imagine how that would feel', since it recognizes that the other person's experiences and feelings are individual and profound.

### 2. Avoid platitudes

We all have a tendency to grasp for something that sounds wise and comforting when we don't know what to say. Remember that *one size does not fit all*, so any 'meaningful' phrases you have heard before are probably a bad idea. For example, if someone tells you that their partner has died, do *not* say:

- Plenty more fish in the sea!
- Every cloud has a silver lining!
- Time's the greatest healer!

Typically, these lines are delivered with inappropriate cheer and result in the loss of rapport.

### 3. It's not what you say, but how you say it

So what *do* you say? Well, apart from falling back on clichés, you can say almost anything and it will work, if you say it compassionately. To get the right tone and make it meaningful, there's no point in using phrases that you wouldn't use in everyday life; so take note of your response the next time a close friend tells you something difficult or painful. Your own natural response will be better than anything you can memorize from a book. Generally, the simpler the better, e.g. 'That's awful' is often more meaningful than 'I must say, that sounds as though it must have been utterly awful for you'.

### 4. Depression doesn't make people stupid

There's a tendency to point out obvious 'quick-fixes,' which can feel patronising, e.g.

> **Carrie:** *(sobbing)* Then he beats me 'til I do what he says. He says I'm a useless girlfriend and he wishes he'd never met me . . .
>
> **You:** You should leave him. *I'd* never put up with that!

Explaining how *you* would have easily dealt with their problems makes people feel that you think they're stupid. If it were *that* simple, they'd probably have done it by now.

## 5. Don't fear the tear

It's OK if people cry; it may even be therapeutic. You haven't done anything wrong, so you don't need to apologize or stop them crying; simply recognize that they are upset and let them be upset. People are more likely to open up to you if you can cope with their sadness than if they think they are distressing you and feel they must 'protect' you from the full force of their feelings.

## 6. Slow down

Because of psychomotor retardation and difficult subject matter, this is unlikely to be a fast-paced conversation. Set aside plenty of time for your interview and allow lots of time for answers; learning to tolerate silence is essential. Open questions are still the rule, unless someone is *very* psychomotor retarded, when you may need to switch earlier to closed questions if simple *yes* or *no* answers (or nodding or shaking their head) may be all they can manage.

## 7. Don't shout

People with depression often speak softly, so you're more likely to mirror them if you aim low. Additionally, they may have hyperacusis (everything sounds uncomfortably loud), which can make a slightly loud voice unbearable.

## 8. Saying it's *OK* won't make it OK

Depressed patients often make negative statements about themselves. It can be very tempting to try to convince your patient otherwise, e.g.

> **Beth:** I'm useless. *(Or fat, stupid, ugly, guilty, etc.)*
>
> **You:** No you're not!
>
> **B:** How would you know?!

Your patient is not looking for a debate; they are trying to tell you how they feel! Telling them they're wrong won't make them feel any better. Instead, try reflecting back the underlying message, e.g. 'You don't like yourself at the moment'. Let them realize that you understand and are not dismissing their views. That can be difficult in an interview, so a simpler response might be, e.g. 'It must be horrible to feel like that'. You can also ask *why* they hold these views.

## The interview

• = example of question; * = question that links to other parts of the history.

Remember that two or more core symptoms must be present for at least 2 weeks for a diagnosis.

## Mood

- **How have you been feeling recently?**
- Have you been feeling sad or tearful?
- Have you been more anxious or snappy than normal?
- Which bit of the day feels the worst/do you dread the most? (diurnal variation)
- * You've been low for a year. Did something happen a year ago?

## Anergia

- **What are your energy levels like at the moment?**
- Have you been feeling worn out or tired all the time?
- How is it affecting you? (work/childcare etc.)

## Anhedonia

- **Are you able to enjoy things like you used to?**
- Have you lost interest in things you used to do?
- * Do you still enjoy work (*or* hobbies . . . relationships . . . )?
- * Can you still enjoy spending time with friends or family?

## Sleep

- **How's your sleep been lately?**
- Which part of the night is the problem (falling asleep/staying asleep/waking early)?
- * How does that affect your energy levels?

## Appetite

- **What's your appetite been like recently?**
- Has it caused a change in your weight? How much, roughly?
- Have you noticed your clothes getting baggy (or tight)?
- * Can you be bothered (or have the energy) to cook for yourself?

## Libido

- **When people feel low like this, they can lose their sex drive. Is this a problem for you?**

Both depression *and* antidepressants cause sexual dysfunction, but most people won't discuss this unless you've built a rapport *and* asked directly.

## Concentration/memory/thinking

- **How's your concentration been?**
- Can you focus enough to read a whole page (or watch a whole TV programme)?

- Have you become more forgetful recently?
- Can you remember details, say, after reading the paper?
- Does your thinking feel more muddled or slowed down than usual?

## Helpless

- Do you think that there's anything you can do to improve this situation?
- * What about your family, friends, or the doctors . . . ? Do you think they can help?

## Worthless

- What do you think of yourself, as a person?
- How would you compare yourself to other people?
- Can you think of something you're proud of? (Anything *at all*?)

## Guilt

- Why do you think you've had such a hard time recently?
- Do you blame yourself for . . . ?
- Do you feel like you've let people down?

## Hopeless

- (You've said how everything feels bad now.) How do you see the future?
- Could things change for the better?
- * Is it ever *so* bad you wish you were dead?

## Suicidal ideation (see Suicide Reality for more, p.63)

- Things have been awful recently. Is it ever so bad that you want to die?

## Psychotic symptoms (see Schizophrenia Reality for more, p.83)

- Have you had any thoughts that people have been ganging up against you?
- Have you seen or heard anything recently that has struck you as strange or frightening?

If you believed you were worthless, which would make you question this the most?
- A total stranger telling you that you were worthwhile, or
- A total stranger taking time to listen to everything you had to say.

# 1. Depression history (15 minutes)

## Candidate's instructions

Mr Rahul Kapoor is 19 years old and a second-year dental student. He presents with low energy.

You are a final year medical student attached to the GP practice. Please interview Rahul with a view to making a psychiatric diagnosis.

## Patient's brief

### Key characteristics

- I'm softly spoken and monotonous.
- I'm emotionally flat and feel sad.
- I'm uncomfortable, making poor eye contact, and crossing my arms as I speak.
- I want to 'get this fixed' but don't really want to admit that I'm depressed.

Though I've always been a hard-working student, I've been feeling drained for the past three months. Everything's an effort. My concentration's gone and I have to keep re-reading the same paragraph to understand it. I feel like nothing's going in. My memory's terrible—I worry I just don't have the ability to learn the things I need to pass. I study late into the night (go to bed about 1am, though I couldn't sleep before then anyway) and wake up feeling exhausted when my alarm goes at 6am. I try to get 2 hours' reading in before lectures or clinics at 9am. I know I'm pushing myself hard, but since failing my exams last year I've lost a lot of confidence in my own ability. I'm in the bottom 5% of students, and I've got to compensate for my low intelligence with hard work. I don't have time to cook and I'm not hungry often. I might have lost weight.

I used to enjoy dentistry. I wanted to go into maxillo-facial surgery and knew I needed top grades; I suppose this made everything challenging and interesting. Now, studies seem boring—I guess because I've done it all before. Right now, I can't even see myself graduating, let alone doing max-fax work. I was a member of the photography society, but I don't enjoy it enough to put the time aside, and I feel guilty when I'm doing things other than studying. I broke up with my girlfriend, Priya, a month ago, since I'd lost interest in all aspects of our relationship (including sex). I felt I was holding her back and making her miserable. Apart from the study group I attend every evening, I don't really socialize anymore.

The final term was hard, last year. My father was diagnosed with prostate cancer and I returned to India to support my family while he was undergoing treatment. He died just before my exams. He'd saved so much money for me to come to the UK and study; he was so proud of me and I've let him down and wasted his money. My family were very disappointed when they heard I'd have to re-sit, but they are certain that I will pass. It puts the pressure on.

I'm not suicidal, but I just want this all to be over. Sometimes I daydream . . . It would be good to die heroically, save someone from being hit by a car or something. Everyone would remember me well, not see me as a failure.

### Other history

- I have no medical problems and take no medication.
- I've never had mental health problems, though my mother had a breakdown many years ago.
- I've never smoked and don't drink or use drugs.

### Questions

Can you rule out anaemia, diabetes, and hypothyroidism? I know they cause tiredness.

### Worries

I'm worried you'll tell the university I'm depressed and it'll affect my future career—if I have one.

## 2. Psychotic depression history (15 minutes)

### Candidate's instructions

Miss Annette Bristow is a 26-year-old accountant who underwent a termination of pregnancy two months ago, following the identification of 'severe abnormalities' at her 12-week scan. Her boyfriend, Mark, has brought her to casualty. He is worried that Annette is now not eating or drinking.

You are a final year medical student attached to the psychiatrist on call. Please take a mood disorder history.

### Patient's brief

#### Key characteristics

- My voice is quiet and monotonous but not slowed.
- I am agitated and desperate to 'right my wrongdoing'.
- I make poor eye contact and am distracted at times by demons' voices.
- I am not aware that I am behaving oddly.

Mark and I were trying for a baby for two years. A good mother would have kept him and loved him . . . But I am bad through and through; I'm a murderer. I told the doctors to kill my baby because he was disabled. When he died, he tore the cord between us and my life began to drain away. The doctors didn't take his corpse from my womb because they knew I should be punished for what I made them do. I know this because I smell his corpse rotting inside me; it's so strong I don't know how Mark can't smell it. I'm becoming his grave . . . my organs are rotting and becoming earth over his corpse. I have no womb, just earth. I have no bowels, just earth. I'll soon be completely dead. *You* can't see it, because the death is from the inside, out.

I realized this was happening about two weeks ago. Before that (following the termination) I was sad and cried a lot. I cut my legs to punish myself. Then the tears stopped and I hardly needed the toilet because my body was dying. I haven't eaten in a week—there's no point. I last drank yesterday, but there's no point in this either— where would it go? I stay awake at night, praying for my baby's soul. I've no energy, but that's because I'm dying. I don't deserve to enjoy anything. My brain is dying too and everything is slowing to a standstill so I can't remember things or think clearly.

I came willingly to hospital today because I need the doctors to open me up and exhume his corpse. They must hand him to the priests for a proper burial so that he can be blessed and properly buried. They won't need an anaesthetic; my nerves are already earth, so I won't feel it. If the doctors won't open me up, I will do it myself . . .

The skin barely holds in the soil so it won't take much to open me up; I could do it easily with a sharp knife. I hear children calling: 'You're too frightened to die! You'll never free the baby!' They are always with me like black whispers. They scare me, but all this will soon pass.

### Other history

- My mother suffered postnatal depression.
- I was depressed and used to cut myself with scissors as a teenager, but never tried to kill myself.
- I smoked 20 cigarettes a day until two years ago. I don't drink and never used drugs.

- I am physically fit.
- I don't have any friends now. I don't deserve them or their sympathy.

### Questions

When can you perform the operation?

### Worries

That I'll die before the baby can be freed and his soul will go to Hell.

# REALITY: MANIA

## General approach: tips, tricks, and cautionary tales

### 1. Set boundaries

When manic, people may become disinhibited, which can result in rude, irritable, sexualized, or aggressive behaviour. The most important thing is your safety (see Safety, p.17). As a medical student, it really *doesn't* matter if you can't get the history, so don't feel that you have to 'bravely' continue with unsafe situations.

You need to be the responsible boundary-setter. To do this, you should know where your boundaries lie *before* you start, otherwise you and your patient will feel confused. Although we usually give patients the option of being called by their first name, in mania it is often best to remain formal, since disinhibited patients may misinterpret even mild informality as flirtation. It makes sense that a manic patient who was addressed informally by an attractive young medical student might think that romance was in the air. Later being 'rejected' by the student might provoke outrage at being unfairly 'teased'.

Everyone has their own boundaries, but both you and your patient should expect that there will be:

- no flirting
- no touching (unless 'safe'/clinical)
- no threatening or abusive behaviour.

Often, people don't jump straight to breaching boundaries —they commonly test them first to see what you will allow, e.g. complimenting you on your good looks or

briefly touching your hand. Don't reinforce the behaviour, e.g. by giggling or returning the compliment. Be aware of your own body language and don't give out the wrong signals, e.g. sitting too close, making coy eye contact.

### 2. Match your defences

You shouldn't run from the room if your patient cheekily winks at you, but *match* the level of your defence to that of the 'attack': a small infringement should result in a small (but definite) defence; a big threat requires a big defence. For example:

- Ignore or distract if very low level (just the once; don't tolerate repeated 'low-level' boundary pushes).
- Increase the distance, e.g. lean backwards/move your chair back.
- Say NO!
- If you feel threatened, make your excuses and leave.

Recognize that you are vulnerable and ensure that you have the support of experienced staff if patients make you feel uncomfortable or threatened. Safety is paramount!

### 3. Saying 'No'

Telling another adult that their behaviour is inappropriate can feel awkward. However, it feels much *less* awkward than dealing with an 'incident'! Explain what they are doing and why they must stop. Then say what you will do if it happens again (e.g. end the interview). If it *does* happen again, do as you said you'd do; don't go back on your word. For example:

**Dan Davis:** *(touching your knee, suddenly)* Sexy legs!

**You:** *(moving out of reach)* Please don't touch me, Mr Davis —it's not appropriate.

**DD:** I just wanted to see what it felt like.

**Y:** I don't want to be touched. If you do it again, we'll stop the interview. OK?

**DD:** OK. So, as you were saying *(playfully tries to grab you)*.

**Y:** No, Mr Davis. I said not to touch me, but you're making me feel uncomfortable, so I'm stopping the interview. *(getting up to leave)*

**DD:** I'll be good! Please . . . ?

**Y:** We can arrange to talk another time. Thank you.

It's firm, but fair!

## 4. Focus on them

Although it probably doesn't matter whether a manic patient knows if you can drive (for example), even quite innocent questions can pave the way to inappropriate ones, such as whether or not you are a virgin! Cut the questioning off early on, and turn the focus back on them, e.g.

* I'm here to talk about *you*. I'm really interested in what you said about [insert subject]

In mania, people tend to be distractible *and* enjoy talking about themselves and their own interests, which is why this often works. If it doesn't work, just politely explain that you're there in a professional capacity and won't talk about yourself.

## 5. Rudeness and verbal abuse

As a medical student, try to view verbal abuse (and disinhibited behaviour) a little like haematemesis: an important but unpleasant symptom *and* a sign that you should not be dealing with the patient by yourself. Don't take it personally!

Disinhibited and irritable manic people can be rude and verbally abusive. That does *not* mean that it is acceptable for you to receive any form of verbal abuse —whether or not it progresses to a physical attack. Lay down your boundaries and end the interview if you feel uncomfortable, returning only with experienced staff. As a qualified doctor, you may have to tolerate some abuse while managing *unwell* patients, but don't suffer it from people who are disrespectful when well.

## 6. The runaway conversation

Because of pressure of speech and flight of ideas, conversations can turn into hefty monologues. Initially, let your patient talk uninterrupted for a little while; if you cut them off early, you'll start an immediate power-struggle. As they talk, glean as much information as possible, looking for themes as they arise and making a mental note to refer back to them. Then:

* Take control of the conversation firmly but politely by steering back to something they've said that you would like to hear more about.
* Keep questions short (or you'll lose their concentration). Use closed questions more than usual.
* Use reflection.
* Summarize or clarify to show that you've understood; then change direction. For example:

**Dan Davis:** . . . By that time, I could heal any disease and the power was just oozing out of me. The songs I was writing! People were drawn to me—and my sexy body! I heard Madonna calling to me, begging me to write songs for her and to teach her my holy message of . . .

**You:** You could heal? *[Redirection]*

**DD:** Yes! Anything at all—anything you could think of! Better than modern medicine!

**Y:** When did that start? *[Short question]*

**DD:** About three weeks ago. It was so exciting I can hardly explain how I felt! I didn't realize I had anything like this going on until God told me I could heal and . . .

**Y:** God told you? *[Reflection]*

**DD:** Yes!

**Y:** Did anyone else hear Him? *[Closed question]*

**DD:** No! Just me!

**Y:** It's a lot to take in! Let me check I've got it so far. Three weeks ago, God said you could heal and that's when you got these healing powers. Right? *[Summary]*

**DD:** Right!

**Y:** Anything like this ever happened before? *[Redirection]*

## 7. Don't mirror!

Mania is contagious and it is very easy to be drawn in to the excitement and action! Whereas usually you try to gently mirror people to enhance rapport, in mania it is better to do the opposite and remain calm. If you become impatient or frustrated, or talk loudly and quickly across your patient, mirroring will make the situation rapidly spiral out of control. So, sit still and speak calmly; stay interested, but don't become excited or annoyed. Your patient may mirror *you* and calm down a little.

## 8. Humility and irritability

However intelligent you are, a manic patient may find your relative 'slowness' and attention to 'meaningless details' rather tiresome. By recognizing this and being a little humble, you can make the conversation more palatable. For example:

> **Dan Davis:** I could cure HIV just using myself, no chemicals needed. I do exactly what it says on the tin and I'm no tin pot doctor! Can't you see now why they all wanted my songs?
>
> **You:** I'm not sure I followed the connection at the end there. I know I sound a bit slow and annoying, but could you explain more about people wanting your songs?

## The interview

You are unlikely to get a fully manic patient in an OSCE, simply because it disrupts the whole exam! Collateral histories are more common. Nevertheless, you should try to interview such people on the wards.

### Mood

- **How have you been feeling recently?**
- Are you happier or more cheerful than usual?
- Do other people irritate you more easily these days?
- \* When did you start feeling like this? What happened around then?

### Increased energy

- **What are your energy levels like at the moment?**
- \* Have you always had this much energy?
- \* How are you spending your new-found energy?

### Interests/enjoyment

- **You seem interested in so many different things—are these *new* interests?**
- \* You must have a lot of energy to do so much . . .
- \* You're so busy . . . ! When do you find time to sleep/eat/work?
- \* How do you concentrate on so many things at once?

### Sleep

- **How's your sleep been lately?**
- How has it changed . . . ?
- \* How does that affect your energy levels?
- \* You haven't slept in a week? You must be exhausted!

### Libido

- **Have you noticed a change in your sex drive, as well as your energy?**

### Concentration/thought

- **How's your concentration been?**
- Can you focus enough to read or to watch a whole TV programme?
- Do you find your thoughts jump about a lot?
- Are your thoughts racing?
- I can hardly keep up! Do you always think so quickly?
- \* You've so many ideas—where do they come from?

### Self-worth

- **What do you think of yourself, as a person?**
- How would you compare yourself with other people?
- What are you most proud of/best at? (See *Psychotic symptoms*, below)
- \* Would you say that you're more daring than other people? (Risks)

### Hope

- **You seem such a positive person . . . How do you see things turning out?**

### Psychotic symptoms (see Schizophrenia Reality for more, p.83)

#### Delusions

- Do you have any special talents or powers?
- Does your life have a mission or special purpose?
- Have you seen or heard anything in the news that had a special meaning for you?

#### Hallucinations

- Has anyone important or famous spoken to you recently?
- (You seem a very sensitive person.) Do you pick up on things other people can't see or hear?

### Risk/impulsivity

- Have you been in any trouble recently?
- Have you been doing things you wouldn't usually dare to do (drugs/sex/gambling etc.)?
- Have you been spending a lot more than usual?
- What happens when people irritate you?

> ➜ Don't take it for granted that people with mania are enjoying themselves. As well as feeling irritable and angry, people sometimes feel tearful, scared, and out of control. Recognizing these feelings can help people to feel calmer and better able to talk to you.

## Candidate's instructions

Miss Sally Bateman is a 22-year-old secretary who was admitted to a psychiatric ward five days ago under Section 2 of the Mental Health Act 2007.

You are a fourth-year medical student and the ward psychiatrist has asked you to take a mood disorder history.

## Patient's brief

### Key characteristics

- I speak very quickly and jump between subjects, sometimes bursting into song.
- I'm distractible and restless, pacing and moving about.
- I'm over-familiar and ask questions of the student/try to touch them or flirt with them.
- I can suddenly and briefly become irritable, giggly, or tearful.
- I'm wearing brightly coloured clothes and sunglasses (despite being indoors).
- At times, I hear the voice of The Narrator and may answer him.

About two weeks ago I got the feeling something amazing was going to happen! I hadn't slept properly for a few days but still had loads of energy. I was getting so much done at work that I had time to paint my office purple! My manager was amazed and gave me the afternoon off as a reward. It was a nice change, what with my boyfriend leaving me the week before. Bastard cheated on me. Well, we'll see who's laughing now.

I bought a magazine on the way home and there was an article about a new reality TV series looking for contestants with beauty, brains, personality, and heaps of talent. It *had* to be me! I bought new outfits, saw a voice coach and personal trainer. I used my savings . . . It's only a few thousand but an important investment! People started staring at me in the streets, and the paparazzi were everywhere on mopeds; cameras were put up in the shops to film me . . . I love the attention—I kiss my fans and give them cash handouts. I even had (unprotected) sex with a fan who recognized me in the street! I show off my moves and sing the songs I'm writing! I've got more ideas than ever before, coming out so fast I can barely keep up with them! I sometimes hear The Narrator's voice, you know? '8.46am, Sally shimmies at some fans who are disguised as tramps.' I'm not sure how I hear it, but it's got to be a microchip or a widget or a digit or a fidget or something.

A week ago I was doing a striptease in the supermarket when the TV company staged a police pick-up! (It's all actors, of course, but what a treat!) Anyway, I've ended up in this 'hospital' and it's just amazing! The cameras are everywhere and I've already given them plenty to watch!

There's a cute guy here—Juan. He's the *Juan* for me! *Juan*, two three four five . . . I grabbed him into the shower and was about to give him the time of his life when the staff stopped us. I put up a good fight for the cameras and had a cry afterwards (got to keep the general public on side). I don't need to sleep! I think it's something the TV company's put in the water, to keep me awake so I don't bore the viewers. I practise my singing and dance routines throughout the night. I feel *great*! The best I've ever felt! After I win this competition I'll get the Christmas No. 1. I'm designing my own line of clothing to complement my new perfume, which I'm calling *Sex*. Would you like my autograph?

### Other history

- Depression two years ago, treated with antidepressants.
- No medical problems.
- They've started me on lithium but it's for show—just a sugar pill. No other medications.
- I was drinking quite a bit before I came in, champagne mostly! No drugs.
- No-one in my family has psychiatric problems

### Questions

Do you have a boyfriend/girlfriend?

### Worries

I think the nurses are jealous of me and might want me off the programme (*starts crying*).

# NEXT STEPS

## Poor rehabilitation following a heart attack

You are the junior doctor on a cardiology team. Mr Jacobs is a 74-year-old man who was admitted to your ward in a dishevelled state two weeks ago, following a myocardial infarction. He has a history of congestive cardiac failure and stroke. The team are frustrated because he is not making the expected progress in his rehabilitation programme and presents as withdrawn and unmotivated. You note that his wife died three months ago.

At the multidisciplinary team meeting, someone proposes that Mr Jacobs should be discharged to a nursing home.

1. What could be wrong with Mr Jacobs (differential diagnosis)?
2. How would you manage this situation before making plans about his discharge?

### Issues
- Diagnosis
- Assessment, including risk assessment
- Management—in hospital and longer term

### Differential diagnosis
This includes depressive disorder, a bereavement reaction, adjustment disorder, dementia, or delirium. These diagnoses are not mutually exclusive.

### Management
Prepare to interview Mr Jacobs by reviewing his medical and any past psychiatric notes. Speak with other members of your team regarding their opinions and observations of Mr Jacobs and call his GP to find out more of his history and how he had been coping before this admission to hospital. When taking a history from Mr Jacobs ask about symptoms of depression and discuss his bereavement in more detail. Sensitively explore specific risk factors for pathological grief, e.g. what the marriage was like, the circumstances of his wife's death, and how he has been since she died. Ask about alcohol and drug use, past psychiatric history, and relevant family history of psychiatric disorder. Your personal history should explore his background and how he has coped with loss events and adversity in the past. A social history will give some clues regarding how he was coping with activities of daily living (ADLs) and important social contacts for practical help and psychological support.

Your mental state examination includes a description of his mood, consideration of any psychotic symptoms, and an assessment of his cognitive function, such as the Mini-Mental State Examination (MMSE) (p.16). Evidence of clouding of consciousness during this assessment will suggest a current delirium. You should ask Mr Jacobs what he understands about the current situation and what he wants in the short and longer term.

Perform a risk assessment; in particular, consider the risk of suicide, self-harm, and accidental injury or neglect if he were discharged home without being able to manage safely. Seek Mr Jacobs' consent to speak with a close relative or friend for collateral information. This is particularly helpful in considering how he has coped since the loss of his wife and whether there was evidence of cognitive impairment prior to her death.

If Mr Jacobs is suffering a depressive episode of moderate severity with no evidence of comorbid disorder, further investigations and management should include a full physical examination and appropriate blood tests, and you could consider using a standardized rating scale for depression, e.g. the Hospital Anxiety and Depression Scale (HADS). Mr Jacobs will also need an OT assessment of his functional ability both in the hospital and in his home environment. This will help to inform your risk assessment should he return home. Management will include giving psychological therapy, such as CBT. If an antidepressant is appropriate, consider safety with regard to cardiac side effects; an SSRI should be used first line. Follow-up by GP or community mental health services will be needed, depending on his response to treatment on the medical ward.

> This scenario isn't unusual. In the 6 months after the loss of a spouse there is a significant increase in mortality from a variety of sources, such as heart disease, cancer, suicide, and accidents. Depression affects as many as 35% of people in Mr Jacobs' position. Normal and pathological bereavements benefit from social support and counselling organizations, e.g. Cruse Bereavement Care. An abnormal reaction will need further psychological input.

## Film list

### Depression

*The Hours* (2002)
*About a Boy* (2002) (Marcus's mother, Fiona)
*Breaking the Waves* (1998)

### Mania/BPAD

*Mr Jones* (1993)
*The Mask* (1994)
*The Devil and Daniel Johnson* (2005)

## Books

### Depression

Diski, J. (1986) *Nothing Natural*. London: Virago. *Nothing Natural* explores depression and relationship problems—hailed and simultaneously reviled by critics for controversially including sections on female masochism.

Diski, J. (1994). *Monkey's Uncle*. London: Phoenix. This follows Charlotte's breakdown after the death of her daughter, and includes an illuminating look at therapist–patient problems.

Lewis, G. (2002). *Sunbathing in the Rain*. London: Harper Perennial. A funny, honest account of depression that includes a plethora of useful suggestions of what works—and what doesn't.

Plath, S. (1971) *The Bell Jar*. London: HarperCollins. Plath's semi-autobiographical account of depression demonstrates the waxing and waning nature of the disease with tense clarity.

Styron, W. (1992) *Darkness Visible*. London: Vintage. Astoundingly frank and insightful autobiographical account of award-winning author William Styron's (*Sophie's Choice*), descent into depression with concomitant anxiety—includes the simple but deep description of depression as 'the despair beyond despair'.

### BPAD

Campbell, B.M. (2005). *72 Hour Hold*. New York: Anchor Books, 2006. This novel explores the woefully insufficient support available for carers of young people with BPAD, leading to the search for alternative, illegal treatment programmes. Issues of ethnic bias and stigma are included.

Jamison, K.R. (1995). *An Unquiet Mind: A Memoir of Moods and Madness*. London: Picador. Autobiographical account of BPAD by an eminent psychologist. She explores the agonies of living with BPAD and attempting to maintain her clinical reputation amidst the stigmatizing views of colleagues.

Jeffrey, D. (2008). *Finding Jericho*. Brentwood: Chipmunkapublishing. Fictional text on BPAD, written by a mental health professional. Very suitable for a child or adolescent whose parent or close relative has BPAD; easily understandable and non-stigmatizing.

Walker, A. (1993). *Possessing the Secret of Joy*. London: Vintage. Walker's sequel to *The Color Purple* examines Tashi's migration to the USA from Africa. It explores the problems of defining BPAD within a Western framework, and how this falls short of understanding her cultural heritage.

## Quotes

Something has happened to me, this vital spark has stopped burning—I go to a dinner table now and I don't say a word, just sit there like a dodo . . . The most important thing I say is 'good evening' and then I go quiet.
**Spike Milligan**

You want to go home, back to the womb. You watch the world bang door after door in your face, numbly, bitterly. You have forgotten the secret you knew, once, ah, once, of being joyous, of laughing, of opening doors.
**Sylvia Plath, *Journal, 18 November 1952***

Eeyore, the old grey Donkey, stood by the side of the stream, and looked at himself in the water. 'Pathetic', he said. 'That's what it is. Pathetic.'
**A.A. Milne, *Winnie the Pooh***

## Note

1. Rowling, J.K. (1999) *Harry Potter and the Prisoner of Azkaban*. London: Bloomsbury. Copyright © J.K. Rowling 1999.

## References/Further reading

Beck, A.T., Rush, A.J., Shaw, B.F., *et al*. (1979) *Cognitive Therapy of Depression*. New York: Wiley.

Blackburn, I.M., Euson, K., and Bishop, S. (1986) A two-year naturalistic follow-up of depressed patients treated with cognitive therapy, pharmacotherapy and a combination of both. *Journal of Affective Disorders*, **10**, 67–75.

Brown, G.W. and Harris, T.O. (1978) *Social Origins of Depression: A Study of Psychiatric Disorder in Women*. London: Tavistock Press.

Cade, J.F.J. (1949) Lithium salts in the treatment of psychotic excitement. *Medical Journal of Australia*, **2**, 349–52.

Cadoret, R.J. (1978) Evidence for genetic inheritance of primary affective disorder in adoptees. *American Journal of Psychiatry*, **135**, 463–6.

Caspi, A., Sugden, K., and Moffitt, T.E. (2003) Influence of life stress on depression: moderation by a polymorphism in the 5-HTT gene. *Science*, **301**, 386–9.

Gilbert, P. (1997) *Overcoming Depression: A Self-Help Guide Using Cognitive-Behavioural Techniques*. London: Robinson Press.

Hawton, K., Salkovskis, P., Kirk, J., and Clark, D. (1996) *Cognitive Behaviour Therapy for Psychiatric Problems: A Practical Guide*. Oxford: Oxford Medical Publications.

Holmes, T.H. and Rahe, R.H. (1967) The social readjustment rating scale. *Journal of Psychomatic Research*, **11**, 213–17.

Jamison, K.R. (1995) *An Unquiet Mind: A Memoir of Moods and Madness*. London: Picador.

Jamison, K.R. (1996) *Touched with Fire: Manic–Depressive Illness and the Artistic Temperament*. New York: Simon & Schuster.

Kessler, R.C., Berglund, P.A., Demler, O., *et al.* (2005a) Lifetime prevalence and age-of-onset distributions of DSM-IV disorders in the National Comorbidity Survey Replication (NCS-R). *Archives of General Psychiatry*, **62**, 593–602.

Kessler, R.C., Chiu, W.T., Demler, O., and Walters, E.E. (2005b) Prevalence, severity, and comorbidity of twelve-month DSM-IV disorders in the National Comorbidity Survey Replication (NCS-R). *Archives of General Psychiatry*, **62**, 617–27.

McGuffin, P., Rijsdijk, F., Andrew, M., *et al.* (2003) The heritability of bipolar affective disorder and the genetic relationship to unipolar depression. *Archives of General Psychiatry*, **60**, 497–502.

Maier, S.F. and Seligman, M.E.P. (1976) Learned helplessness: theory and evidence. *Journal of Experimental Psychology: General*, **105**, 3–46.

Paykel, E.S. (1994) Life events, social support and depression. *Acta Psychiatrica Scandinavica Supplementum*, **377**, 50–8.

Rush, A.J., Trivedi, M.H., Wisniewski, S.R., *et al.* (2006) Acute and longer-term outcomes in depressed outpatients requiring one or several treatment steps: A STAR*D Report *American Journal of Psychiatry*, **163**, 1905–17.

Sartorius, N. (2001) The economic and social burden of depression. *Journal of Clinical Psychiatry*, **62** (Suppl 15), 8–11.

Smith, L.A., Cornelius, V., Warnock, A., *et al.* (2007) Effectiveness of mood stabilizers and antipsychotics in the maintenance phase of bipolar disorder: a systematic review of randomized controlled trials. *Bipolar Disorder*, **9**, 394–412.

Souery, D., Amsterdam, J., Montigny, C., *et al.* (1999) Treatment resistant depression: methodological overview and operational criteria. *European Neuropsychopharmacology*, **9**, 83–91.

Treuer, T., Oruc, L., Loza, N., *et al.* (2007) Acute phase results from STORM, a multicountry observational study of bipolar disorder treatment and outcomes. *Psychiatria Danubina*, **19**, 282–95.

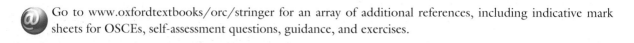 Go to www.oxfordtextbooks/orc/stringer for an array of additional references, including indicative mark sheets for OSCEs, self-assessment questions, guidance, and exercises.

# 8 Suicide and self-harm

*Jack Nathan*

## True or False? Test your existing knowledge—answers in the chapter and online

1. Rates of suicide are highest in social classes IV and V.

2. The suicide rate is lower during war times.

3. Up to 60% of people who kill themselves have self-harmed in the past.

4. Following government interventions, including limiting paracetamol pack sizes and installing catalytic converters, the suicide rate in the UK has decreased.

5. The issue of organ donation should be avoided following a completed suicide.

6. Paracetamol overdose should be treated with activated charcoal if blood paracetamol levels are significantly elevated.

7. The majority of patients who present to hospital following self-harm should be admitted to minimise risk of completed suicide.

8. SSRIs are the safest antidepressants where there is a risk of overdose.

9. Asking a patient directly about suicidal thoughts can trigger a suicide attempt.

10. The Mental Health Act is required to treat the physical complications of self-harm against a patient's will.

## Contents

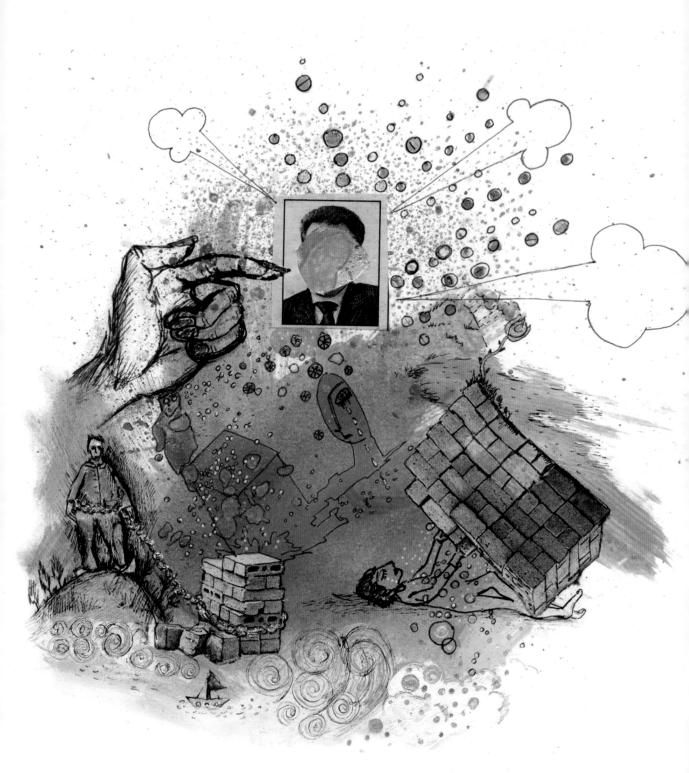

# PRINCIPLES

Dearest, I feel certain that I am going mad again. I feel we can't go through another of those terrible times. And I shan't recover this time. I begin to hear voices, and I can't concentrate. So I am doing what seems the best thing to do [ . . . ] What I want to say is I owe all the happiness of my life to you. You have been entirely patient with me and incredibly good. I want to say that—everybody knows it. If anybody could have saved me it would have been you. Everything has gone from me but the certainty of your goodness. I can't go on spoiling your life any longer. I don't think two people could have been happier than we have been.

Virginia Woolf[1]

## Introduction

Doctors are supposed to treat patients who are 'victims' of ill health, trying their best to recover. The model breaks down when patients deliberately harm themselves or do not *want* to get better. Staff may feel ambivalent or even hostile towards patients who are perceived as 'bad' because they have broken their side of the doctor–patient contract, provoking negative attitudes and even unprofessional behaviour in otherwise caring professionals.

This chapter aims to provide an understanding of suicide and self-harm that addresses these uncomfortable feelings, enabling you to work professionally and compassionately with these patients.

### Definitions

- **Suicide** is any act that deliberately brings about one's own death.

- **Self-harm** is any act intentionally causing physical injury to the body, but not resulting in death. Although some of these may represent attempted suicide, many have little or no suicidal intent and may have very clear alternative reasons for their actions. Methods include self-cutting, burning, and poisoning (overdoses). The term *deliberate self-harm* is avoided because of the derogatory implication of the term 'deliberate' and user group objections.

➡️ Terminology can hide meaning. Always explain *what* your patient did and *why* they did it. A superficial thigh laceration without suicidal intent is *very* different from a near-fatal hanging, although both are strictly 'self-harm'.

## Suicide

### Epidemiology

One per cent of all deaths are suicides, representing a million deaths worldwide each year. Globally, the suicide rate has increased in the past 50 years from 10 to 16 per 100 000. Suicide is one of the top ten causes of death in *every* country. There is a sevenfold difference between the highest (Finland, Russia) and lowest (Italy, Ireland) rates, although this may partly be due to under-reporting in Catholic countries. Rates in the UK are the lowest ever recorded (8.5 per 100 000), possibly reflecting government measures to prevent suicide since 1997.

The elderly (over 65s) and younger (15–30 years) age groups are at highest risk of suicide. It is second only to road accidents as a cause of death in men aged 15–24 years, and overall men are three to four times more likely than women to die by suicide in the UK. This is partly due to the method chosen: men use more violent methods, e.g. hanging, shooting.

### Aetiology

Numerous factors may interact and result in suicide.

#### A. Social causes

1. **Life events and stress** Suicide is often preceded by life events, especially bereavement and other losses. Childhood adversity such as abuse or neglectful parenting may predispose individuals to suicide many years later.

2. **Social class** Social classes I and V are at the highest risk of suicide; in contrast, classes IV and V are at highest risk of self-harm.

3. **Social isolation** People who die by suicide are more likely to be *isolated, divorced, widowed, single, unemployed,* or *living alone*. Social cohesion is a protective factor. The suicide rate decreases during wars (Stengel 1964), presumably because the suicidal impulse is subsumed by a sense of being connected to other people in resisting a common enemy.

4. **Occupation** Certain stressful jobs, with access to lethal means (e.g. drugs and firearms), have higher rates of suicide: vets, pharmacists, dentists, farmers, and doctors.

### B. Mental health causes

Nine out of ten individuals who die by suicide have a major mental illness at the time of death.

1. **Previous suicide attempt: lifetime risk 10–15%** Non-fatal self-harm with clear suicidal intent is the strongest predictor of eventual suicide (Suominen *et al.* 2004).

2. **Previous self-harm: lifetime risk 3–5%** Up to 60% of people who kill themselves have previously self-harmed, regardless of the suicidal intent (Zahl and Hawton 2004).

3. **Depression: lifetime risk 15%** Up to 80% of people who die by suicide are depressed. Depressed patients at highest risk of suicide tend to:
   - be older, single
   - have previously self-harmed
   - experience recurrent suicidal thoughts
   - suffer insomnia or weight changes
   - feel extremely hopeless, worthless, or guilty (McGirr *et al.* 2007).

➤ The risk of suicide *increases* as a severely depressed person begins to recover—gaining the energy and motivation to act on suicidal ideas.

4. **Schizophrenia: lifetime risk 10%** Particularly vulnerable are young ambitious patients, early in their illness, with insight into the severity of their diagnosis. Command hallucinations may place people at extra risk.

5. **Substance misuse** Alcohol dependence carries a lifetime risk of suicide of 3–4%. Alcohol and drug abuse also increase the risk of suicide.

6. **Personality disorders** Up to half the people who die by suicide have a personality disorder.

### C. Physical health problems

Chronic, painful, and terminal illnesses increase the risk of suicide.

### D. Family history

The risk of suicide is increased by having a family history of mental illness or suicide. These factors are independent of each other.

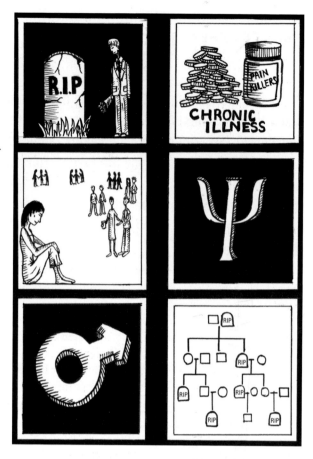

FIGURE 8.1 Risk factors for suicide

## Suicide prevention strategies

As noted earlier, government interventions at a national level appear to have lowered the UK suicide rate. Strategies include:

- limiting pack sizes of paracetamol
- installing barriers at suicide 'hotspots' and providing a free telephone for calling the Samaritans
- catalytic converters (these have decreased the suicide rate from inhaling car exhaust fumes).

➤ It is not always a good sign when an agitated patient suddenly appears calm: they may have made the decision to die and therefore be at peace.

## Following a suicide

Death is never the end of the story. As well as the protocols and reviews that follow a suicide, there is usually a group of people about to suffer one of the most traumatic forms of bereavement. If you are involved in the care of someone who has died by suicide, you may need to speak to their family and friends. Beforehand, gain all the facts you can about the death, including:

- names of key staff involved
- suicide method

- injuries sustained
- treatments given
- whether they were conscious when found
- any 'final words'.

Be clear and compassionate in your explanation: keep to the facts and remember that people may not be able to cope with hearing *every detail* all at once. Be aware that the bereaved often feel that the death was their fault or that they should have prevented it—allowing discussion of these feelings may help. Encourage people to take a companion when identifying the body, and to let friends and family support them in the aftermath; this is a very hard time to be alone. Don't avoid the topic of organ donation (if relevant) since this might be the only positive outcome for the bereaved. Make them aware of services that may help (e.g. hospital chaplains, counsellors, charities such as SOBS (Survivors of Bereavement by Suicide)). Discuss any protocol of which you are aware (e.g. the coroner is involved in all suspected suicides, which may postpone the funeral). Depending on your involvement, time commitments, and the family's wishes, you might meet with the family at a later point.

Remember that *you* and other staff may need emotional support afterwards. For example, the GP receptionist who was unable to offer the person an appointment on the day they died may feel overwhelmed with guilt.

 For every suicide, six people suffer intense grief reactions (Clark and Goldney 2000).

## Self-harm

Although self-harm is an umbrella term for all non-fatal self-injury, it is clinically important to distinguish the potentially lethal acts of attempted suicide (e.g. hanging, shooting) from painful but usually non-lethal methods of self-harm where there is commonly no conscious intention to die, rather the hope is to escape an intolerable situation.

Self-cutting is the most common form of self-harm, although overdoses present more often to hospitals.

---

**BOX 8.1** Reasons for self-harm

- Avoiding more dangerous self-harm or suicide
- Self-punishment (e.g. for being fat, stupid, etc.)
- Suicide attempt
- Substituting psychological distress with physical pain
- Overcoming numbness
- To change intolerable situations (often relationship issues)

---

Other methods include burning, bruising, and self-stabbing. The reasons for self-harm are complex and personal. A fairly common explanation for self-cutting is that a sense of pressure or tension grows as emotions build up. Self-harm 'releases' the tension and a sense of calm or mild elation takes over, either at the point of cutting or upon seeing blood. Many people self-harm secretly and hide their scars; the common view that this is simply 'attention-seeking' behaviour is outdated.

### Epidemiology

The lifetime risk of self-harm is 7–13%. It is more common in children and adolescents (unlike suicide) and probably under-reported. Women are more likely than men to present in casualty, although actual rates may be similar.

### Aetiology

Self-harm is associated with diagnoses of affective disorder and personality disorder (Haw *et al.* 2001). Substance abuse and borderline and dissocial personality disorders are also at higher risk due to impulsivity. Past childhood abuse (including sexual abuse) and current domestic violence are common associations. There may be a culture of self-harm among some adolescents.

### Theories of self-harm

Childhood ideally provides a 'validating environment' where parents take their child's experiences seriously and speak to them in a way that helps to manage intense emotions. This provides the basis for people to learn to 'mentalize'—to reflect on and process emotional experiences. When childhood is traumatic, abusive, or neglectful, there is little space for reflection and thought, and emotional experiences can only be dealt with by action. This may evolve into self-harm as a way of dealing with difficult emotions when the ability to mentalize is poorly developed or damaged.

Something so trivial left me cold,
You went out of the room to be alone
Rejection, pain, hate,
Slap, punch *without thought*.
Excerpt from a poem by a patient who self-harmed

Although it looks destructive, self-harm may represent a coping strategy: attacking only a part of the body (representing the condemned self), thereby securing survival of the person. Self-injury can retrieve a sense of separate identity in states of mind where the boundary between self and other is felt to dissolve or be violated. Implicit in all these ideas of self-harm is a relationship between parts of the self, or between the self and other, in which there is such unmodulated emotion that it cannot be expressed in words alone.

## Management

Because of the high risk of suicide and the intense levels of distress experienced by those who self-harm, every self-harming patient must be taken seriously. As noted, we may become impatient with people who deliberately harm themselves, and we may inadvertently show revulsion at the sight of self-mutilation. Additionally, people who self-harm often dislike themselves and may provoke us to share their negative perception. Good management depends on building rapport with patients who have self-harmed to understand their actions.

Studies show that self-harming people attending casualty are ignored and made to wait in public areas. They can feel judged, rejected, and even punished for their willed 'badness', including being offered less analgesia for pain (Horrocks *et al.* 2003).

### 1. Physical treatment

The physical consequences of self-harm must be dealt with swiftly. Patients who wish to leave before this must have their capacity assessed first. If they lack capacity they should be treated in their best interests. Treatment depends on the method used and resultant damage and includes:

- Overdoses (dependent on the substance)
  - Activated charcoal—decreases gut absorption of some substances, e.g. antidepressants
  - 'Antidotes' e.g. *N*-acetyl cysteine treats paracetamol overdose
- Lacerations
  - Superficial cuts: suture/close with Steristrips
  - Plastic surgery for deep cuts with nerve or tendon damage
  - Adequate analgesia *must* be given while suturing lacerations

### 2. Risk assessment

The involvement of a specialist with psychiatric experience is important at this point. Where possible, risk factors should be addressed through initial and follow-up interventions. In addition to the risk factors already described above, certain aspects of the attempt should be regarded as a sign of greater risk:

- Careful planning (duration and attention to detail)
- Final acts in anticipation of death (e.g. writing wills)
- Isolation at the time of the act
- Precautions taken to prevent discovery (e.g. locking doors)
- Writing a suicide note
- Definite intent to die (rather than to change, or temporarily escape, a situation)
- Believing the method to be lethal (even if it wasn't)
- Violent method (e.g. shooting, hanging, jumping in front of a train)
- Ongoing wish to die/regret that the attempt failed

The clinician should err on the side of caution when making a risk assessment and remember that even seemingly 'low-risk' patients kill themselves.

>> *Details on how to assess suicide risk are given in the Reality section (p.63).*

Patients who seriously wish to kill themselves may deliberately deny their intentions.

### 3. Immediate interventions

The immediate risk must be managed. If the patient is at high risk of suicide they may be admitted to a psychiatric ward for their own safety. This enables close observation in a safer environment as well as further assessment and treatment of underlying problems such as depression or schizophrenia. Some people can be safely managed at home, especially if they do not feel suicidal, have supportive friends or family around them, and are willing to seek help if they experience suicidal ideation. Any immediate stressors or risk factors that *can* be addressed should be addressed with a problem-solving approach (e.g. accessing a hostel placement for someone who has been evicted). A plan should be made to deal with future suicidal ideation or thoughts of self-harm, including who they will tell and how they will get help (e.g. by coming straight to hospital).

After an episode of self-harm a patient reported how an A&E staff member accused her in a public area of 'being selfish' and asking if 'she was doing the same to her children'.

### 4. Follow-up interventions

Follow-up should be arranged for within a week of the self-harm or discharge from an inpatient ward (NICE 2004). This may be via a community mental health team, an outpatient clinic, a GP or counsellor. Swift and detailed communication between all involved clinical parties is essential.

Underlying disorders (such as depression) must be treated. If antidepressants are required, SSRIs are the safest in case of overdose, although prescriptions should still be kept short and reviewed regularly to try and prevent stockpiling for an overdose.

The severity of the injury/overdose may not reflect the degree of distress experienced.

Longer-term psychological therapies that have been shown to decrease repeated self-harm include CBT-based therapies (e.g. dialectical behaviour therapy), mentalization-based treatment in a day hospital setting, and transference-focused psychotherapy.

**Thirty per cent of all suicides occur within three months of discharge from psychiatric wards (Department of Health 2001).**

### 5. Coping strategies

It is often useful to discuss alternative ways of dealing with painful moods and situations. These might include distraction techniques and mood-raising activities such as exercise or writing. Additionally, there are strategies that some patients find helpful in decreasing or preventing self-harm (Box 8.2). Be aware that these measures may seem patronizing to someone who is seriously addicted to self-harm.

Somewhat controversially, if people cannot or *do not want to stop* self-harming, there is still scope for harm reduction to make the process safer, e.g. not sharing blades, learning basic first aid, and cleaning the skin before cutting. Giving information does not mean you are endorsing self-harm, but take care not to lapse into *condoning* it (Pengelly *et al.* 2008).

### Prognosis

In the year following an episode of self-harm, one in six people will self-harm again. The risk of completed suicide is 50–100 times that of the general population. Despite the best management possible, there will always be some people who kill themselves. For some though, the attempt may be a turning point in their lives, and a successful recovery is made.

---

**BOX 8.2** Strategies to decrease or avoid self-harming

**Prevention**

- Put tablets and sharp objects out of reach and sight to avoid cueing.
- Avoid self-harm 'triggering' images (e.g. self-harm photographs online).
- Stay in public places or with supportive people when tempted to self-harm.
- Call a friend/support line (keep contact numbers to hand).
- Avoid drugs and alcohol.

**Alternatives to painful, damaging self-harm**

- Squeeze ice cubes/plunge fingers into ice cream.
- Snap a rubber band around the wrist.
- Bite into something strongly flavoured, e.g. ginger root, a lemon.

**Alternatives to drawing blood**

- Put red food dye on the dull side of a knife and draw it across the skin.
- Use a washable red pen to mark the skin instead of cutting it.

---

# REALITY

---

## General approach: tips, tricks, and cautionary tales

### 1. Be aware that your patient has probably had a bad day

Your mindset when you go in will set the tone for the whole interview. If you expect your patient to be deliberately unpleasant or 'attention-seeking', the interview will go badly. People don't hurt themselves when life is going well. Be mindful and recognize this early on, e.g.

- I understand x has happened . . . Have you been having a tough time recently?

### 2. Bear the unbearable

When people try to harm themselves, they often have extremely unpleasant feelings, thoughts, or memories with which they feel unable to cope. If *you* can bear to hear these things you will communicate the idea that they are not alone in their situation. As long as someone can cope with those feelings, there's hope that something can be done. The moment you interrupt, become distracted or dismissive, or give the impression that you are in a hurry, you're saying that you can't bear their problems and they must cope alone.

**Remember that however difficult the encounter, the very presence of your patient communicates (perhaps unconsciously) their desire to be helped.**

### 3. Don't minimize distress

When people try to kill themselves, they usually feel that their problems are serious and insoluble. It will not help to tell them: 'Don't worry . . . it'll be OK' or 'It's not as bad as you think'. It will make them feel as though you are not taking their problems seriously. Likewise, challenging their story too actively (e.g. disputing how many tablets they have taken by saying, 'Well your paracetamol levels were OK') detracts from their story and almost challenges them to 'do it properly next time'.

### 4. You are *not* the parent; the patient is *not* your child!

It's easy to slip into being *parental* towards patients, especially if (at some level) you feel that they 'need' parenting or they interact with you as though you *are* their parent. Your patient is not a child to be told off (e.g. 'That was stupid of you') or 'looked after' (e.g. 'You poor thing, I must help you!'). Outside of this consultation they are many things to many other people—possibly a parent themselves, or someone's partner or manager.

### 5. Address ambivalence

Following very dangerous self-harm or a statement about wanting to die, patients can feel that they have crossed a 'point of no return', making it difficult to think or talk about a change in direction away from suicide or death. You can address this by recognizing that they *may* be a bit ambivalent about dying, e.g. 'Part of you wanted to die and maybe a part didn't . . . ?' Remember, that the act may also have 'cured' a problem (at least temporarily) by changing the person's circumstances, and this may offer a way forward.

### 6. Don't take it personally ('Transference', see p.229)

Your patient may be angry or rude. Remember that this probably isn't *in response to you*—especially if you haven't even had a chance to upset them yet! It can feel confusing and unfair, when you are trying your best to treat them well. Retaliating makes things *much* worse. Instead, acknowledge the anger and work with it:

- I can see that you're angry and upset. I'd like to try and help you, and part of that is understanding what's made you feel like this.

Remember that your patient is there in part *because* they have interpersonal difficulties: these problems are a central issue, rather than an irritating side effect.

### 7. Recognize *your* feelings and don't throw them back at the patient ('Countertransference', see p.229)

We feel a lot of emotions in response to patients, but it's not professional to display them all during the consultation since, although they are natural and often very understandable, they may not be appropriate. Try to identify the feelings that the patient evokes in you and consider where they come from, rather than simply *reacting* to them. You will start to understand something about this person and what happens when they interact with people, since it is likely that they sometimes make other people feel this way too (probably making life very difficult for them). Don't fall into the trap of adding your distress to theirs, as this reinforces their sense of being 'bad', worthless, and beyond help.

### 8. Don't start by asking *why* they self-harm

Not everyone can explain exactly why they self-harm, and the reasons may be deeply personal. Starting with 'Why do you cut yourself?' can be overwhelming. Find out what happened and how they were feeling *first*. Once you have gained rapport, you might ask, 'How does cutting yourself help you?' This may get you to the point of understanding *why*.

### 9. Consider the act as a form of communication

Your patient won't expect you to be emotionally cold, and will watch your reactions closely. Do respond to the harm, but don't get distracted by the gory side so that you miss the underlying 'message'. For example:

**Helen:** Look! *(showing cuts)* I cut down to the bone and needed surgery!

**You:** That looks painful! Things must have felt really bad for you to cut yourself so deeply.

 Asking a patient about suicide does not increase the risk of suicide, so don't be afraid to mention it.

### 10. Manage your own feelings

Dealing with suicide attempts and self-harm can stir up your emotions. It can help to talk over your experiences with a friend, supervisor, or consultant. We all need support sometimes.

➡ It is a myth that people who talk about suicide won't kill themselves. They do. Take any expression of suicidal thoughts very seriously.

## The interview

### A. Assessing for suicidal thoughts and plans

If your patient has not presented with self-harm, assessing suicidal thoughts can feel awkward. Rather than asking out of the blue 'Do you want to kill yourself?', try broaching the subject with a sequence of questions. For example:

- How do you see your future?
- Do you ever feel hopeless about the future?
- Do you ever wish you were dead?
- Have you ever thought about trying to end your life?
- Have you ever made plans or actually tried to kill yourself?
- Do you have current plans to kill yourself?

Obviously, don't keep pushing if there are clearly no suicidal ideas!

If someone has already talked about current distress, you can start with something that recognizes that their experiences are stressful and that desperation is *not* abnormal.

- Many people who have been through what you've gone through might feel that life just wasn't worth living. Do you ever feel that way?
- It wouldn't surprise me if all these things made you sometimes feel very desperate—even suicidal. Do you ever feel like that? *Tell me about that . . .*

Don't be content with a simple *no*; double check and be more direct:

- So, let me just check . . . Have you *ever* felt like harming or killing yourself?

Once you have established that there are suicidal thoughts . . .

- What thoughts have you been having?
- Have you made any definite plans? What?
- Have you taken any steps towards this yet? (e.g. buying tablets, making a will)
- Is there anything stopping you from doing this?
- What could push you over the edge/be so unbearable that you might resort to this?
- Have you told anyone about how desperate you feel?

Gain *all* your patient's plans (means, timing, etc.) and assess for risk factors, as below.

## B. Risk assessment following self-harm

There are four main points to this history:

1. **The story**
2. **Now**
3. **Future**
4. **Risk factors**

### 1. The story

This starts with the stressors leading up to their first thought of self-harm. There may be a 'final straw' event that precipitated the act. Begin with an open question, e.g.

- You've been through a lot today. It may be hard to talk about, but could you tell me what happened?
- What *first* made you think of killing (or harming) yourself?
- What was the final straw?
- Did you have any big problems or worries? (work, relationships, money, health . . . )

Encourage your patient to narrate the whole episode from then until now, without gaps in the story. Then recap and ask questions to fill in missing details. Impulsive acts can be recounted very swiftly and seem almost a blur in the patient's mind. If so, try slowing down the act by asking plenty of step-by-step questions.

### Degree of planning

- How long were you planning this?
- Tell me about the preparations . . .
- Did you put your affairs in order beforehand? (e.g. writing a will, saying goodbye to people?)
- Did you tell anyone you were feeling suicidal?

### The act

- Talk me through exactly what you did . . .

### Precautions

- Did you do anything to make sure people couldn't interrupt you? e.g. locking doors, telling people you were somewhere else . . . ?
- Were you alone?

### Method—find out all the details, e.g.

- What tablets were they? How many? Did you take every tablet you had?
- Did you drink any alcohol or take any drugs with them?

### Purpose

- Did you hope that this would kill you, or did you hope for something else?
- A big part of you wanted to die. Was there a small part of you that wanted to live?

### Certainty

- At the time, how sure were you that this would kill you?
- Did you think that anyone could save you if they found you?
- Did you write a note? What did it say?

 Try to see the suicide note if there was one.

### Discovery (What went 'wrong'?)

- How did you end up coming to hospital? (It sounds as though you planned things very carefully.)
- Were you found or did you get help yourself?
- How do you feel about that?

**When taking self-cutting histories try asking:**

- What was going on immediately before you cut yourself?
- What mood were you in just before you cut? (e.g. boredom, frustration, rejection?)
- How did you feel immediately after you cut yourself?

### 2. Now

- Looking back, how do you feel about trying to harm yourself?
- Do you regret trying to kill yourself?
- Do you regret *failing* to kill yourself?
- How do you feel about being alive?
- Do you still wish you were dead?
- Has anything changed, or are your problems still as bad as before?

### 3. Future

- How do you see the future?
- Do you have any plans to harm or kill yourself? (assessment, as per section A)
- Can you think of anything that would make life easier for you?
- What will you do if [stressor] happens (or happens again)?

### 4. Risk factors

**Past psychiatric history**

- Have you tried to harm or kill yourself before?
- Have you ever seen a psychiatrist or been treated for depression?

**Support**

- Do you have friends you can talk to about your worries?

**Screen for:**

- Current depression (mood, energy, anhedonia) and hopelessness
- Current use of drugs and alcohol
- Problems with relationships, work, recent losses, physical ill health

The result of the interview should be an assessment of the risk of suicide and future self-harm: both immediately and longer term. This can be described as *low, medium,* or *high* and you should give some thought to how this risk could be decreased through management. Ultimately, the most important question for you and the patient will be whether they are safe to go home today—or whether they need to stay in hospital.

Towards the end of a good interview you may be able to do something therapeutic with impulsive patients, e.g. 'So next time, what could you do instead of reaching for that razor blade/bottle of pills?'

As a medical student, you should *never* send people home (although you may give a valuable view on their risk, following your assessment). As a junior doctor, always spread the responsibility by discussing fully with your seniors, and get a psychiatric opinion.

## 1. Risk assessment following self-harm (15 minutes)

### Candidate's instructions

Anthony Fowler is a 19-year-old pet shop assistant who was brought to casualty by his father, who discovered him cutting himself.

You are a medical student in casualty. The liaison psychiatric nurse has asked you to assess the risk of suicide in this patient, and will ask you two questions when you finish your assessment.

### Examiner's questions

1. What level is the *immediate risk of suicide* for this patient?
2. Will you send him home?

### Patient's brief

*Key characteristics*

- This is pointless.
- I'm sarcastic and angry.
- I feel depressed but just want to get on with it, my way.
- I won't show my cuts—I don't need an audience.

It's Dad's fault and he knows it: this whole *caring father thing* isn't fooling anyone. I cut myself today. So? I've been cutting for years. He's been too wrapped up in himself to notice. I'm not about to give him Father of the Year award just because he drags me to hospital. Today, my manager had a go at me for not cleaning out the rodent cages properly. Not my fault—I was doing someone a favour; it wasn't even my job! He had a go at me in front of *everyone*. I was so angry I just walked out.

All I could think about was cutting myself. I felt everything building up—anger, hate, everything. It took an hour to walk home, and I just went straight upstairs and got my stuff out. I use a sharp Stanley knife. I get excited as I build up to it, but I'm patient and don't rush; it feels best that way. As I cut, I focus on the blood bulging along the edges of skin and it calms me. It's like I'm treating myself to something—the rush is amazing. I always clean the blade before and bandage up afterwards. Today I cut my chest (I allowed myself five cuts) and was about to start taping up when Dad walked in. He went ballistic when he saw the blood and starting yelling, calling me a freak. He *literally* dragged me to the car, screaming all the way to hospital. Never asked me why.

I wasn't trying to kill myself. I know I'd be better off dead, but I wouldn't do anything about it. I've tried to kill myself before and it just made things worse . . . First when I was 14 (Mum walked out on us) I cut my wrists, thinking it would kill me but of course it didn't. It made me feel better and I've been doing it since. Second time was when Dad kicked me out, at 16. I took an overdose and ended up in casualty. Social Services put me in care and the child psychiatrists counselled me for a year. They said I had depression but weren't interested after I dropped out of college. I've been bored and depressed for years—nothing helps. I *enjoy* cutting and talking to people online and in cutting forums. I've got no energy, but I never have had. I feel useless, but I'm good with animals so it's not too bad.

I've been living with Dad for a year. He beat me when I was a kid, but he doesn't much now he needs my rent. I can't see a future, but I guess one day I'll just die or be killed. I'm not going to kill myself—Dad would think he'd won. I'll keep cutting; it's my right to do what I want with my body.

### Other history

- I had asthma as a kid but grew out of it—I'm otherwise fit and well.
- I smoke 20 cigarettes a day. I don't drink, but smoke weed (cannabis) most evenings. No other drugs.
- Dad's an alcoholic. Mum died of breast cancer just after she walked out on us.

### Questions

When can I go home?
If I didn't cut, how would I handle my stress?

### Worries

You're not going to admit me, are you?

## 2. Assess suicide risk following self-harm (15 minutes)

### Candidate's instructions

Scarlet Gillespie is a 25-year-old single mum and freelance DJ. She was admitted to A&E following an overdose yesterday and is medically cleared for discharge.

You are a final year medical student working in casualty. The casualty doctor has asked you to assess suicide risk and will ask you two questions when you finish your assessment.

### Examiner's questions

1. What level is the risk for this patient?
2. Can she go home?

### Patient's brief

*Key characteristics*

- I'm not keen to talk.
- Although I deny wanting to die, my plan is to go home and kill myself. I don't admit this initially and lie if needed.
- Nothing has changed. There's no point living.

Two months back I got stranded in town, about 3am. I rang my best friend, Dee. She was worried about me and came to get me but never turned up. She died in an accident on the way. It wouldn't have happened if I hadn't called her out. I've been depressed and suicidal since . . . I lie awake every night thinking about her . . . It leaves me drained. I can't work, just sit around the house. Mum's had to babysit Erica (my 4-year-old)—I couldn't cope with her . . . No kid should have to see her mum in such a state.

About three weeks ago, I started seriously thinking about killing myself. I tried to put it out my mind, but I couldn't. I wanted everything to *just stop* and not to have to think anymore. Two weeks ago I started getting tablets. My GP's nice: he gave me a month of antidepressants and two weeks of sleeping pills. I bought four packets of paracetamol from different shops so people wouldn't get suspicious. I knew I needed to provide for Erica when I was gone, so I sorted out my will with Mum as Erica's legal guardian.

Last week I told Mum I'd start DJing again. I spent good times with her and Erica—made sure they knew how much I loved them. Mum came round to look after Erica about 7pm yesterday. I took the train into town like I was going to a gig, but I booked into a hotel instead. I locked the door and wrote a letter to Mum and Erica, explaining that I was sorry, but couldn't go on. I took the tablets with water: 28 Prozac; 14 Valium (10mg); three packs of paracetamol (36 tablets). I was sure I'd taken enough to kill myself but woke up in hospital. Some maintenance man got his rooms mixed up and found me by accident, unconscious. He called an ambulance 'just in time'. I've had all my treatments now and just need to go home.

### The lie

I'd never do this again. I'm glad I was found and regret everything that happened; it was so stupid.

- If asked about how things have changed, I go silent.
- If asked what I have to live for, I say, 'Erica needs me' (but don't believe it).

### The reality (only revealed with careful and compassionate questioning)

My heart sank when I woke up: *I'm still here*. There's nothing to live for. Nothing can bring Dee back. Erica doesn't need me—Mum does a better job than I do anyway. I'm going to jump in front of a train.

### Other history

- No medical problems. Recently started on fluoxetine 20mg every morning.
- I've never tried suicide before. I got depressed when Dad killed himself 10 years ago.
- I don't drink, smoke, take drugs.
- I've got friends but not to talk to, not like Dee.

### Questions

Can I go home?

### Worries

The doctors might put me in a mental hospital.

# NEXT STEPS

## Refusal of treatment following self-harm

You are a casualty officer about to assess Duncan Moore, a 22-year-old man bought to A&E by ambulance after jumping off the second floor of a car park. He appears to have suffered lower limb fractures, but the paramedic reports there is no evidence of head injury or damage to internal organs. Since admission, Duncan has appeared very tense and anxious, and has refused to give any personal details. He has also been muttering to himself and laughing for no apparent reason. Although he allowed basic observations (temperature, BP, pulse, SaO$_2$), he has already stated that he won't undergo any X-rays because he knows the government will use the X-ray machine to stop his heart beating.

1. What would be your immediate management of this situation?
2. What are the likely longer term needs of this gentleman?

### Issues

- Diagnosis
- Risk assessment
- Immediate management: medical, refusal of X-ray
- Further management

## Immediate management

You must ensure that Duncan is physically stable and that there are no urgent medical needs to be addressed. A short focused assessment is then needed, to perform a mental state examination (MSE) and a psychiatric history. A detailed description of the suicide attempt may ascertain that Duncan was suffering distressing persecutory delusions or auditory hallucinations that commanded him to jump. You should identify affective symptoms (e.g. depression) and consider the possible causes of a psychotic episode. In the absence of prior contact with psychiatric services, the most likely diagnosis is that of an acute and transient psychotic episode or drug-induced psychosis. You must ask about previous episodes of self-harm or suicide attempts.

You should assess Duncan's capacity to refuse medical treatment. He appears to be refusing the X-ray because of persecutory delusions which prevent him from *understanding* the nature of the proposed investigation. If this is the case, he lacks capacity. You should discuss the options fully with him and discover whether he might agree to the X-ray if accompanied by someone he trusts who may be able to reassure him. If he still refuses, the X-ray will have to take place under the MCA (p.28) as you have a duty of care and this is certainly in his best interests. If he becomes acutely agitated or aggressive in response to this course of action, rapid tranquillization may be required to calm him (e.g. lorazepam 1–2mg orally or by intramuscular injection).

Your risk assessment includes the risk of harm to self, which is *high*. You should also consider the risk of harming others and the risk of self-neglect and vulnerability to abuse by others.

## Short-term needs

Duncan will need to see a psychiatrist for further assessment and management once his acute medical issues have been dealt with. He will need treatment for his acute psychotic episode. Depending on his injuries, this may be started on the orthopaedic ward, or if physically fit for discharge, the psychiatrist will probably arrange admission to a psychiatric ward. If he is not willing to be admitted to the psychiatric ward or attempts to leave the orthopaedic ward, a Mental Health Act assessment will be required.

The process of risk assessment is ongoing; this will dictate the level of nursing and observation required. Timely treatment with an atypical antipsychotic should bring about a resolution of psychotic symptoms, at which point the risk of suicide should be much reduced. The risk of suicide following recovery from a first episode of psychosis should be assessed—this can increase as insight is gained.

> Did you miss a head injury? Although the paramedics report that there was no evidence of head injury, every patient must receive a full medical examination—particularly following a fall from height. A head injury may cause psychotic symptoms or be masked by them. It is easy to assume that a patient's symptoms are psychiatric in origin, simply because they are 'a psychiatric patient'.

### Film list

**Suicide**
*The Bridge* (2006)
*The Hours* (2002)
*The Virgin Suicides* (1999)
*It's a Wonderful Life* (1946)

**Self-harm**
*Thirteen* (2003)

**Books**

Coelho, P. (1998) *Veronika Decides to Die*. London: Harper Collins, 2000. Philosophical text, beginning with Veronika's suicide attempt and admission to a psychiatric unit; in which she meditates on the meaning of life and, indeed, the meaning of death.

Kettlewell, C. (1999) *Skin Game: A Memoir*. New York: St Martin's Griffin. Autobiographical narrative examining self-harm in the form of cutting.

Ray, R. (1998) *A Certain Age*. London: Penguin. Brilliant book written from the perspective of a 13-year old girl who becomes enmeshed in a relationship with a much older man and begins to cut herself as a result. A Frank examination of self-harm, including the lack of realization of the severity of self-harm, and the lack of a necessarily major trigger for the act.

Runyon, B. (2004) *The Burn Journals*. London: Penguin, 2006. Diary of author Brent Runyon following his almost accidental suicide attempt at the age of 14, during which he sustained major burns and required intensive rehabilitation.

### Quotes

Down on the ocean floor
That's where I'm heading for
Hold on to a sinking stone
Until the worst is known
Nobody wants to think about it
Nobody wants to talk about it
Nobody protects you
***Nobody Wants To***—Crowded House

Frances and Courtney, I'll be at your altar. Please keep going Courtney, for Frances. For her life which will be so much happier without me. I LOVE YOU. I LOVE YOU.
**Kurt Cobain,** *suicide note*

> ...just as a little bit of knowledge is a dangerous thing, a little bit of energy, in the hands of someone hell-bent on suicide, is a very dangerous thing.
> **Elizabeth Wurtzel, *Prozac Nation***
>
> Self-harming keeps me alive
> **Anonymous patient**

## Note

1. Virginia Woolf (1882–1941): writer, key figure in the intellectual 'Bloomsbury Group'. Woolf wrote this note to her husband, Leonard, before drowning herself in the River Ouse.

## References/Further reading

Bateman, A. and Fonagy, P. (2004) *Psychotherapy for Borderline Personality Disorder: Mentalisation-Based Treatment.* Oxford University Press.

Bouch, J. and Marshall, J.J. (2005) Suicide risk: structured professional judgement. *Advances in Psychiatric Treatment*, **11**, 84–91.

Clark, S.E. and Goldney, R.D. (2000) The impact of suicide on relatives and friends. In: *The International Handbook of Suicide and Attempted Suicide* (eds K. Hawton and K. van Heeringen), pp. 467–84. Chichester: John Wiley.

Department of Health (2001) *Safety First. Five-Year Report of the National Confidential Inquiry into Suicide and Homicide by People with Mental Illness.* London: Department of Health.

Favazza, A.R. (1992) *Bodies Under Siege: Self-mutilation and Body Modification in Culture and Psychiatry.* Baltimore, MD: Johns Hopkins University Press.

Haw, C., Hawton, K., Houston, K., and Townsend, E. (2001) Psychiatric and personality disorders in deliberate self-harm patients. *British Journal of Psychiatry*, **178**, 48–54.

Horrocks, J., Price, S., House, A., and Owens, D. (2003) Self-injury attendances in the accident and emergency department: clinical database study. *British Journal of Psychiatry*, **183**, 34–49.

Main, T. (1989) *The Ailment and Other Psychoanalytic Essays.* London: Free Association. The Ailment is a classic paper on splits and conflicts within staff aroused by working with self-harming and suicidal patients.

McGirr, A., Renaud, J., Seguin, M., *et al.* (2007) An examination of DSM-IV depressive symptoms and risk of suicide completion in major depressive disorder: a psychological autopsy study. *Journal of Affective Disorders*, **97**, 203–9.

McLean, D. and Nathan, J. (2007) Treatment of personality disorder: limit setting and the use of benign authority. *British Journal of Psychotherapy*, **23**, 231–46.

Nathan, J. (2006) Self-harm: a strategy for survival and nodal point of change. *Advances in Psychiatric Treatment*, **12**, 329–37.

NICE (2004) *Self-harm: The Short-term Physical and Psychological Management and Secondary Prevention of Self-harm in Primary and Secondary Care* (CG16). London: NICE.

Pengelly, N., Ford, B., Blenkiron, P., and Reilly, S. (2008) Harm minimisation after repeated self-harm: development of a trust handbook. *Psychiatric Bulletin*, **32**, 60–3.

Stengel, E. (1964) *Suicide and Attempted Suicide.* Harmondsworth: Penguin Books.

Suominen, K., Isometsä, E., Suokas, J., *et al.* (2004) Completed suicide after a suicide attempt: a 37-year follow-up study. *American Journal of Psychiatry*, **161**, 562–3.

Zahl, D.L. and Hawton, K. (2004) Repetition of deliberate self-harm and subsequent suicide risk: long-term follow-up study of 11 583 patients. *British Journal of Psychiatry*, **185**, 70–5.

 Go to www.oxfordtextbooks/orc/stringer for an array of additional references, including indicative mark sheets for OSCEs, self-assessment questions, guidance, and exercises.

# 9 Schizophrenia

*Ajay Bhatnagar, Naveen Sharma, Noreen Jakeman, and Michelle Butterworth*

## True or False? Test your existing knowledge—answers in the chapter and online

1. A hallucination is the misperception of a stimulus.

2. People with schizophrenia are more likely to be born in December than June.

3. The incidence of schizophrenia is twice as high in urban than rural areas.

4. Persecutory delusions are one of Schneider's first rank symptoms of schizophrenia.

5. Haloperidol has fewer extrapyramidal side effects than clozapine.

6. Neuroleptic malignant syndrome is an antipsychotic side effect characterised by hyperkinesia and clonus.

7. 1 in 10 people with schizophrenia continue to be seriously and continuously disabled by it.

8. Late onset predicts poor prognosis in schizophrenia.

9. Temporarily colluding with delusions is an important aspect of a primary interview.

10. When assessing the risk of violence, past behaviour should not be seen as predicting future behaviour.

## Contents

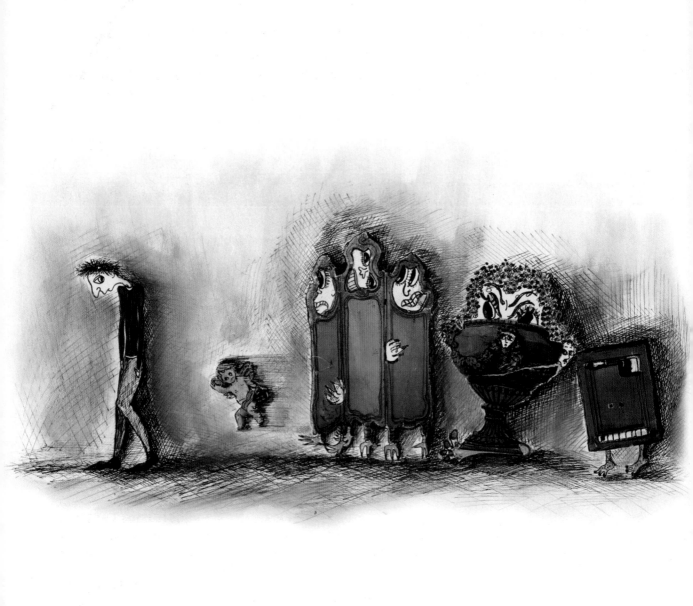

# PRINCIPLES

*Was it there? Again that awful uncertainty—I would seem to have it, then it was gone. I sat hunched on the bed, clutching myself around the shins, my forehead on my knees. Did I have it? Was there gas? Was it seeping from my* groin*? I lifted my head and turned it helplessly from side to side. Gas from my groin? It was at that moment that I became aware of the noise in the attic overhead, quiet laughter followed by a sort of bump—then there was silence again.*

Patrick McGrath—*Spider*[1]

## Introduction

Schizophrenia is a greatly stigmatized and misunderstood illness. This stigma is reflected historically: patients who would now be diagnosed with schizophrenia were regarded as being possessed by demons or afflicted with 'madness' as a divine punishment for their sins. Years on, the ignorance and fear persist: the media condemn people with schizophrenia as dangerous criminals and the general public wrongly believes that they have split personalities. This stigma may be partly due to the unsettling effect that the illness has on those who witness it.

Schizophrenia is a *psychotic* illness. In psychosis, people lose touch with reality, experiencing hallucinations and delusions.

- **Hallucination**: a perception in the absence of a stimulus, i.e. hearing, seeing, smelling, touching or tasting something that isn't there.
- **Delusion**: a fixed, false belief, held despite rational argument or evidence to the contrary. It cannot be explained by the patient's cultural, religious, or educational background.

This chapter aims to help you understand the experience of people with schizophrenia—and to overcome the stigma that may interfere with the quality of your care.

---

**BOX 9.1** What's in a name?

The name *schizophrenia* was coined by the psychiatrist Eugene Bleuler, and is derived from the Greek *skhizein* ('to split') and *phrēn* ('mind'). Around this time, the expression '*splitting of the mind or its function*' was often used to explain abnormal behaviour. Schizophrenia has nothing to do with having a 'split personality'.

---

## Epidemiology

The lifetime risk of developing schizophrenia is ~1%. Onset is typically from 15 to 45 years, with men affected earlier and more severely than women. Overall men and women are affected equally.

 Although extremely rare, schizophrenia *can* present in childhood, often associated with developmental delay.

## Aetiology

Schizophrenia has a complex multifactorial aetiology.

### Genetics

There is good evidence for a genetic basis to schizophrenia. The lifetime risk increases from 1% to 10% for first-degree relatives of people with schizophrenia; and 48% for a child whose parents are both affected (Tsuang *et al.* 2001). Monozygotic twin concordance is 40–50%, whereas for dizygotes it is 10–20% (Cardno *et al.* 1999). Adoption studies show that children of people with schizophrenia, raised in families without schizophrenia, remain at high risk of the disorder.

Numerous genetic loci are currently under investigation, though it is unlikely that a single 'schizophrenia gene' exists (van Haren *et al.* 2008). Instead, multiple *susceptibility* genes probably interact, each making someone slightly more likely to develop schizophrenia. Genes may code for symptom clusters (e.g. psychotic, depressive, or manic symptoms), creating an overlap between genes that contribute to a spectrum of psychotic disorders: schizophrenia, schizoaffective psychosis, and affective psychosis.

### Obstetric complications

Maternal prenatal malnutrition or viral infections increase the risk of schizophrenia, as do pre-eclampsia, low birth weight, and emergency Caesarean section. These may reflect underlying genetic abnormalities, or hypoxic brain damage.

Rates of schizophrenia are higher in people born in the winter (January–March in the northern hemisphere), when viral infections are rife.

## Substance misuse

Substances such as cannabis, amphetamines, cocaine, and LSD can produce psychotic symptoms. Cannabis does not *cause* schizophrenia in itself but increases the overall risk, contributing to the development of the disorder in susceptible people (Henquet *et al.* 2005). The enzyme catechol-*O*-methyl transferase (COMT) breaks down dopamine. There are two alleles coding for the COMT gene: Val and Met. The Val allele increases the risk of schizophrenia in cannabis users: people who are Val–Val have the highest risk, those who are Met–Met have the lowest risk, and heterozygotes have intermediate risk (Caspi *et al.* 2005). Of course, people don't know their genotype before smoking cannabis . . .

The types of cannabis that people use is also important. *Skunk* is a particularly dangerous form for those vulnerable to schizophrenia, since it has higher concentrations of tetrahydrocannabinol, the chemical in cannabis most associated with psychosis.

Smoking cannabis more than 50 times *as a teenager* makes you six times more likely to develop schizophrenia (Andreason *et al.* 1988). Adolescents are very vulnerable since their brains are still developing.

## Social disadvantage

Higher prevalence of schizophrenia among adults of lower socio-economic status is not reflected in their status at birth, suggesting that the downward 'drift' is due to the illness, and results from social isolation and unemployment.

## Urban life and birth

The prevalence of schizophrenia is twice as high in urban than rural areas. This may be due to drift or to stress specific to the urban environment.

## Migration and ethnicity

First- and second-generation immigrants have an average threefold increase in the risk of schizophrenia compared with indigenous populations (Cantor-Graae and Selten 2005). These rates seem to vary with ethnicity, with Black Caribbean and Black African populations showing the highest rates (a 4 to 6-fold increase compared to the White British population) (Fearon *et al.* 2006). This is neither fully understood, nor explained by preferential migration, diagnostic bias, higher rates of schizophrenia in the country of origin, or lower social class.

## Expressed emotion (EE)

Close contact with highly critical or over-involved relatives doubles the risk of relapse in the 9–18 months following

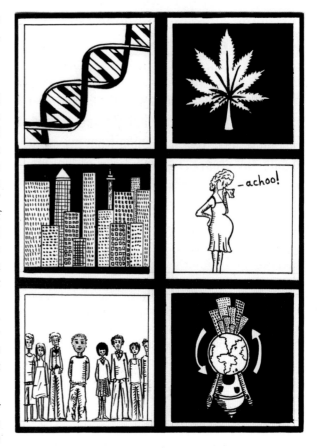

FIGURE 9.1 Risk factors for schizophrenia

discharge from hospital. This 'high expressed emotion' does not *cause* schizophrenia (Kavanagh 1992).

## Premorbid personality

Premorbid schizoid personality precedes schizophrenia in up to a quarter of cases. Schizotypal disorder[2] is more commonly associated with schizophrenia, possibly due to a shared genetic basis.

## Adverse life experience

Sexual or physical abuse in childhood or adulthood increases the risk of schizophrenia (Read *et al.* 2005). Psychological treatments to address these may be an important part of management.

## Main theories

### Neurodevelopmental theories

Studies show brain changes in some people with schizophrenia, notably enlarged ventricles with overall smaller and lighter brains (Johnstone *et al.* 1976). There is no gliosis at post-mortem, which may indicate that changes occur before adulthood. Brain changes are also suggested by lower pre-morbid IQ, and particular deficits in learning, memory, and executive function (Heinrichs and Zakzanis 1998).

Schizophrenia can therefore be viewed as a neuro-developmental disorder. Initial brain abnormalities, whether from genetic origin or early brain damage, may be imperceptible at first, but progress as the brain matures through ongoing myelination and synaptic pruning. The maturation, together with other risk factors (e.g. cannabis), may allow functional and connectivity abnormalities to evolve until overt schizophrenic symptoms emerge (Weinberger 1995).

## Neurotransmitter theories

The *dopamine hypothesis* states that schizophrenia is a result of dopamine overactivity in certain areas of the brain (van Praag 1977). *Positive* symptoms (hallucinations and delusions) are thought to result from excess dopamine in the *mesolimbic* tracts. By contrast, *negative* symptoms (e.g. apathy, social withdrawal) may result from dopamine underactivity in the *mesocortical* tracts.

Evidence for this includes:

- All known effective antipsychotics are dopamine antagonists (dopamine receptor blockers).
- Antipsychotics work better against positive, rather than negative, symptoms.
- Dopaminergic agents like amphetamine, cocaine, L-dopa, and bromocriptine can all induce psychosis, symptomatically indistinguishable from schizophrenia.

Dopamine is not the whole story, otherwise antipsychotics would cure all psychoses, which they don't. Hence there is also room for theories involving serotonergic overactivity (Meltzer *et al.* 2003) and glutamate dysregulation (Tuominen *et al.* 2005).

## Psychological theories

Cognitive models propose subtle defects of thinking such as the tendency to jump to conclusions without adequately examining contradictory evidence, leading to delusions. Alternatively, fear of madness may prompt the defences of denial and rationalization, resulting in a delusional system to explain persecutory voices.

## Clinical picture

The clinical picture in schizophrenia can be divided into three stages:

- at-risk mental state (*prodrome*)
- acute phase: *positive* symptoms are hallucinations and delusions
- chronic phase: *negative* symptoms reflect things that are *lost* in schizophrenia (e.g. motivation).

## The at-risk mental state (ARM)

People who develop the *ARM* are at high risk of developing full-blown psychosis. The older term, *prodrome*, is losing popularity since it wrongly suggests that psychosis is inevitable.

The ARM consists of low-grade symptoms such as social withdrawal and loss of interest in work, study, and relationships, without any frank psychotic symptoms. Typically, the picture is of someone in their late teens or early twenties who has dropped out of college or work after a period of increasing absences. They often seem 'distant', giving no reason for isolating themselves in their bedroom. They may deny vague psychotic symptoms for fear of their significance.

> The ARM can be hard to distinguish from depression, substance misuse, or *normal teenage behaviour!*

## Acute phase

The acute phase has the most striking and florid psychotic features: delusions and hallucinations. Thinking is disturbed, resulting in muddled speech, and behaviour may be withdrawn, overactive, or bizarre.

> Negative symptoms such as a marked decrease in self-care, social withdrawal, and anhedonia can also present in the acute phase.

Many patients experience hallucinations, often auditory in nature. Of particular diagnostic significance are:

- Voices discussing or arguing about the patient, e.g.
  - 1st voice: 'No-one likes her.'
  - 2nd voice: 'Yeah . . . It's because she's ugly.'
- Voices giving a running commentary on the patient's actions, e.g.
  - 'He's going into the bedroom now. He's taking off his shoes . . .'
- *Thought echo*: the voices say the patient's thoughts aloud, e.g.
  - Patient thinks: *I'm hungry.*
  - Voice: 'I'm hungry.'

Delusions can be of any kind, but are often persecutory. The most diagnostically significant are:

- *Delusional perception*. This is a two-stage process whereby a real perception is then interpreted in a delusional way, e.g.
  - 'The traffic lights changed to green and I knew I was Queen of Ireland!'
- *Passivity*: belief that movement, sensation, emotion, or impulse are controlled by an outside force, e.g.
  - 'He makes my eyes go round and round and I can't keep them still.'

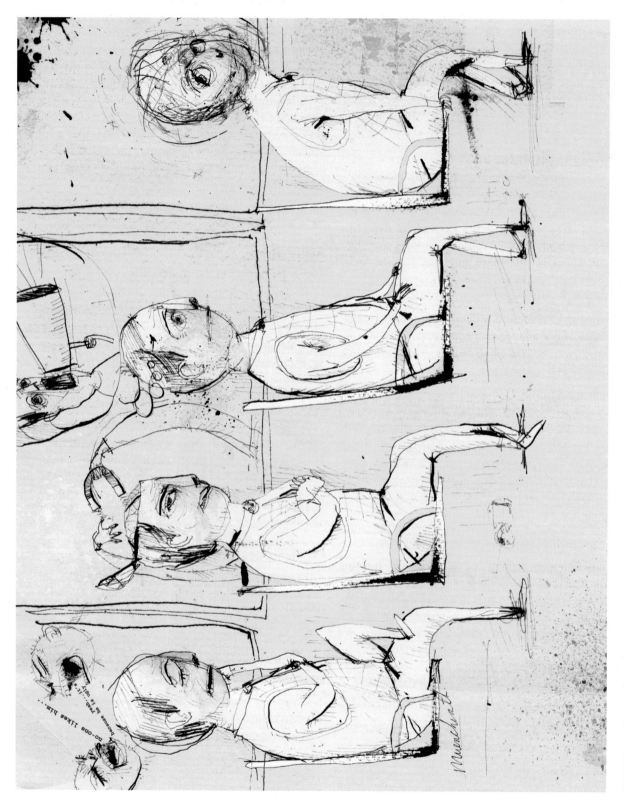

**FIGURE 9.2** Some of the first-rank symptoms of schizophrenia. How would your concentration be affected if you were experiencing these symptoms while studying?

- *Thought interference*: the patient believes that their thoughts are under the control of something or someone else.

  – *Thought withdrawal*—thoughts are removed from the patient's mind, e.g. 'The old man uses an invisible fishing line to pluck the thoughts from my head!'

  – *Thought insertion*—thoughts are placed directly into the patient's mind, e.g. 'She uses magnets to push her thoughts in. They suddenly pop up from nowhere. I know they're not mine—they feel completely different to mine.'

  – *Thought broadcasting*: thoughts are broadcast to others so that people can know what they are thinking, e.g. 'As I think, my thoughts flash up on a website. Anyone who logs on can read what I'm thinking.'

Formal thought disorder is when thoughts become disconnected (loosening of associations). Vagueness may progress to very disjointed speech that is hard to follow and apparently senseless. Poverty of thought and thought blocking may also occur.

➜ In word salad, words become so disconnected from each other that a sentence is nonsensical. *Limerick and alter prep lemon enlist if light subsonic thrum ginger*. It is diagnosed more often than it is heard!

---

**BOX 9.2** Schizophrenia in Britain: the first clear description

James Tilly Matthews was a London tea merchant who travelled to France in the 1790s, aiming to dispel the threat of war between England and revolutionary France. He gained the trust of the French government with his *own* set of peace terms but was later arrested under suspicion of being a spy. Following his release, he returned to England, consumed

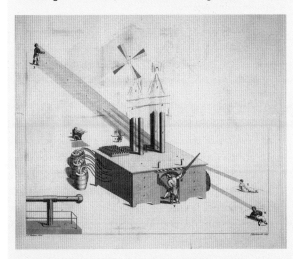

**FIGURE 9.3** The Air Loom (courtesy of the Bodleian Library)

---

by conspiracy theories, and in 1797 was committed to the Bethlem Hospital after shouting 'Treason!' from the Public Gallery of the House of Commons.

Two independent doctors later agreed he was sane, prompting the Bethlem's apothecary, John Haslam, to describe Tilly's beliefs in his book *Illustrations of Madness*. This was both a bid to prove Tilly's insanity *and* support his own view of medicine for the mentally ill as a new specialty.

Tilly drew the illustration, which shows the 'Air Loom' being operated. He believed that a gang acted as 'active worriers'. 'Bill the King' was the ringleader, 'Glove Woman' operated the machine, and 'Sir Archy' was a 'common liar' who communicated with James through 'brain sayings'.

The Air Loom had a powerful hold over Tilly and ran on a mixture of foul substances like 'male and female seminal fluid' and 'gaz (sic) from the anus of the horse'. Tilly described what we would now consider first-rank symptoms, for example, 'Laugh Making' (Made Affect) and 'Kiteing' (Thought Insertion), e.g.

> As boys raise a kite in the air, so these wretches, by means of the Air Loom and magnetic impregnations, contrive to lift into the brain some particular idea, which floats and undulates in the intellect for hours together [. . . the victim] is, during the whole time, conscious that the kited idea is extraneous, and does not belong to the train of his own cogitations. (J. Haslam, *Illustrations of Madness*)

Although Tilly was ultimately decreed both insane and dangerous, he provided architectural designs that contributed to the new Bethlem Hospital. His final year was spent in a more pleasant private asylum, book-keeping and gardening for a doctor who regarded him as entirely sane.

His case illustrates classic first-rank symptoms as well as the controversy regarding illness and dangerousness—issues still relevant today.

---

## Chronic phase

Some patients' psychoses become 'burnt-out' after a few years. Rather than becoming well, they enter a chronic phase of prominent negative symptoms which may last indefinitely and be immensely disabling. These symptoms are:

- apathy—the opposite of enthusiasm; loss of motivation
- blunted affect—decreased reactivity of mood
- anhedonia—the inability to enjoy interests/activities
- social withdrawal
- poverty of thought and speech.

These may manifest as a lack of attention to personal hygiene and care, a limited repertoire of daily activities, and social isolation. There may also be residual and less prominent 'positive symptoms', e.g. the person may still have the same persecutory delusional thoughts but seem less distressed and affected by them.

➡ Depression and antipsychotic side effects both resemble the chronic phase, but are often *much* easier to treat. Don't overlook them, since treatment can give your patient a new lease of life.

## Subtypes of schizophrenia

Schizophrenic presentations can be divided into subtypes based on the most prominent symptoms. Don't get too tied up in this though, since patterns may overlap and individual presentations can change over time.

### Paranoid

The most common type—it is exemplified by the acute phase description above and the main symptoms are prominent *delusions and hallucinations.*

### Catatonic

This is dominated by *psychomotor disturbance.* Abnormalities include:

- *Stupor*—a state of being immobile, mute, and unresponsive, despite appearing to be conscious (eyes are open and will follow people around the room).
- *Excitement*—periods of extreme and apparently purposeless motor hyperactivity.
- *Posturing*—assuming and maintaining inappropriate or bizarre positions.
- *Rigidity*—holding a rigid posture against efforts to be moved.
- *Waxy flexibility*—the patient's limbs offer minimal resistance to being placed in odd positions which are maintained for unusually lengthy periods (*cataplexy*).
- *Automatic obedience*—to any instructions.
- *Perseveration*—inappropriate repetition of words or movements:

**You:** Where were you born?

**Stephen:** Sidcup.

**Y:** What was your father's job?

**S:** Sidcup.

**Y:** Um . . . Your father's *job?*

**S:** Sidcup.

Catatonia is now rare in developed countries, probably due to the availability of antipsychotics and active rehabilitation programmes.

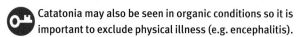

🔑 Catatonia may also be seen in organic conditions so it is important to exclude physical illness (e.g. encephalitis).

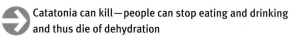

➡ Catatonia can kill—people can stop eating and drinking and thus die of dehydration

### Hebephrenic

Onset is between the ages 15 and 25 years. The predominant features are *disorganized and chaotic* mood, behaviour, and speech. Affect is often shallow or inappropriate, and the patient's behaviour feels aimless. Delusions and hallucinations are not prominent.

### Simple

*Negative* features only, without ever having had positive psychotic symptoms.

### Residual

Prominent *negative* symptoms are all that remain after delusions and hallucinations subside.

## Diagnosis

Schneider described first-rank symptoms that are suggestive of schizophrenia in the absence of organic disorder. However, they are neither necessary nor sufficient to make the diagnosis, as they can occur in mania and delirium, and may be absent in schizophrenia. Symptoms should be present for one month before making the diagnosis.

---

**BOX 9.3** Schneider's first-rank symptoms

................................................................

*Delusional perception*
*Passivity*
*Delusions of thought interference*

- Thought insertion
- Thought withdrawal
- Thought broadcasting

*Auditory hallucinations*

- Thought echo
- 'Third person' (voices discussing or arguing about the patient)
- Running commentary

---

## Differential diagnoses

1. **Organic**: physical causes of psychosis must be excluded before diagnosing schizophrenia.
   (a) *Substance misuse* Since people are usually young at first presentation, substance misuse is the most practical first differential to be excluded. Drug intoxication and alcohol withdrawal can produce psychotic symptoms. Common drugs include amphetamine, cocaine, LSD, Ecstasy, ketamine, and phencyclidine.
   (b) *Dementia* (especially in elderly patients).
   (c) *Delirium* (especially in elderly patients).
   (d) *Epilepsy* (especially temporal lobe epilepsy).

(e) *Medication side effect*, e.g. steroids, dopamine agonists.

(f) *Other*, e.g. brain tumour, stroke, HIV, Wilson's disease, porphyria, neurosyphilis.

2. **Acute and transient psychotic episode** can appear identical to schizophrenia, but resolves completely *within a few months*. It can be stress related.

3. **Mood disorder**: both depression and mania, if severe enough, produce psychotic symptoms. Schizophrenia should not be diagnosed in the presence of striking mood disturbance unless the schizophrenic symptoms clearly came first.

4. **Schizoaffective disorder** is diagnosed if both schizophrenic and affective symptoms develop together and are roughly evenly balanced, to the extent that one set of symptoms cannot be said to be more important than the other.

5. **Persistent delusional disorder** describes delusions with few if any hallucinations.

6. **Schizotypal disorder** is a lifelong state of eccentricity with abnormal thoughts and affect which is regarded as a personality disorder in DSM-IV. Patients may be suspicious, cold, and aloof with rather odd ideas, without showing definite symptoms of schizophrenia (though some eventually do develop schizophrenia).

➔ A drug-free inpatient admission may clarify the diagnosis if someone is psychotic while using drugs.

➔ New psychotic symptoms in older people are *far* more likely to represent delirium or dementia than schizophrenia.

## Investigations

A full physical examination and investigations are important in excluding an organic cause *and* in making a general assessment of physical health before starting medical treatment.

1. Blood tests: FBC, TFTs, U&E, LFT, CRP, fasting G. Consider HIV testing, syphilis serology. Lipids should be checked before starting long-term antipsychotics.

2. MSU.

3. Urine drug screen.

4. CT scan—only to rule out any organic pathology if *suspected*. Routine imaging is not indicated.

5. EEG—if epilepsy or another organic cause are suspected, e.g. by visual hallucinations, confusion.

6. Symptom rating scales may help to assess severity and monitor response to treatment.

7. OT assessment of activities of daily living.

8. Social work assessment of housing, finances, and carers' needs.

9. Collateral history.

## Management

A biopsychosocial approach is taken, involving:

- biological therapies including drug treatment with antipsychotics
- psychological therapies
- social interventions.

---

**BOX 9.4** Early Intervention Services

.................................................................................................

The duration of untreated psychosis (DUP) is the time delay from the *first ever* clear-cut psychotic symptom until the start of the *first ever effective treatment*. Psychosis itself is *toxic*—the longer the DUP, the greater the damage to the person's cognitive abilities, insight, and social situation (e.g. dropping out of school, work, relationships). The sooner effective treatment can be started, the better the prognosis. This has led to Early Intervention Services being set up with the specific aim of engaging patients with very early symptoms. Patients are offered antipsychotics and psychosocial interventions with the aim of keeping the DUP below three months.

---

## Antipsychotics

Antipsychotics are dopamine antagonists; they block postsynaptic D2 receptors. In general, the greater the affinity, the more effective they are in treating positive symptoms, caused by dopamine excess. Extrapyramidal side effects (EPSEs), due to generalized dopamine blockade, are inevitable at higher doses of all antipsychotics, although newer 'atypicals' are more selective, reducing the risk of EPSEs at therapeutic doses. Blockade of other neurotransmitters produces a variety of side effects (see below).

### Typical antipsychotics

These are the older drugs, such as chlorpromazine, haloperidol, and depot preparations like flupentixol decanoate. They tend to cause distressing EPSEs at normal treatment doses. Despite this, they are still widely used because they are effective, cheap, and provide depot options. Depots are long-acting injections that are useful for patients who have difficulties taking daily tablets.

### Atypical antipsychotics

Although these newer medications cause fewer EPSEs and generally do not increase prolactin levels, they are certainly not free of side effects. All atypicals block dopamine receptors, but they also block serotonin 5-$HT_2$ receptors. This combination of receptor blockades makes their effectiveness and side-effect profile different from typical antipsychotics. Examples include: olanzapine, risperidone, quetiapine, aripiprazole, amisulpride, and clozapine. Risperidone is available as a depot injection.

Consider starting an atypical when:

- choosing first-line treatment in newly diagnosed schizophrenia
- there are unacceptable side-effects from typical antipsychotics
- relapse occurs on a typical antipsychotic (NICE 2002).

Where possible, the choice of medication should be made in collaboration with the patient. To reach the lowest dose that controls symptoms, titrate the drug against symptoms and side effects, allowing time at each dose for the drug to reach therapeutic levels. Avoid using more than one antipsychotic as multiple drugs increase risk and widen the side-effect profile.

## Side effects of antipsychotics

1. *Extrapyramidal side effects* (EPSEs) (see Table 9.1):
   - dystonia
   - akathisia
   - parkinsonism
   - tardive dyskinesia.
2. *Hyperprolactinaemia*—this causes:
   - galactorrhoea, amenorrhoea, gynaecomastia, and hypogonadism
   - sexual dysfunction
   - increased risk of osteoporosis.

3. *Weight gain*—especially olanzapine and clozapine.
4. *Sedation.*
5. *Increased risk of diabetes.*
6. *Dyslipidaemia* (raised triglycerides and cholesterol).
7. *Anticholinergic side effects*, e.g.
   - dry mouth, blurred vision, constipation, urinary retention, and tachycardia.
8. *Arrhythmias.*
9. *Seizures* by reducing the seizure threshold. Clozapine has the greatest risk of this.
10. *Neuroleptic malignant syndrome* (see Box 9.5).

---

**BOX 9.5** Neuroleptic malignant syndrome (NMS)

- A rare but life-threatening side effect of antipsychotics.
- Usually triggered by a new antipsychotic or dose increase.
- Thought to be an idiosyncratic response to dopamine antagonism.
- Symptoms: muscle stiffness and rigidity, altered consciousness, and disturbance of the autonomic nervous system (fever, tachycardia, and labile BP).
- Raised creatine kinase and white cell count.
- Treatment: stop antipsychotics immediately and get urgent medical treatment, often in an intensive care unit.
- Death may occur from a range of causes, e.g. acute renal failure secondary to skeletal muscle breakdown (rhabdomyolysis).

---

**TABLE 9.1** Extrapyramidal side effects

| Type of EPSE | Onset | Symptoms | Treatment |
|---|---|---|---|
| Dystonia | Early, sometimes within hours | An involuntary, painful, sustained muscle spasm, e.g. torticollis: neck twists to one side oculogyric crisis: eyes twist up and can't look down | Anticholinergic (e.g. procyclidine) |
| Akathisia | Hours to weeks | An unpleasant subjective feeling of restlessness; patients often have to pace about or jiggle their legs to cope with it | Decrease dose/change antipsychotic Add propranolol or benzodiazepines |
| Parkinsonism | Days to weeks | A triad of: resting tremor rigidity (experienced as stiffness) bradykinesia Patients may have mask-like facies and a shuffling gait | Decrease dose/change antipsychotic Try an anticholinergic (e.g. procyclidine) but review frequently and do not prescibe prophylactically |
| Tardive dyskinesia | Months or years | Rhythmic involuntary movements of the mouth, face, limbs, and trunk which are very distressing Patients may grimace, or make chewing and sucking movements with their mouth and tongue | Stop antipsychotic or reduce dose if possible (though problems may worsen initially). Avoid anticholinergics since they often worsen the problem. Switch to an atypical or clozapine Often irreversible |

**→** People with schizophrenia have increased rates of smoking, obesity, hypertension, cardiac disease, diabetes, and dyslipidaemia. Add antipsychotics, and you have a potent recipe for premature death.

### Monitoring

Anyone prescribed an antipsychotic long term needs regular monitoring and review. Basic monitoring includes:

- BMI and waist circumference.
- Blood pressure.
- FBC, LFTs, U&Es, glucose tolerance test (fasting glucose or $HbA_{1C}$ if not possible), lipids.
- Some may need:
  - prolactin levels—if hyperprolactinaemia is suspected or likely (e.g. risperidone)
  - ECGs—important in middle-aged to elderly people and in those on high-dose antipsychotics or clozapine —to monitor the QTc interval.

### Clozapine

*Treatment resistance* is the failure to respond to two or more antipsychotics, at least one of which is an atypical, each given at a therapeutic dose for at least six weeks. Clozapine is the first-line drug for treatment-resistant (or 'refractory') schizophrenia. It can work when everything else has failed (Kane *et al.* 1998), but has *the potentially fatal complication of agranulocytosis in 0.7% of patients*. Its use requires weekly blood tests to detect early signs of neutropenia. This occurs in 3% of patients and means that clozapine must be stopped. In the absence of problems, tests are gradually reduced to once a month.

The sooner an effective treatment is started, the better the patient's prognosis; hence, if other treatments fail, a trial of clozapine should follow promptly—despite the unpleasant blood tests. This potentially improves the quality of life through symptom reduction, and reduces the suicide risk in such patients. Some patients do not respond well even to clozapine and require augmentation with other medications.

**→** When admitting a patient on clozapine to a medical ward, seek advice regarding doses and blood monitoring from a psychiatrist or pharmacist as soon as possible.

## Psychological management

A number of psychological approaches have been adopted for the treatment of schizophrenia, and the following interventions may be available.

### Cognitive behavioural therapy (CBT)

CBT is now recognized as an integral part of treatment that should ideally be offered to all patients proactively (Cormac *et al.* 2002). The general principles of CBT apply (see p.37), and a particular emphasis is placed on reality testing. As noted earlier, people with schizophrenia have a tendency to jump to conclusions without questioning the validity of their beliefs. In CBT, the therapist aims to gently challenge the patient's beliefs, aiding awareness of illogical thinking, e.g. 'I'm a bit confused by that. If the Prime Minister is stalking you all day, how does he find the time to run the country and appear on TV?' The patient is encouraged to think about the evidence for and against a belief and to consider alternative explanations.

As well as improving self-esteem and problem-solving, CBT may help patients to cope with troublesome hallucinations and delusions.

### Family therapy

Family therapy can reduce relapse rates (Pharoah *et al.* 2006). The effects of high expressed emotion can be ameliorated through communication skills training, education about schizophrenia, problem-solving, and helping patients to expand their social network, as well as taking time out from their families.

### Concordance therapy

This is a collaborative approach where the patient is encouraged to consider the pros and cons of the management, improving their understanding of their treatment needs.

**→** Psychodynamic theory conceptualizes the patient's symptoms and behaviour as a conflict between the psychotic and non-psychotic parts of the personality. This can be a helpful idea for staff and families as they face the limitations imposed by the illness.

## Social approaches

These may include admission to hospital for observation, treatment, or refuge, but are also concerned with practical needs like benefits, housing, training, and education. *Social skills training* is primarily aimed at improving interpersonal skills. Using methods such as role-play, the patients develop improved confidence and skills in their day-to-day functioning in the community (Kopelowicz *et al.* 2006).

Schizophrenia is no longer a social death sentence; patients are not 'looked after' in asylums for the rest of their lives, but encouraged to develop the skills to care for themselves in the least restrictive environment possible. Rehabilitation psychiatry focuses on the patient's quality of life, overcoming disability where possible and accepting limitations where not. It is a long-term approach, addressing such varied needs as:

- accessing education, training, or employment
- skills, e.g. budgeting and cooking

**TABLE 9.2** Management summary

| | Biological | Psychological | Social |
|---|---|---|---|
| Immediate | Exclude organic cause<br>Start (atypical) antipsychotic | Reassurance<br>Education<br>Supportive counselling | Carer support and psycho-education |
| Medium term | Continue medications<br>Monitor for side effects, physical health, and concordance | CBT<br>Family therapy<br>Concordance therapy | Address housing and financial issues<br>Carer assessment and support |
| Long term | Treatment resistance: start clozapine<br>Concordance problems: try depot | | Social skills training<br>Rehabilitation:<br>   housing, education, work, recreation, etc.<br>Day centres |

- housing, e.g. supported accommodation, independent flats
- accessing social activities
- developing personal skills, e.g. creative writing.

## Risk assessment

Contrary to popular belief, people with schizophrenia are a greater risk to themselves than to others.

### Risk to self

This includes suicide, self-neglect, social decline, and victimization by others. The lifetime risk of suicide is 10%, ten times that of the general population. Intelligent young men with good premorbid functioning are especially vulnerable. Risk is highest in the early years after diagnosis, following first admission, or where there are depressive symptoms.

### Risk to others

Only a small subgroup of people with schizophrenia are more likely to be violent than members of the general population; they account for less than 10% of violent crimes in the UK. In some cases, violence is a direct response to persecutory delusions or command hallucinations. Factors that increase the risk of violence are:

- past history of violence
- substance misuse
- acute psychotic symptoms
- non-concordance with treatment
- access to weapons
- specific threats to a victim
- comorbid personality disorder (dissocial, emotionally unstable, or paranoid) or psychopathy.

### Risk from others

In general, the community is a greater threat *to* people with schizophrenia than they are to it. Patients are at increased risk of being victims of crime, and in one study were at least 14 times more likely to be the victim of a violent crime than to be arrested for one (Brekke *et al.* 2001).

**!** A particularly worrying scenario might be a man with persecutory delusions and command hallucinations living with his highly critical mother, with whom he spends all his time in face-to-face contact. Add in substance misuse and non-concordance with medication and the risk would become even higher!

## Prognosis

A quarter of patients recover and experience no further difficulties after a single episode. Two-thirds remain liable to relapse or continue to have symptoms. One in ten will be seriously and continuously disabled. However,

**TABLE 9.3** Prognostic indicators in schizophrenia

| Factor | Prognosis | |
|---|---|---|
| | Good | Poor |
| Sex | Female | Male |
| Onset | Later, acute | Early, insidious |
| DUP | <3 months | >3 months |
| Premorbid IQ | High | Low |
| Prominent symptoms | Affective (mood) | Negative |
| Social support | Good | Poor/social withdrawal |
| Concordant with medication | Yes | No |
| Family history | No | Yes |
| Precipitating features | Yes | No |
| Substance misuse | No | Yes (especially cannabis) |

the prognosis of schizophrenia varies between patients, depending on numerous factors.

The relative mortality of patients with schizophrenia is more than twice that of the general population, with significantly higher rates among males than females because of their increased rates of accidents and suicide.

Poor physical health contributes to the high mortality rates.

> It can be easy to avoid or forget the physical needs of patients with schizophrenia—but they are *more likely* than the general population to need your medical attention.

# REALITY: SCHIZOPHRENIA AND PSYCHOSIS

## General approach: tips, tricks, and cautionary tales

### 1. Stop thinking 'This person is mad'

You and your patient have different realities that feel equally true. If you have the attitude that your reality is right and theirs is wrong, you will seem arrogant and difficult to talk to. Instead, listen to the story with the recognition that your day has probably been fairly average by comparison, and you are lucky that this is the case. If you *had* been stalked, poisoned, and talked about, it would be a relief to discuss this with someone who wasn't staring at you in smug disbelief.

### 2. Gain trust

Paranoia makes few exceptions: medical students are as suspect as anyone else. If your patient is suspicious of you and your motives, don't become defensive—this only makes you look shiftier! Be open about who you are and what you want from them. Explain confidentiality and try to understand what they are most worried about. If they really don't want to talk, that's fine. They may change their mind if they see you working well with other patients on the ward.

### 3. Be curious

Let your curiosity carry you through the history; don't change the subject as soon as you think you've discovered a 'psychotic symptom'. As mentioned previously (p.21), if a friend told you that someone had followed them home, you would be full of logical questions—and a history is no different from an ordinary conversation in this sense.

### 4. Respond!

Empathize, suspend your disbelief, and *respond* appropriately to what your patient says. Here is an example of what *not* to do:

**Ralph:** I realized they were gassing me to take my organs for their experiments. I woke last night and heard them say, 'You take his head and I'll have the eyes!'

**You:** OK. Do you have any allergies?

### 5. The balancing act

There is a line to walk between colluding with your patient and disagreeing with them. This is particularly difficult when patients ask, '*You* believe me, don't you?' Lying and saying that you *do* believe their delusions can create all kinds of problems. At the same time, it is unhelpful to say, 'Of course not—you're delusional'.

Try holding the point of view that you don't believe it, but you *do* believe that *they* believe it. Sometimes you can deflect the question, for example by refocusing on the emotional side of the patient's story; at other times, you must answer more directly.

**Ralph:** You *do* believe me, don't you?

**You:**

- I haven't been through what you've been through, but I can see it's really frightening you.
- I know you're not lying, Ralph. What do your family think about it?
- I come from a medical background—I think stress has a lot to do with what you're experiencing. What do you think about that?

Never argue—you won't 'cure' people with arguments and they won't like you if you try.

### 6. Don't say 'think'

Remember that people are certain about their delusions. They are often sensitive to the word *think* when you describe their thoughts, e.g.

**You:** So for the last three weeks you've been thinking people have been gassing you and . . .

**Ralph:** I don't *think*—I *know*! You don't believe me! Why can't you take me seriously?

You are trying to let your patient know that you have understood their experience; you are not telling your consultant about it. Try instead:

**You:** So for the last three weeks you've been terrified because people have been gassing you and trying to steal your organs.

**Ralph:** Right.

## 7. Don't talk about The Voices

Similarly, don't call auditory hallucinations *voices* unless your patient does. Many people associate 'hearing voices' with mental illness, and your patient may not see their experiences as a sign of illness. Use their terminology: if they call their voices 'the police' then you should too (e.g. 'What do *the police* say to you?').

## The interview

### General screening questions

#### Starting out

- I'd like to ask you some questions. Some of them might sound a little strange, but please don't worry—these are routine questions that I ask all my patients.
- Sometimes when people are stressed they can have strange experiences. Has anything strange or unusual happened to you?
- Has anything scared or upset you?
- Has anything happened you find hard to explain?
- How have you been getting on with other people recently?
- Have you been troubled by people you don't actually know?

Sometimes the most helpful question is:

- Why *are* the doctors keeping you here?

### Asking about delusions

#### Persecutory

- Is anyone trying to *make life difficult* for you?
  - e.g. follow/spy/hurt/watch/trick/poison . . . you?
- Have you got people around who you can trust?
- Have other people been acting suspiciously?

### Delusions of reference

- Have people been saying or doing things with a special meaning, just for you?
- Has anything in the news seemed to be meant for you or about you?

### Delusional perception

- Did something happen which alerted you to what was going on?
- Were you ever given 'a sign'?

### Passivity

- Are you in full control of everything you do and feel?
- Do you ever feel as if you are controlled by someone else, almost as if they have a remote control for you? (. . . like you're a robot/character in a computer game?)

### Thought interference

📖 If your patient *has* experienced thought interference, they will often be surprised that you could know about it and sometimes relieved to tell you. If they haven't, they'll look puzzled.

- Are you completely in control of all your thoughts?
- Can anyone mess with (*or* interfere with) the thoughts in your head?

#### *Insertion*

- Do you ever feel like the thoughts in your head don't belong to you?
- Can anyone put *their* thoughts into your head without even talking to you?

#### *Withdrawal*

- Can anyone steal/take/pluck thoughts from your head?

#### *Broadcasting*

- Do you ever feel like other people know what you're thinking?
  - . . . even if they're nowhere near you? How?
  - . . . as if your head can't keep your thoughts safe inside it anymore? How?

📖 Ask for examples of thought interference, e.g. 'Mum *puts thoughts in my head*. She'll say we're having chips for dinner, then I really want chips'. This is not thought insertion.

### Grandiose

- How do you see the future?
- Do you have any special talents or abilities that other people don't have?
- Have you got a special purpose or mission in life?

### Nihilistic

- Do you ever feel as though you're doomed?
- Are you worried about your body . . . ? (not working/not existing/being blocked or rotten)

## Asking about hallucinations

### General

- (You seem like a sensitive person.) Can you hear/see things other people don't notice?
- Have you seen or heard anything that's worried you recently?

### If they are distracted (e.g. glancing about/mumbling) ask why . . .

- Is something making it hard for you to concentrate?
- Can you hear or see something?

### Auditory

- Have you ever heard strange noises or voices when you thought you were alone?
- Do people talk behind your back or gossip about you?
- Have you heard people talking, but can't work out where they are?
  - I'm a bit confused. I know you can hear other people talking right now, but I can't. Why do you think that is?'

#### Voices

- Do you know who's speaking?
- What do they say?
  - Is it just one person, or more than one? Who is it?
  - Do they talk *to* you or *about* you?
  - Do you hear them talking to each other about you?
  - Do they ever describe everything you do, just as you do it?
  - Do they make comments about what you're doing?
  - Do they ever say your thoughts aloud?
  - Do they ever tell you to *do* things?
- Can you hear them now?

### Visual

- Have you seen anything recently that seemed frightening or hard to explain?
- Have you ever seen ghosts/spirits/visions?
- Have you seen animals/insects/people that others can't see?

### Somatic/tactile

- Have you had any funny feelings in your body?
- Any strange feelings on or just under your skin? (e.g. like insects crawling?)
- Do you ever get strange feelings in your insides/organs?
  - . . . As if they're being twisted/stretched/squeezed?

### Gustatory/olfactory

- Have you noticed any strange tastes or smells that have worried you?
- Does food taste normal to you?

## Test conviction

Follow the story as mentioned in general tips. You need to *gently* test how strongly they hold their beliefs. This isn't about trying to prove them wrong.

- Why is this happening to *you*?
- How do you explain what's been happening?
- How do you *know for sure* this is going on?
- Have you been able to gather any evidence or proof? (e.g. for the police)
- What do your family/friends think?
- Why do you think they don't agree with you?
- Sometimes people's minds can play tricks on them (under stress). Could that possibly be true in your case?
- Could this be an elaborate hoax/a trick/a nasty joke?

Be aware that *someone* might share your patient's delusional view! In *folie à deux*, two people with a close relationship develop a shared delusion.

## Assess risk

Think about suicide and violence:

- You've put up with a lot so far. Have you done anything about it?
- What will you do if it goes on?
- What would make you defend yourself/do something about it?
- Do you worry that you might lose your temper with x?

Always find out any plans, access to weapons, victims, etc.

If command hallucinations/passivity/thought insertion:

- What do they want you to do?
- Do you think that you or anyone else might be hurt by what they want you to do?
- Can you resist, or do you have to do what they want?
- What do you think will happen if you don't do *x*?

Don't assume that everything you hear is delusional; psychosis does not prevent people from having real adverse experiences. Although your patient may be paranoid, their neighbours really *might* be harassing them and making their life miserable.

## Candidate's instructions

Miss Rita Olsworth is a 45-year-old woman, well known to psychiatric services with a diagnosis of treatment-resistant paranoid schizophrenia. She has attended the Community Mental Health Team today after an argument with her neighbours.

You are a third-year medical student attached to the team. The consultant has asked that you take a history of psychosis.

## Patient's instructions

*Key characteristics*

- I'm scruffy, in baggy, stained clothes; my hair is a mess.
- I slump in my chair and look distracted throughout the interview.
- I'm angry and talk loudly, sometimes rambling off the topic.
- I'm preoccupied with my hair and touch it often to feel its thickness.

No-one's taking me seriously. I came here to see Polly (my care coordinator) to get them evicted but she hasn't done anything more than say she'll see me every day—what good's that gonna do? The *ASBOs*[3] want me out so they can have my flat. They started leaving rubbish bags on my balcony a month ago. It attracts the rats. Why should I have rats? I dragged the bags up to their floor and left them there, but they kept coming back—new ones every week! Today I told them what I thought of them. They called the police and I said that was fine because they could sort it out but all the police did was have a go at me. They're so scared of ASBOs they won't do anything.

ASBOs walk about on the estate doing V-signs at my flat. I do V-signs back—and shout at them! They make signals with their cars—park them in special lines so the number plates show which room I'm in (kitchen, bathroom, or bedroom). I know it because they move their cars when I move rooms. For two weeks, they've been tapping my phone and talking about me when I pick the receiver up: 'Rita's on the phone again . . . now she's looking for a knife to cut the lines'. They know it makes me angry—and they're now talking so loudly, I can hear them even when I'm not on the phone.

I went shopping and left my home unprotected, a month ago. They got in and put something in my shampoo and my hair started falling out—big clumps in my hairbrush and in the shower! Mario (my boyfriend) said I was being silly, but I know what's happening—polonium poisoning! Radioactivity! I can't wash my hair—a second dose would kill! They're still getting in: putting dirt round the bath and fiddling with my food (it tastes funny). I've left Mario guarding things, but I need to get home in case they sneak in. I'm angry, not depressed and wouldn't let them make me suicidal. I wouldn't hurt them, but I'll keep doing V-signs and I'm going to dump *my* rubbish on *their* balcony—see how they like it!

*Other history*

- I'm not schizophrenic. Doctors say I am and drug me up so things won't bother me so much.
- They've sectioned me lots and I've been in and out of hospital since I was 20.
- I was in a hostel until I got my own flat two years ago. The ASBOs were bastards just after I moved in, but it got sorted out and they've been good 'til now.
- I take clozapine morning and night. *[If asked . . . ]* I haven't taken it for two months—it was making me fat and tired and I was always dribbling.
- My mum and dad met in a mental hospital after their breakdowns.
- Mario lives at my old hostel. He's getting his own flat soon and we'll move in together.
- I smoke 40 fags a day. I drink a couple of pints down the pub sometimes, but don't use drugs.
- I have high blood pressure and diabetes. I take medicines and go to the diabetic clinic.

*Questions*

Can you help me get them evicted?

*Worries*

I don't want to go back into hospital just because no-one believes me again.

## Candidate's instructions

You are a medical student on a general adult psychiatric ward. Mrs Banton is the mother of a patient you know well (David, 19 years). She has some questions about her son's diagnosis of schizophrenia and has asked to meet with you. David has given permission to speak to his mother, and his consultant is happy for you to do this.

Explain schizophrenia to Mrs Banton.

## Relative's instructions

### Key characteristics

* I feel confused and guilty about David's illness.

* I have a strong faith and become angry if this is dismissed.

* I understand medical ideas if explained well. I don't always agree with them.

We've all been so worried about David. He was always a good Christian boy, and never did drugs or got into trouble. Then a few weeks ago he told us demons were talking about him and calling him to Hell. He had to do what they said, cutting up his clothes and tearing pages out of books. He stopped eating because the demons had cursed his food and he said that he would be sinning if he ate it. He stopped washing and was very frightened by lots of things but could not tell us what was happening—he just used to say, 'It's not for you to know, Mum'. He said that his Dad had been replaced by a demon in disguise and attacked him with a chair. Since his admission, David has been taking a medicine beginning with O *[recognize the name if the student prompts olanzapine]*. At church we pray for David to be free of the demons and he is now nearly back to normal. My older brother was also demon-possessed and I can see similarities between him and David.

### Questions

The doctors say he has schizophrenia, but David doesn't have split personality. Is the diagnosis wrong?

What is schizophrenia? What causes it?

How is schizophrenia treated? How does the medicine work? Are there side effects?

He can't stay in hospital for ever. What will happen next?

Will David get better? Will he ever get back to college?

### Worries

This is my fault (either my sins are being punished or I have given him bad genes).

Maybe it goes against God's will for him to take tablets. Prayer should be enough.

---

 Guidelines for the information to be imparted are included with the Mark Sheet on the ORC.

The medical model is only one way of making sense of mental illness—religious (and other) beliefs are a different framework. A family may believe that demons are the problem but that their son is better with medication *and* prayer.

### BOX 9.6 Giving information

* Gain the patient's permission before speaking to their family.
* Check what is already known and what the person wants to know.
* Understand the relative's explanatory model (their views on cause, appropriate treatment, etc.).
* Use *chunking and checking* (Silverman *et al.* 2004): give a small chunk of information; then check it has been understood before proceeding to the next chunk.
* Pitch the information to the level of your audience and avoid medical jargon.
* Empathize and acknowledge relatives' feelings (guilt is common).
* Help retention by summarizing main points, offering written information and follow-up meetings.

# NEXT STEPS

## Seizures on clozapine

You are a junior doctor on a general medical team. Yesterday you admitted Mr Dennis O'Brien, a 42-year-old man, following two generalized tonic–clonic seizures. Dennis has no past medical history, though he has a diagnosis of paranoid schizophrenia and takes clozapine 250mg mane, 400mg nocte. His keyworker took him to hospital yesterday and explained that the clozapine was recently increased after Dennis' persecutory delusions had become more prominent following the death of his mother.

Dennis was diagnosed aged 21. His first admission followed an attack on a stranger in a café; he had been convinced that the man was controlling his movements by the way he used his cutlery. Dennis moved from forensic to rehabilitation services and currently lives in a 24-hour staffed hostel.

Since admission to the medical ward, Dennis has been quiet and shown no signs of aggression or resistance to his care and treatment. The staff nurse, Richard, calls you, requesting PRN antipsychotic medication for Dennis. Richard thinks that Dennis could become dangerous on the ward, since he has just complained that a female patient was trying to steal things from his bedside cabinet.

1. How would you handle this request for you to prescribe?
2. How will you continue to manage Dennis while he is under your care?

## Issues

- Risk assessment
- Assessment and management of current mental state and seizures

## Request for PRN medication

Your assessment will involve gathering information from the following people to help you decide what to do:

- **Ward nursing staff** Listen to the concerns of Richard and his colleagues, finding out what has been happening on the ward and *why* they think Dennis would benefit from additional antipsychotics. This will help to inform your risk assessment. Ask whether the other patient *might have* been interfering with Dennis's locker (it certainly happens!).

- **Community psychiatric team** Request that the team fax over a copy of Dennis's current care plan and last discharge summary to inform your management and risk assessment. Find out how Dennis usually presents, the reasons for increasing clozapine, and warning signs of relapse. If Dennis's persecutory delusions are chronic, they may have little effect on his behaviour, making his risk no greater than usual.

- **Dennis** Ask Dennis to explain the situation with the female patient. Perform a mental state examination, looking particularly for signs of psychosis or depression; remember that Dennis is at risk of relapse, secondary to bereavement or seizures. Review his physical examination and investigations so far.

Perform a risk assessment, looking at the risk to self and others. Table 9.4 will help you to think about current factors affecting the risk assessment

You need to consider whether the request for more medication is influenced by Dennis's current mental state and risk, or if it is based entirely on fears relating to his diagnosis of schizophrenia and past history of violence. If the latter, you should decrease fear and stigma by explaining schizophrenia and the logic of your risk assessment. Well-informed staff will be better able to alert you to any changes in the risk assessment, e.g. if Dennis appears intoxicated.

Should you decide that rapid tranquillization *is* required, be very clear about *what* medication you will prescribe, *when* it will be used, *why* you are prescribing, *how* it will be given safely, and *who* will monitor the effects and

**TABLE 9.4** Risk assessment

| Current factors | History |
|---|---|
| • Current mental state, e.g. command hallucinations, persecutory delusions, passivity | • History of self-harm and suicide attempts |
| • Stated intent/threats to harm someone | • History of violence to others |
| • Concerns expressed by family/carers | • Past psychiatric history |
| • Disengagement from services/non-concordance with medication | |
| • Drug and alcohol misuse | |
| • Weapon carrying | |
| • Social isolation | |
| • Homelessness | |

side effects. A short-acting oral benzodiazepine (e.g. lorazepam 1–2mg) would be safer than antipsychotics, which will lower Dennis's seizure threshold.

## Further management

This will require investigation of the seizures and liaison with a psychiatrist to ensure that treatment is optimized and risks minimized. The seizures may be due to the recent increase in clozapine, since it decreases the seizure threshold—it is usually recommended that anti-convulsants are given prophylactically at higher doses of clozapine. However, clozapine may have nothing to do with the seizures, so Dennis should receive a standard set of investigations. Good communication between the community team, Dennis, his family, and ward staff is essential in monitoring Dennis' health and risk.

➡ Remember that Dennis is on clozapine because basic antipsychotics are *not* effective for him; additional antipsychotics will cause additional side effects, without affecting treatment-resistant symptoms.

**Film list**
*Revolution #9* (2003)
*A Beautiful Mind* (2001)—NB: visual hallucinations are unusual in schizophrenia.
*K-PAX* (2001)—persistent delusional disorder or . . . ?
*Benny and Joon* (1993)

**Books**
Amis, M. (1987) *Insight at Flame Lake*. In: *Einstein's Monsters*. London: Vintage, 2003. Charts the relapse of schizophrenia in Dan; narrated through alternating diaries of Dan and his uncle, and takes a critical look at clinical and lay notions of insight.

Crawford, P. (2002) *Nothing Purple, Nothing Black*. Lewes: Book Guild, 2002. Beautiful novel exploring schizophrenia. Crystal is taken out of the asylum during the move to community care but is completely unable to cope. Relapse involves command hallucinations and sheer terror.

Diski, J. (1990) *Then Again*. London: Vintage, 1991. Early onset psychosis in the character of Katya. Her mother's struggle to accept and understand her illness is sensitively portrayed—a striking feature of this novel is the graphic but not sensationalized account of the vulnerability of psychotic individuals represented through Katya's rape and self-harm.

McGrath, P. (1990) *Spider*. London: Penguin, 2002. An accurate and compelling fictional description of schizophrenia. Includes olfactory and auditory hallucinations, and nihilistic delusions.

Perkins Gilman, C. (1892) *The Yellow Wallpaper*. New York: Dover Publications, 1997. Account of the historical use of 'rest cure' for mental illness. One of the key images throughout the book is the barred yellow wallpaper through which the narrator begins to claw, finally gaining freedom at the cost of complete psychosis—often used as a feminist text.

Schiller, L. and Bennett, A. (1994) *The Quiet Room: A Journey Out of the Torment of Madness*. New York: Warner, 1996. Autobiographical account of psychosis told from several perspectives—the patient, doctors, parents, brothers, friends—useful because of its examination of the impact of psychosis on the whole family and social network.

**Quotes**
Because something is happening here
But you don't know what it is
Do you, Mister Jones?
*Ballad of a Thin Man*—Bob Dylan

Could there be wires in the walls? I had contemplated often, with distressing inconclusiveness, that there might be no other earthly reason for their taking me to the toilet, as they did now and then, and leaving me there for hours, except for the purpose of spying on me in isolation.
**Paul Sayer, *Comforts of Madness***

I read the Bible every day
Trying to keep the demons at bay
Thank God when the sun goes down I don't blow away
***I Told Him That My Dog Wouldn't Run*—Patty Larkin**

## Notes

1. McGrath, P (1990) *Spider*. London: Penguin, 2002, p.30.
2. DSM-IV treats schizotypal disorder as a personality disorder; ICD-10 classifies it with schizophrenia and other psychoses.
3. ASBO = Anti Social Behaviour Order—a civil order in the UK to prevent people from behaving antisocially.

## References/Further reading

Andreason, S., Allebeck, P., Engstrom, A., and Rydberg, U. (1988) Cannabis and schizophrenia: a longitudinal study of Swedish conscripts. *Lancet*, **ii**, 1483–6.

Brekke, J.S., Prindle, C., Bae, S.W., and Long J.D. (2001) Risks for individuals with schizophrenia who are living in the community. *Psychiatric Services*, **52**, 1358–66.

Cantor-Graae, E. and Selten, J.-P. (2005) Schizophrenia and migration: a meta-analysis and review. *American Journal of Psychiatry*, **162**, 12–24.

Cardno, A., Marshak, J., Coid, B., *et al.* (1999) Relationships between symptom dimensions and genetic liability to psychotic disorders in the Maudsley Twin Psychosis Series. *Archives of General Psychiatry*, **56**, 162–8.

Caspi, A., Moffitt, T.E., Cannon, M., *et al.* (2005) Moderation of the effect of adolescent-onset cannabis use on adult psychosis by a functional polymorphism in the catechol-*O*-methyltransferase gene: longitudinal evidence of a gene × environment interaction. *Biological Psychiatry* **57**, 1117–27.

Cormac, I., Jones, C., and Campbell, C. (2002) Cognitive behaviour therapy for schizophrenia. *Cochrane Database of Systematic Reviews*, **1**, CD000524.

Fearon, P., Kirkbride, J.B., Morgan, C., *et al.* (2006) Incidence of schizophrenia and other psychoses in ethnic minority groups: results from the MRC AESOP Study. *Psychological Medicine*, **36**, 1541–50.

Frith, C.D. (1992) *The Cognitive Neuropsychology of Schizophrenia*. Hove: Erlbaum.

Haslam, J. (1988) *Illustrations of Madness* (Facsimile edition), Tavistock Classic Reprints in the History of Psychiatry. London: Routledge.

Heinrichs, R.W. and Zakzanis, K.K. (1998) Neurocognitive deficit in schizophrenia: a quantitative review of the evidence. *Neuropsychology*, **12**, 426–45.

Henquet, C., Murray, R., Linszen, D., and van Os, J. (2005) The environment and schizophrenia: the role of cannabis use. *Schizophrenia Bulletin*, **31**, 608–12.

Johnstone, E.C., Crow, T.J., and Frith, C.D. (1976) Cerebral ventricular size and cognitive impairment in chronic schizophrenia. *Lancet*, **ii**, 924–6.

Kane, J., Honigfeld, G., Singer, J., and Meltzer, H. (1998) Clozapine for the treatment-resistant schizophrenic. *Archives of General Psychiatry*, **45**, 789–96.

Kavanagh, D.J. (1992) Recent developments in expressed emotion and schizophrenia. *British Journal of Psychiatry*, **160**, 601–20.

Kopelowicz, A., Liberman, R.P., and Zarate, R. (2006) Recent advances in social skills training for schizophrenia. *Schizophrenia Bulletin*, **32** (Suppl 1), S12–23.

Leff, J. and Vaughn, C. (1981) The role of maintenance therapy and relatives' expressed emotion in relapse of schizophrenia: a two-year follow-up. *British Journal of Psychiatry*, **139**, 102–4.

Link, B.G., Stueve, A., and Phelan, J. (1998) Psychotic symptoms and violent behaviors: probing the components of 'threat/control-override' symptoms. *Social Psychiatry and Psychiatric Epidemiology*, **33**, S55–60.

McGorry, P.D. and Jackson, H.J. (1999) *The Recognition and Management of Early Psychosis: A Preventive Approach*. Cambridge University Press.

Meltzer, H.Y., Li, Z., Kaneda, Y., and Ichikawa, J. (2003) Serotonin receptors: their key role in drugs to treat schizophrenia. *Progress in Neuropsychopharmacological and Biological Psychiatry*, **27**, 1159–72.

NICE (2002) *Guidance on the Use of Newer (Atypical) Antipsychotic Drugs for the Treatment of Schizophrenia. Technology Appraisal No. 43*. London: National Institute for Clinical Excellence.

Pharoah, F., Mari, J., Rathbone, J., and Wong, W. (2006) Family intervention for schizophrenia *Cochrane Database of Systematic Reviews*, Issue 4.

Read, J., van Os, J., Morrison, A.P., *et al.* (2005) Childhood trauma, psychosis and schizophrenia: a literature review and clinical implications. *Acta Psychiatrica Scandinavica*, **112**, 330–50.

Silverman, J., Kurtz, S.M., and Draper, J. (2004) *Skills for Communicating with Patients* (2nd edn). Oxford: Radcliffe.

Tsuang, M., Stone, W.S., and Faraone, S.V. (2001) Genes, environment and schizophrenia. *British Journal of Psychiatry*, **178**, s18–24.

Tuominen, H.J., Tiihonen, J., and Wahlbeck, K. (2005) Glutamatergic drugs for schizophrenia: a systematic review and meta-analysis. *Schizophrenia Research*, **72**, 225–34.

van Haren, N.E., Bakker, S.C., and Kahn, R.S. (2008) Genes and structural brain imaging in schizophrenia. *Current Opinion in Psychiatry*, **21**, 161–7.

van Praag, H.M. (1977) The significance of dopamine for the mode of action of neuroleptics and the pathogenesis of schizophrenia. *British Journal of Psychiatry*, **130**, 463–74.

Weinberger, D.R. (1995) From neuropathology to neurodevelopment. *Lancet*, **346**, 552–7.

 Go to www.oxfordtextbooks/orc/stringer for an array of additional references, including indicative mark sheets for OSCEs, self-assessment questions, guidance, and exercises.

# 10 Substance misuse psychiatry

*Michelle Butterworth and Saman Saidi*

## True or False? Test your existing knowledge—answers in the chapter and online

1. Middle-aged men are the heaviest drinkers.

2. 75% of the predisposition to alcohol dependency is inherited.

3. The maximum safe daily alcohol intake for women is 2–3 units.

4. Alcohol is a CNS stimulant, inhibiting the GABA system.

5. Dual diagnosis refers to a drug misuse problem combined with alcohol dependency.

6. Snowballing is the use of crack with cocaine.

7. Synaesthesia is the experience of a sensation in another modality.

8. Hallucinogens are commonly smoked.

9. The CAGE screening questionnaire only relates to alcohol.

10. A 28 year old man becomes aggressive and acutely confused 72 hours after a drink-driving accident in which he suffered multiple fractures. Rapid tranquillisation with benzodiazepines is the first step in managing his aggressive behaviour.

## Contents

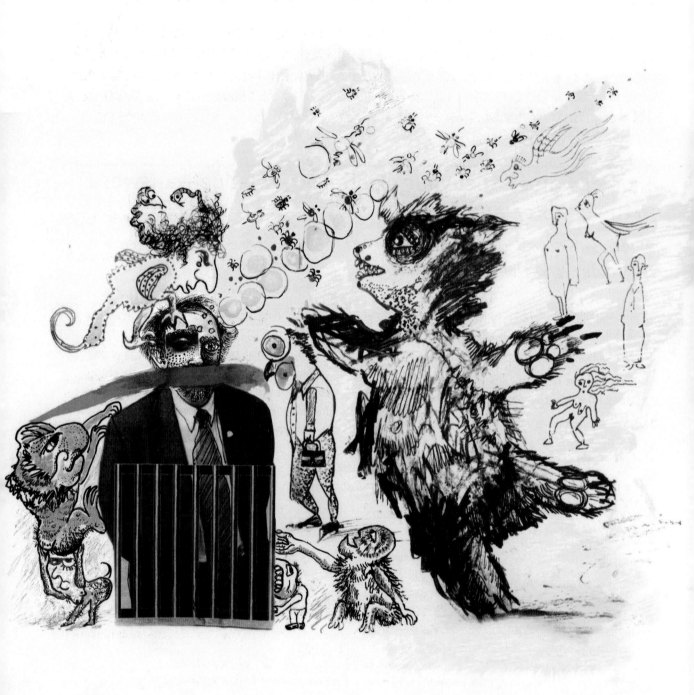

# PRINCIPLES

Sherlock Holmes took his bottle from the corner of the mantelpiece, and his hypodermic syringe from its neat morrocco case. With his long, white, nervous fingers he adjusted the delicate needle and rolled back his left shirtcuff. For some little time his eyes rested thoughtfully upon the sinewy forearm and wrist, all dotted and scarred with inumerable puncture marks. Finally he thrust the sharp point home, pressed down the tiny piston, and sank back into the velvet-lined armchair with a long sigh of satisfaction.

'Which is it today', I asked, 'morphine or cocaine?' . . .

'It is cocaine', he said, 'a seven percent solution, would you care to try it?'

*The Sign of Four*—Arthur Conan Doyle[1]

## Introduction

As is typical of 'sensation-seeking' personalities, Sherlock Holmes used drugs to alleviate boredom. Some people use drugs to 'treat' psychiatric symptoms, e.g. using cannabis to reduce anxiety. Others use drugs because of peer pressure or ease of availability. Whatever the reason, some people reach a point where they feel unable to function or feel 'normal' without drugs.

## Overview of substance misuse

Substance misuse describes a pattern of substance use causing physical, mental, social, or occupational dysfunction. This can be divided into the following categories:

- **Intoxication** is a transient state of emotional and behavioural change following drug use. It is dose dependent and time limited.
- **Harmful use** is a pattern of use likely to cause physical or psychological damage.
- **Dependency** denotes 'a cluster of physiological, behavioural and cognitive symptoms in which the use of a substance takes on a much higher priority than other behaviours that once had greater value' (ICD-10) (see Table 10.1).
- **Withdrawal** is a transient state occurring while readjusting to lower levels of the drug in the body.

## Epidemiology

Young males (late teens to early twenties) are the heaviest drinkers, though alcohol misuse has increased in women over the past decade. The male-to-female ratios are:

- 2:1 for alcohol disorders
- 4:1 for substance misuse disorders (Crome 1997).

Prevalence rates are shown in Table 10.2. Substance misuse is highly comorbid with mental illness.

Binge drinking in males and females is becoming a recognized phenomenon, distinct from alcohol addiction. *Recreational* drug use is increasingly common and, while risky, may not constitute a disorder.

## Main theories of dependence

### Learning theories

#### Classical (Pavlovian) conditioning

Pavlov's famous experiment showed that by presenting the natural stimulus for salivation (food) together with the sound of a bell, dogs are conditioned to salivate to the bell alone. In substance misuse, cravings become conditioned to 'cues' (e.g. needles for heroin users), so the cue itself can trigger craving, causing drug-seeking behaviour.

#### Operant (Skinnerian) conditioning

- Operant conditioning depends on repetitive behaviours having predictable outcomes.
- Behaviours that are rewarded are repeated (positive reinforcement). For example:
  - A rat will keep pressing a lever that supplies food.
  - A drug providing pleasure will be used again.
- Behaviours are also repeated if they relieve unpleasant experiences (negative reinforcement). For example:

**TABLE 10.1** Features of dependency

| Dependency feature | Explanation | Example |
|---|---|---|
| Tolerance | Larger doses required to gain the same effect as previously. | An opiate-dependent person may easily inject enough heroin to kill a non-tolerant person |
| Compulsion | Strong desire to use the substance. | *Craving* the next cigarette. |
| Withdrawal | Physiological withdrawal state when the substance is stopped/decreased, seen by: (a) The characteristic withdrawal syndrome for the substance, *or* (b) Substance use to prevent or relieve withdrawal symptoms | (a) Alcohol withdrawal fits (b) Early morning drinking |
| Problems controlling use | Difficulties controlling starting, stopping, or amounts used | It becomes hard to say *No* |
| Continued use despite harm | Despite clear problems caused by the substance, the person can't stop using | Injecting heroin despite developing abscesses |
| Salience (primacy) | Obtaining and using the substance becomes so important that other interests are neglected | Not eating because the money is needed for cocaine |
| Reinstatement after abstinence | Tendency to return to the previous pattern and level of use after a period of abstinence | Someone who stops smoking for a year may return quickly to their previous 20/day habit after smoking one cigarette |
| Narrowing of the repertoire | Loss of variation in use of the substance | A dependent drinker drinks the same amount of the same drink in the same way every day |

**TABLE 10.2** Prevalence of substance misuse

| Disorder | 12 month prevalence[a] | Lifetime prevalence[b] |
|---|---|---|
| Alcohol dependence | 1.3% | 5.4% |
| Drug dependence | 0.4% | 3.0% |
| Any substance misuse disorder | 3.8% | 14.6% |

[a]Kessler *et al.* 2005b
[b]Kessler *et al.* 2005a

– A rat will keep pressing a lever that ends an electric shock.

– A drug will be used again if it relieves unpleasant feelings, either by ending withdrawal or by providing a temporary escape from painful consciousness.

### Social learning theory (vicarious learning)

We learn by copying the behaviours of others; substance misuse can result from peer pressure.

**Some American soldiers became dependent on heroin during the Vietnam War. On returning to the USA, many gave up heroin almost effortlessly—the loss of cues removed much of the withdrawal phenomena (Robins 1993).**

## Neurobiological models

All drugs of abuse affect the dopaminergic 'reward' pathway in the brain. This pathway starts in the ventral tegmental area and projects onto the prefrontal cortex and limbic system (the 'emotional' brain).

- The prefrontal cortex has a role in motivation and planning.
- Dopamine release in the nucleus accumbens is central to the sensation of pleasure, which is important in reward.

Cocaine and amphetamine block dopamine reuptake, increasing synaptic dopamine levels, and causing a pleasurable sensation. Alcohol and opiates also increase dopamine and affect other neurotransmitters.

## Alcohol

### Aetiology

#### Genetics

Twin studies suggest that 25–50% of the predisposition to alcohol dependence is inherited. This is supported by adoption studies, which show that adopted-out sons of alcohol-dependent fathers have a fourfold increased risk of alcohol dependence.

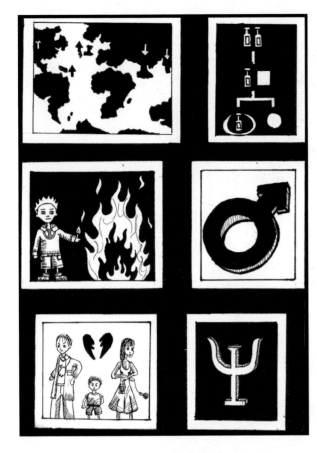

FIGURE 10.1  Risk factors for alcohol misuse

Ethanol is metabolized to acetaldehyde, which is then broken down by aldehyde dehydrogenase. In East Asian populations, a less effective variant enzyme occurs. Acetaldehyde accumulates, causing flushing, palpitations, and nausea (the 'flush reaction'). This probably contributes to the lower rates of alcohol dependency among East Asians.

## Occupation

Alcohol misuse is associated with certain occupations, e.g. publicans, journalists, doctors, the armed forces, and the entertainment industry. Stressful work and socially sanctioned drinking combine to increase risk.

## Social background

There is often a history of a difficult childhood, with parental separation. Educational achievement is com-

monly poor and there may be evidence of juvenile delinquency.

### Psychiatric illness

Substance misuse is associated with personality disorders, mania, depression, and anxiety disorders (particularly social phobia).

 **If you and your patient swapped the first 10 years of your lives, would you still be the medic?**

## Clinical presentation

### Intoxication

Alcohol causes relaxation and euphoria, though at higher levels people may become irritable, aggressive, weepy, morose, and disinhibited. Impulsivity and poor judgement can make people take risks and behave irresponsibly. Speech becomes slurred, the gait ataxic, and there may be increasing sedation, confusion, and even coma.

### Withdrawal

As alcohol levels fall, withdrawal symptoms occur. Headache, nausea, retching and vomiting, tremor, and sweating are all typical. Insomnia is often problematic and

**TABLE 10.3**  Levels of alcohol consumption

| | Safe levels | | Harmful levels | |
|---|---|---|---|---|
| | Units/day | Units/week | Units/day 'binge drinking' | Units/week |
| Women | 2–3 | 14 | >6 | >35 |
| Men | 3–4 | 21 | >8 | >50 |

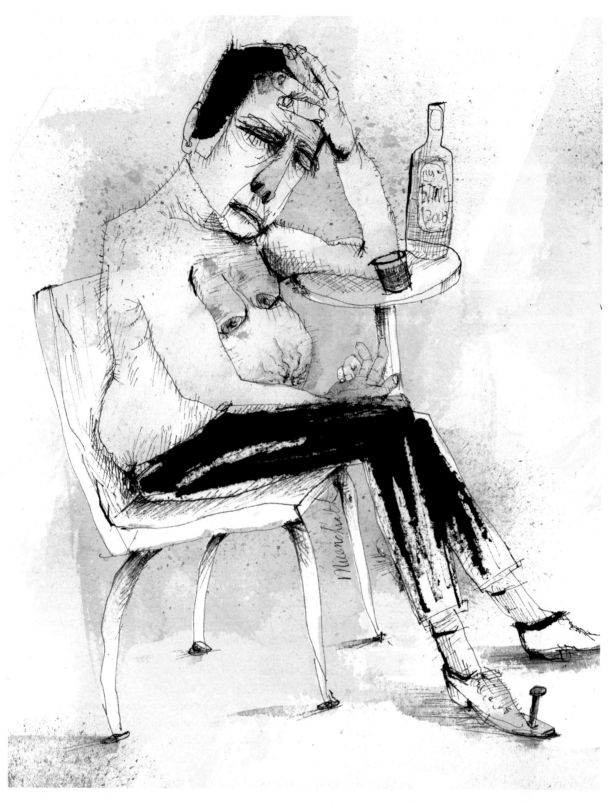

FIGURE 10.2 Can you identify seven clinical signs of alcohol abuse suggested in this drawing? Some signs are indicative of chronic misuse

it may take weeks to regain a normal sleep pattern. Other signs are anxiety, agitation, tachycardia, and hypotension. Alcohol is a CNS depressant, stimulating the GABA inhibitory system to reduce brain excitability. When dependent drinkers suddenly stop drinking, neural pathways become hyper-excitable and seizures can occur. Very severe cases risk delirium tremens (Box 10.2) or even death.

 Don't advise alcohol-dependent people to suddenly *stop* drinking. It is well-meaning but potentially fatal advice.

---

### BOX 10.2 Delirium tremens—a medical emergency

- Onset: ~48 hours into abstinence.
- Duration: 3–4 days.
- Symptoms:
  - confusion
  - hallucinations, especially visual, e.g. animals and people
  - affective changes; extreme fear and hilarity may alternate
  - gross tremor, especially of hands
  - autonomic disturbance: sweating, tachycardia, hypertension, dilated pupils, fever
  - delusions.
- Mortality rate is 5% but rises to 30% if complications occur, e.g. sepsis.
- Urgent medical treatment involves a reducing benzodiazepine regime and parenteral thiamine. Manage potentially fatal dehydration and electrolyte abnormalities.

---

## Complications

### Physical

- **Liver:** alcoholic hepatitis usually occurs after a period of increased intake. Symptoms include malaise, hepatomegaly, and ascites. Liver cirrhosis develops in 10–20% of alcohol-dependent people and complications include ascites and hepatic encephalopathy.
- **Gastrointestinal:** pancreatitis, oesophageal varices, gastritis, and peptic ulceration.
- **Neurological:** peripheral neuropathy, seizures, and dementia.
- **Cancers:** bowel, breast, oesophageal, and liver.
- **Cardiovascular:** hypertension and cardiomyopathy.
- **Head injuries/accidents** while intoxicated; increased risk of subdural haematoma.
- **Fetal alcohol syndrome** (see p.203) affects babies born to mothers who drink during pregnancy.

### Psychological

- **Depression, anxiety, self-harm, and suicide** are increased.
- **Amnesia** (blackouts) due to intoxication.

- **Cognitive impairment** may occur, as either alcoholic dementia or Korsakoff's syndrome (Box 10.3).
- **Alcoholic hallucinosis** is the experience of auditory hallucinations in clear consciousness while drinking alcohol. Hallucinations often have a persecutory or derogatory content.
- **Morbid jealousy** is the overvalued idea or delusion that a partner is unfaithful. It is associated with alcohol dependency, impotence, and violence.

---

### BOX 10.3 Wernicke–Korsakoff syndrome

**Wernicke's encephalopathy**

- Caused by acute thiamine (vitamin B$_1$) deficiency.
- Presents classically with the triad of confusion, ataxia, and ophthalmoplegia.
- A medical emergency! Untreated with parenteral thiamine, it may progress to . . .

**Korsakoff's syndrome (see p.123)**

- This consists of *irreversible* anterograde amnesia (and some retrograde amnesia).
- The patient can register new events, but cannot recall them within a few minutes.
- Patients may confabulate to fill the gaps in their memory.

---

### Social

Alcohol misuse can become a vicious circle: social problems precede alcoholism and are then created and perpetuated by continued misuse. Problems include unemployment, poor attendance and performance at work, domestic violence, separation, and divorce. Law-breaking may occur while intoxicated or, more rarely, to fund addiction, e.g. drink-driving, assault, theft. Children are at increased risk of neglect, abuse, and conduct disorder (see p.215).

## Differential diagnosis

This applies for both alcohol *and* drugs. Substance misuse may coexist with, mask, or be mistaken for other physical and psychiatric illnesses. A substance misuse disorder is more likely if there is a clear temporal relationship between substance use and presentation.

1. **Organic:** when assessing an intoxicated patient, don't assume that confusion, ataxia, or psychotic symptoms are solely due to substance misuse; there may be another physical cause. Be particularly aware of the risk of head injury and subdural haematoma from falls.
2. **Psychiatric illness:** this may be the primary problem or a comorbid problem. Someone with a severe substance misuse problem *and* a severe mental illness is

said to have a *dual diagnosis*. Consider the following in your differential:

- depression/mania
- functional psychosis
- anxiety disorder
- personality disorder.

 **Suicide attempts often include alcohol or drug use. Is your patient suicidal?**

---

**BOX 10.4** Tips for distinguishing substance misuse from psychiatric problems

..........................................................................

- Which problem came first?
- Do the psychiatric symptoms 'fit' with known symptoms of *that* substance?
- Have psychiatric symptoms continued when abstinent?
- Is there a family history or previous diagnosis of the psychiatric illness?

---

## Investigations

1. FBC
   - Alcohol causes a macrocytic anaemia (raised MCV) due to $B_{12}$ deficiency.
2. LFTs
   - γGT rises with recent heavy alcohol use.
   - Raised transaminases suggest hepatocellular damage.
3. Additional investigations are guided by the clinical presentation, e.g. an ECG for chest pain, a urine drug screen (UDS) if you suspect drug misuse, hepatitis screening if intravenous (IV) drug use.

**The AUDIT (Alcohol Use Disorders Identification Test) is a screening tool developed by the WHO (Babor *et al.* 2001). It can help identify alcohol misuse, but does not replace a thorough history.**

## Management

### Assessment and preparation

**Motivation to change**

Readiness and motivation to change are assessed, since they are all-important factors in stopping drinking. The *Stages of Change model* (Prochaska and DiClemente 1982) explains this concept as a stepwise process from carefree, problematic, drinking to maintained abstinence.

- *Pre-contemplation*: the person doesn't see a problem or want to change. They may be in denial, or unaware of the risks.
   - 'Alcoholics are old men, not young women like me!'

- *Contemplation*: the person recognizes the problem but doesn't want to change yet. They may become 'stuck' at this stage due to ambivalence, but it's a good time to work with them because of openness to discussing the pros and cons of change.
   - 'I should cut down, but not today . . . I like drinking too much.'
- *Preparation*: the person is willing to change, planning to do this soon.
   - 'I got the number for Alcoholics Anonymous. I'll stop after my birthday.'
- *Action*: change becomes a reality—the person is actively cutting down or has stopped drinking.
   - 'I'll have a lemonade, please . . .'
- *Maintenance*: the person is able to remain abstinent (or keep to their agreed low level of use). It is often the hardest part: giving up alcohol for a day is easy, lifelong abstinence is not!
   - 'I really crave a beer some nights, but if I distract myself, the feeling passes.'
- *Relapse* is a common problem and part of the overall learning process, rather than a sign of failure. Understanding the triggers for relapse aids the next attempt at abstinence.
   - 'I thought I could have *one* drink, but it led to a binge. I'm a failure!'

Although the Stages of Change model has been applied to many things (e.g. obesity, smoking, safe sex), it is neither perfect nor the whole story (e.g. many smokers stop smoking on a whim and never relapse). Nevertheless, it can help by identifying the kind of support needed, setting realistic goals and meeting the expectations of both therapist and patient. For example, goals might be:

- short term = reduce alcohol consumption
- medium term = undergo detoxification
- long-term = attend college.

**Motivational interviewing** (MI) is a form of counselling which aims to empower the person to change. It works by helping them to recognize the gap between where they are *now* and where they *want* to be, and is based on a supportive but challenging therapeutic relationship.

### Detoxification

Detoxification ('detox') allows metabolism and excretion of the substance while minimizing discomfort. Alcohol detoxification may be *planned*, following a period of preparation, or *unplanned*, e.g. after emergency admission to hospital. Either way, help is needed.

- **Long-acting benzodiazepines** (e.g. chlordiazepoxide) replace alcohol and prevent withdrawal symptoms, including seizures and delirium tremens. They are gradually withdrawn and stopped.
- **Thiamine** (vitamin $B_1$) is prescribed as prophylaxis against Wernicke's encephalopathy. It is best given parenterally (IM or IV) since it is poorly absorbed in the gut.

Community (home) detoxification is used in uncomplicated dependency, using a fixed dosage-reducing regime of benzodiazepines over 5–7 days. Inpatient detoxification is used if there is a history of withdrawal fits, comorbid medical or psychiatric illness, or if the patient lacks someone at home to support and observe them. A symptoms-led assessment is used, where medication is given according to observed withdrawal symptoms. After 24 hours the total dosage given is calculated, guiding the reducing regime prescribed.

### Relapse prevention

- **Psychological** Cognitive behavioural and problem-solving therapies identify causes of use, finding ways to prevent relapse. Group therapy allows experiences and solutions to be shared.
- **Medical** Acamprosate is an anti-craving drug, thought to act in the midbrain. Disulfiram (Antabuse) mimics the 'flush reaction' to alcohol, making drinking highly unpleasant!

### Rehabilitation

Whether as a residential or day programme, the aim is to initiate a complete restructuring of the person's life. Residential (living on-site) options offer a clean break for those whose lives have become submerged in the drinking community and who have few non-drinking contacts. Structured groups focus on aspects of abstinence such as relapse prevention, and there may be skills-based groups (e.g. IT training) or help to access training courses or find employment.

Organizations like Alcoholics Anonymous (AA) can provide essential additional counselling, support, and health information.

## Drugs

### Aetiology

Drug misuse shares many of the social risk factors of alcohol misuse. It also has a genetic element, possibly mediated through risk-taking or self-medication of anxious personality traits.

---

**BOX 10.5** Urine drug screen (UDS)

Although not 100% sensitive, a UDS can detect the presence of drugs for some days after last use:

- Amphetamine   2 days
- Heroin   2 days
- Cocaine   5–7 days
- Methadone   7 days
- Cannabis   Up to 1 month

---

## Opiates

Heroin (diamorphine, *brown, smack, horse, gear, H*) is the most notorious opiate. Others include morphine, pethidine, codeine, and dihydrocodeine (*DF118*). Heroin is a µ (mu) opiate agonist, stimulating brain and spinal cord receptors that are normally acted upon by endogenous endorphins (the body's natural painkillers).

Initially, heroin is usually smoked (*chasing*), but as tolerance builds, people often progress to intravenous (IV) injection. The antecubital fossa is usually the first site used, but with repeated injection the veins become damaged and other sites may be used, e.g. feet, backs of hands, groin. If venous access is difficult, people may inject subcutaneously (SC) (*skin popping*) or intramuscularly (IM). The complications of injecting drug use are summarized in Table 10.4. Pure heroin can be snorted; tablets like dihydrocodeine and codeine are swallowed.

**TABLE 10.4** Complications of IV drug use

| Local complications | Systemic complications |
| --- | --- |
| **Abscess** Injected particles form a nidus of infection under the skin | **Septicaemia** Either from direct injection of bacteria or spread from abscesses or cellulitis |
| **Cellulitis** | **Infective endocarditis** Injected organisms settle on the mitral valve |
| **DVT** Repeated injection into the femoral veins damages the valves, slowing venous return and facilitating blood clotting in the legs | **Blood-borne infections** Hepatitis B & C, HIV, and even syphilis can be transmitted |
| **Emboli** These may cause gangrene, requiring amputation | **Increased risk of overdose** There is less dose-titration than in smoking |

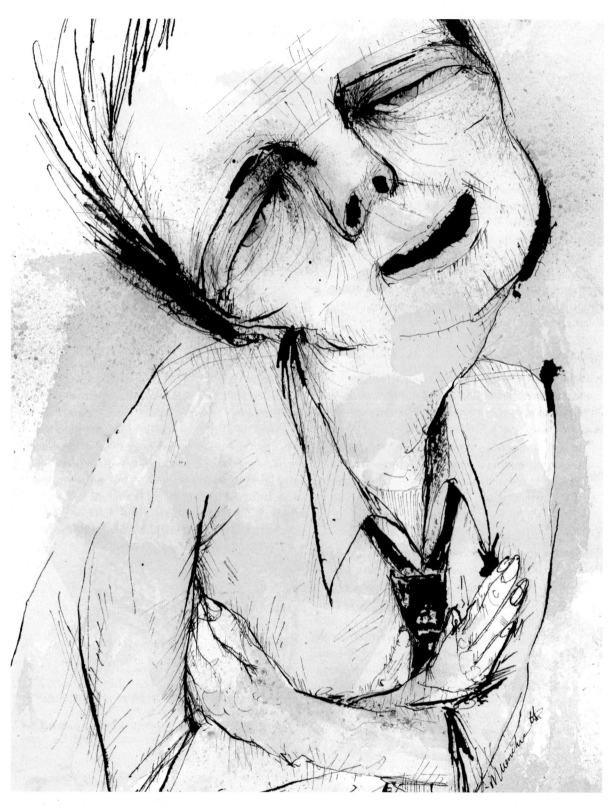

FIGURE 10.3 How does this fit with your view of a 'typical' opiate user?

**BOX 10.6** How heroin is injected

- Heroin is mixed and heated with water, liquefying it for injection.
- A *spoon* (a small container, e.g. bottle cap, actual spoon) is used for the mixing and heating.
- A *cotton* (filter made from a cigarette filter, bit of cotton or lint) is placed in the spoon.
- The heroin is drawn up into the syringe through the cotton, filtering out solid particles that could clog the needle. The heroin is then injected.

Traces of blood can be transferred in needles, cottons, spoons, and the water used for mixing heroin and rinsing used syringes. Sharing *any of these* risks blood-borne infections.

## Clinical presentation

### Intoxication

IV heroin use produces an intense *rush* or *buzz*, with feelings of euphoria, warmth, and well-being. Sedation and analgesia follow, and some people vomit or become dizzy (especially the first time). Bradycardia and respiratory depression occur, and people can die from respiratory failure or aspiration of vomit in overdose. 'Pinpoint' (constricted) pupils are a classic sign of opiate intoxication. Non-IV use results in milder effects. Constipation, anorexia, and decreased libido are side effects.

Naloxone is an opiate antagonist and the antidote for opiate overdose. Beware! After being given naloxone, patients are plunged into immediate withdrawal and will be very distressed.

### Withdrawal

Withdrawal following IV heroin use typically begins around 6 hours after injection; peaking at 36–48 hours. It is extremely unpleasant but rarely life-threatening. Dysphoria, nausea, insomnia, and agitation occur. As the effects on opiate receptors are reversed, everything 'runs' (diarrhoea, vomiting, lacrimation, and rhinorrhoea); the person feels feverish with abdominal cramps and aching joints and muscles. Piloerection causes gooseflesh (hence *going cold turkey* or *clucking*). Patients yawn irresistibly and their pupils dilate.

Funding a habit is expensive and may require theft, fraud, or sex-working.

## Management

The principles outlined in alcohol misuse management apply to opiates and other drugs. *Harm reduction* is another key idea.

**BOX 10.7** Neonatal abstinence syndrome

- Babies born to opiate-dependent mothers suffer withdrawal symptoms.
- Symptoms start within hours of birth and may last several weeks. They include:
  - high-pitched cry
  - restlessness
  - tremor
  - hypertonia, convulsions
  - loose stools, vomiting
  - sweats, fever
  - tachypnoea.
- Treatment involves paediatric opiate preparations, anticonvulsants and supportive measures.
- Opiates also cause intra-uterine growth retardation, low birth weight, and prematurity; sudden infant death syndrome (SIDS) is increased.

### Harm reduction

This is a pragmatic approach to drug use, assessing and minimizing risk, rather than insisting on abstinence. Information and advice on improving the safety of drug use are essential. Intravenous use can be made safer by providing sterile needles via needle exchanges. Additionally, injecting drug users and sex-workers can be offered vaccination and testing for blood-borne viruses, free condoms, and accessible sexual health services.

### Substitute prescribing

Substitute prescribing is 'the deliberate prescribing of drugs in a controlled manner' to 'reduce the use of illicit drugs' or the harm associated with them (Matheson *et al.* 1999). Methadone (liquid) and buprenorphine (sublingual tablet) are oral preparations that replace injectable opiates. Initially taken in a supervised environment, doses are gradually titrated until the patient does not experience withdrawal symptoms. Methadone is a full agonist at opiate receptors with a longer half-life than heroin (so withdrawal is longer but milder). Buprenorphine is a partial agonist at the μ receptor, blocking the euphoric effects of heroin whilst preventing withdrawal symptoms.

Prescribing opiates without reasonable evidence that your patient is a regular opiate user can expose you to allegations of drug dealing! Get a UDS first.

Ideally, the person is slowly weaned off the methadone or buprenorphine over weeks or months. Detoxification may be helped by adjunctive medications such as antidiarrhoeals (loperamide), anti-emetics (metoclopramide)

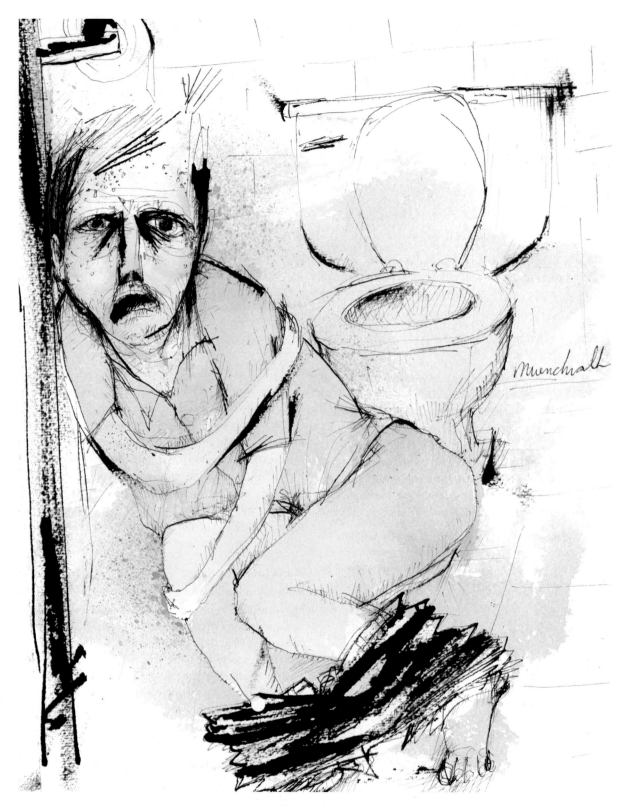

**FIGURE 10.4** A visual mnemonic for the experience of opiate withdrawal. What physical signs of withdrawal can you see? How do you think this person feels?

and non-opiate painkillers. Although complete abstinence is the ultimate goal, it is not always realistic. Some people thrive on substitute prescribing regimes but deteriorate when detoxification is commenced. For these patients, long-term methadone *maintenance* can reduce harm by enabling them to gain stability, e.g. maintain employment.

Naltrexone is an opiate antagonist that blocks opiate receptors and thus the euphoric effects of opiates. It can be given to people who have completed an opiate detoxification as a relapse prevention agent.

## Cannabis

Cannabis is made from the *Cannabis sativa* plant. Different parts of the plant provide different types and varying strengths of the psychoactive compound, delta-9-tetrahydrocannabinol (THC). THC acts on cannabinoid receptors in the brain.

---

**BOX 10.8** Cannabis terminology

..................................................................

- *Blow*, *dope*, *draw*, *ganja*, *hemp*, *marijuana*, *pot*, *wacky-backy*.
- *Grass/weed*: made from dried cannabis leaves, it resembles tightly packed dried herbs.
- *Hash/hashish*: a squidgy, brown-black lump made from the resin and flowers.
- *Skunk* and *sinsemilla* are particularly strong types.

---

Cannabis is usually smoked with tobacco as *spliffs* or *joints*, or smoked in a water pipe (*bong*). It can be eaten in cakes or biscuits, or drunk as a tea. The effects depend greatly on expectation and the original mood state, which tends to be enhanced by the drug. Responses range from relaxation and euphoria to paranoia, anxiety, and panic. Perceptual distortion can occur: time slows down and aesthetic appreciation is enhanced. Hunger pangs (*munchies*) are common and people often seek sweet foods. Nausea and vomiting (*greening*) can occur, especially when used with alcohol. Coordination is affected: users shouldn't drive. Injected conjunctivae (bloodshot eyes), tachycardia, and dry mouth occur. Restlessness and irritability are common after use, although there is no specific physiological withdrawal syndrome.

Early heavy use is particularly likely to precipitate psychosis, potentially leading to schizophrenia in vulnerable people (see p.73). Lethargy and poor motivation are recognized features of chronic heavy use. Smoking aggravates asthma and risks lung disease and cancer.

## Stimulants

Stimulants potentiate the effects of neurotransmitters (dopamine, noradrenaline, sometimes serotonin), increasing energy, alertness, and euphoria, while decreasing the need for sleep. They increase confidence and impulsivity, while impairing judgement—causing risky behaviour. Side effects include cardiac arrhythmias, hypertension, and stroke. Anxiety, panic, and drug-induced psychosis can occur There is often an unpleasant *crash* (period of dysphoria and lethargy) after the substance wears off.

Harm reduction is the main principle of treatment, although short-term benzodiazepines may be offered in an inpatient setting to help with withdrawal anxiety.

### Cocaine (Charlie, coke, snow)

Cocaine hydrochloride is a white powder, usually arranged in lines and sniffed up using a rolled-up bank note (*snorted*). It can also be dissolved and injected.

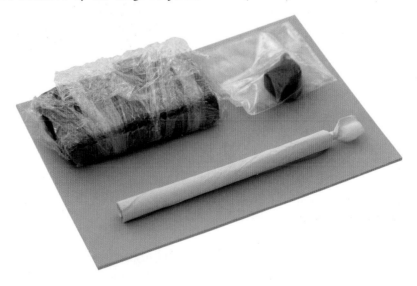

FIGURE 10.5 Cannabis resin. Photo courtesy of Oli Butterworth.

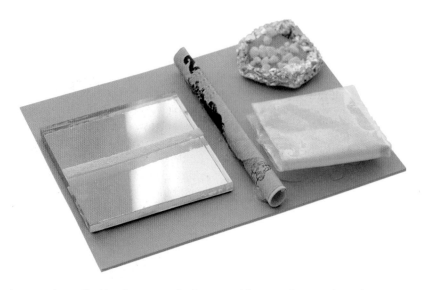

FIGURE 10.6 Cocaine powder, rolled bank note, and mirror used for snorting cocaine. Photo courtesy of Oli Butterworth.

 Cocaine users may experience formication (the sensation of insects crawling on or below the skin), also known as *cocaine bugs*.

 Cocaine is a powerful vasoconstrictor and snorting it damages the nasal mucosa, causing necrosis and septal perforation. Sharing 'snorting equipment' can spread blood-borne infections.

### Crack cocaine (rocks, base, freebase)

Crack is a concentrated smokeable form of cocaine made by heating cocaine in a baking soda solution until the water evaporates, leaving *rocks* of crack which are heated and smoked. Smoking crack produces an almost immediate and extremely intense high, likened to a *whole-body orgasm*. Whereas the high from snorting cocaine may last up to half an hour, smoking crack may only last 5–10 minutes. This on–off effect makes crack highly addictive, leaving users desperate for more.

 The name *crack* comes from the cracking noise made as rocks are heated and smoked.

 *Speedballing/snowballing* is the use of crack with heroin, to produce a bigger rush.

### Amphetamine (speed)

Formed of white powder or tablets, amphetamines can be dissolved and injected; swallowed, or snorted. Some specialist teams use dexamphetamine as a replacement for IV amphetamine dependency, aiming for stabilization and detoxification.

### Khat (quat, chat)

Khat is a mild stimulant, popular in East African communities. It comes as chewable leaves and can cause florid psychosis.

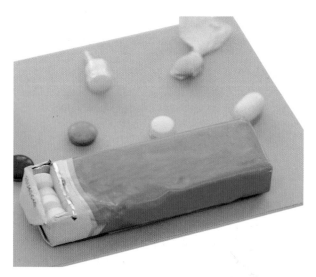

FIGURE 10.7 Ecstasy disguised as sweets. Photo courtesy of Oli Butterworth.

### Ecstasy (3,4-methylenedioxymethamphetamine, E, MDMA)

Ecstasy's chemical structure and action—of serotonin release and reuptake inhibition—make it a cross between a stimulant and a hallucinogen (although hallucinations are rare). Usually taken as a tablet, it can be a white powder; use is usually confined to weekends. As well as stimulant effects, it causes a sense of empathy and closeness to others. Users become very chatty, dance relentlessly, and can show bruxism (tooth-grinding). There may be side effects of nausea, vomiting, and sweating. Death is associated with hyperthermia and dehydration.

## Hallucinogens

Drugs in this group cause visual illusions and hallucinations. Synaesthesia may occur, i.e. the experience of a

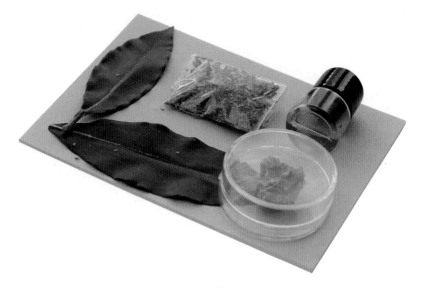

FIGURE 10.8  Khat. Photo courtesy of Oli Butterworth.

sensation in another modality (e.g. hearing a smell). Depersonalization and derealization are fairly common and people sometimes become acutely anxious. *Behavioural toxicity* is the accidental harm that occurs when people act on drug-induced beliefs, e.g. being able to fly.

### LSD (lysergic acid diethylamide, acid)

LSD affects dopamine and serotonin transmitter systems. It is usually impregnated on *tabs* (tiny squares of paper with pictures on them), and ingestion causes *trips* of up to 12 hours' duration, with perceptual changes and euphoria. *Bad trips* are when the experiences become frightening and unpleasant, and sudden *flashbacks* can occur, even years later. Other risks include anxiety, depression, and psychosis.

### Phenylcyclidine (PCP, angel dust)

Phenylcyclidine is becoming increasingly popular. It comes as a liquid or powder that can be snorted or added to a *joint* and smoked, and is associated with violent outbursts and ongoing psychosis.

### Ketamine (Special K)

Ketamine is a powerful veterinary anaesthetic; it prevents the brain's awareness of pain. Because of anaesthesia, people have severely harmed themselves while hallucinating, e.g. pulling out their own teeth.

### Magic mushrooms

Magic mushrooms (e.g. the liberty cap) are eaten or drunk. The greatest risk is of mistakenly eating poisonous mushrooms.

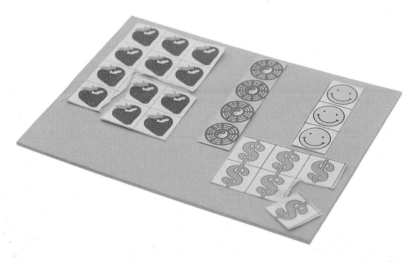

FIGURE 10.9  LSD. Photo courtesy of Oli Butterworth.

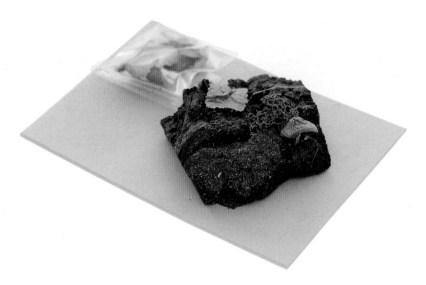

FIGURE 10.10  Magic mushrooms. Photo courtesy of Oli Butterworth.

## Sedatives

Benzodiazepines (*downers, sleepers*) have a sedative effect because they enhance the inhibitory effect of GABA transmission. They are usually swallowed as tablets, but can be dissolved and used IV. Their effects are similar to alcohol, causing a feeling of calm and mild euphoria, with slurred speech, ataxia, and stupor (or even coma) at higher doses. Withdrawal effects are similar to alcohol, e.g. seizures.

Benzodiazepine overdose can be treated with flumazenil, which is a benzodiazepine antagonist.

Barbiturates are rarely seen now. They are more dangerous than benzodiazepines, causing cardiovascular and respiratory collapse.

## Solvents (gases, glue, aerosols)

Solvent abuse is mostly confined to teenagers, who sniff them from an impregnated cloth or sleeve. Gases can be squirted directly into the back of the throat, which may cause swelling and asphyxiation. Solvents can also be sprayed into a plastic bag and placed *over* the head to inhale from within, risking suffocation. Telltale signs are blistering and redness around the mouth and nose. The effects are a little like being drunk, with euphoria, disinhibition, ataxia, nausea, vomiting, and dizziness. Thinking becomes muddled and some people hallucinate. Coma can occur and result in death if vomit is aspirated. A *hangover* can occur afterwards with severe headaches and fatigue.

## Prognosis

Drug and alcohol disorders tend to follow a relapsing and remitting course; people often relapse several times before eventually becoming abstinent. Intravenous drug use, chaotic use, and polydrug use are poor prognostic factors. Abstinence from alcohol is associated with a better outcome than so-called 'controlled drinking' (drinking within healthy limits), which is very difficult to sustain once dependency has developed (Orford and Keddie 1986).

The loss of judgement and increased impulsivity due to intoxication with drugs or alcohol should be taken into consideration when assessing risk of harm to self or others. A few drinks could be the deciding factor in somebody who has been contemplating suicide in the context of a depressive episode.

**TABLE 10.5** Summary of psychoactive drugs

| Drug | Route of administration | Intoxication | Withdrawal |
|------|------------------------|--------------|------------|
| Opiates:<br>  Heroin<br>  Dihydrocodeine<br>  Morphine<br>  Pethidine<br>  Codeine | Smoked<br>IV<br>IM<br>SC<br>Snorted<br>Oral | Euphoria<br>Sedation<br>Analgesia<br>Pinpoint pupils<br>Respiratory depression<br>Bradycardia<br>Death | Everything 'runs':<br>  Diarrhoea<br>  Vomiting<br>  Lacrimation<br>  Rhinorrhoea<br>Dysphoria<br>Nausea<br>Cramps, aches<br>Fever, sweats<br>Insomnia and agitation<br>Yawning<br>Pilo-erection (goose-flesh)<br>Dilated pupils |
| Cannabis | Smoked<br>Eaten<br>Drunk | Relaxation<br>Euphoria<br>Paranoia<br>Anxiety<br>Hunger<br>Perceptual changes | No specific physiological withdrawal syndrome, but agitation and irritability common |
| Stimulants:<br>  Cocaine<br>  Crack<br>  Amphetamine | Snorted<br>Swallowed<br>Smoked | Energy<br>Euphoria<br>Diminished need for sleep<br>Anorexia | 'Crash': depression, lethargy |
| Hallucinogens:<br>  LSD<br>  Magic mushrooms<br>  Ketamine | Swallowed | Visual distortions<br>Hallucinations<br>Synaesthesia | Nil |
| Ecstasy | Swallowed | Stimulant effects with empathic feelings | Lethargy |
| Sedatives:<br>  Benzodiazepines<br>  Barbiturates | Swallowed | Sedation<br>Slurred speech, ataxia<br>Stupor, coma | Similar to alcohol withdrawal, including fits |
| Solvents | Inhaled | Disinhibition<br>Euphoria<br>Hallucinations<br>Dizziness, vomiting<br>Coma | 'Hangover' headache |

# REALITY

## General approach: tips, tricks, and cautionary tales

### 1. No lectures

If your patient has imbibed two bottles of whisky a day for 10 years, you won't be the first person to point out the dangers of their habit, so don't lecture them. They'll switch off and decide you are *Just Like All The Rest*. Be non-judgemental—surprise them with an open mind.

### 2. Don't expect a magic cure

It's highly unlikely that you'll say the magic words that will cure their habit, so don't feel under pressure to offer a life-changing solution to their problems. Relax: just listening is useful.

### 3. On tact and tarrying

Barking 'Tell me what drugs you take!' makes most people a little edgy. A more gentle approach is often appreciated, e.g. if blood tests show a raised γGT and you suspect alcohol excess, gently bring the conversation round to alcohol, giving your patient the chance to raise any concerns they may have themselves:

**You:** Your blood tests suggest your liver's been under stress. Can you think of anything that might have been affecting your liver?

**Sam:** Um . . . no . . .

**Y:** OK. Lots of things can affect the liver, including alcohol. Do you drink alcohol?

**S:** Yes.

**Y:** Could you tell me about that?

However, if you've been asked to take a substance misuse history, *don't* tiptoe around the subject. Use the information you have (in real life or OSCEs) and get on with it:

- I was told you've been using speed. Can you tell me more about this?
- I've been asked to find out about your drinking habits — would that be OK?
- Would you mind telling me about your heroin use?

### 4. Don't bat an eyelid

No matter how shocked you may be by your patient's drug use, don't show it. People close down if they feel they've shocked a doctor, since they presume we've seen *everything*. Although you should be fairly unshockable with regard to drug use, you must still respond to the emotional content. If someone says 'I inject into my legs', find out about this. It becomes shocking (for both of you) if they develop gangrene and need an amputation.

### 5. Clarify and use patient jargon

Street slang varies widely, so don't be afraid to say if you don't understand patient jargon. You'll feel silly for demanding a urine drug screen because your patient was using a Bach Flower Remedy. Clarify their terms, and then use them yourself. For example:

**Tracey:** Cat valium's awesome!

**You:** Sorry, what's cat valium?

**T:** Ketamine.

**Y:** OK . . . How much cat valium do you use?

### 6. Take a hint

Don't ask 'Do you *take* alcohol?' or 'Do you *take* heroin?' People *drink* alcohol. They *smoke*, *use*, or *inject* heroin. To some people, take means steal.

### 7. Never admit to your own substance use

Some students try to 'empathize' with patients by divulging their own substance misuse. Don't—it's inappropriate, and, instead of gaining respect, you'll look like your dad dancing at a wedding. If you *are* using drugs or drinking excessively, you need to deal with these issues in your own time; it won't help your patient to know about them.

 Be professional and remember: you don't have to have a heart attack to be a cardiologist.

In the UK, The Sick Doctors Trust (www.sick-doctors-trust.co.uk) helps doctors with substance misuse problems.

### 8. Don't ignore the signs

If your patient is intoxicated, you're unlikely to have a useful conversation—it's better to come back later. Alternatively, if they are obviously withdrawing, be kind and see if you can make them more comfortable, e.g. by alerting the staff to their symptoms.

## The interview

In a focused history of substance misuse, you should cover four major areas:

1. Current use—TRAP (Type, Route, Amount, Pattern)
2. Current use—dependency and effect on life
3. Past use
4. Future use

You don't need to stick to this order, but it helps provide a structure.

### Current use: TRAP

Discover the full extent of the *TRAP*:

- Do you use any drugs or alcohol?

| | |
|---|---|
| Type of drug | • What do you use? |
| Route of administration | • How do you use it? |
| Amount | • How much do you use? |
| Pattern of use | • How often do you use *x*? |

Although the following examples are for alcohol, the principles work for other substances. Find out whether or not this is daily use. If daily, dependency is more likely. If used daily, try:

- I'd like to get an idea about how much you'd drink in an average day. Can you talk me through the day from your first to your last drink?

If not daily (or they say that there's no such thing as an 'average' day):

- When was the last day you had a drink? Can you take me through *that* day?
- How many days in a week would be like that?

Count up units of alcohol as they tell you about their day. People may describe their substance use in financial terms, and, though tempting to record, it won't necessarily reflect the amount used since prices vary. Always try to understand alcohol in units and drugs in weights.

- Heroin, cocaine and amphetamine are usually sold in grams.
- Cannabis is usually sold in fractions of ounces such as 'eighths' (1/8th of an ounce).

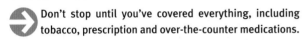 Don't stop until you've covered everything, including tobacco, prescription and over-the-counter medications.

## Current use: dependency and effect on life

You should now be able to focus on the details they gave you and pick out the clues to dependency. Nobody *starts* drinking 50 beers a day—this comes through *tolerance*. If they're drinking daily, the same drink, in the same pubs, they've told you that they have a *narrowed repertoire*—comment on it (e.g. 'It sounds like each day's become very similar?'). If they never just have one drink or can't have an alcohol-free day, this hints at a loss of control. Evidence of tolerance, withdrawal, craving, and use despite harm are probably the most important in a quick exam (e.g. GP clinic/OSCE).

### Tolerance

- Do you need to drink more than you used to, to get the same effects?

### Withdrawal

- How do you feel before your first drink of the day?
- How do you feel if you haven't had a drink for a while?
- What happens when you stop drinking?
- How do you make yourself feel better?' (*use to stop withdrawal symptoms?*)

### Strong desire/compulsion to use

- Do you ever really crave (or desperately want) a drink?

### Difficulties controlling use

- Is it hard to stop drinking, once you've started?
- Do you ever feel like your drinking is out of control?

### Narrowing of repertoire (stereotyped pattern of use)

- Do all your days seem to have the same pattern?

### Effect on life

People usually have good reasons for substance misuse, at least initially. Asking about the 'positives' before you plunge into the negatives lets your patient know that you're not judging them.

- What are the good things about alcohol for you?
- What do you like best about having a drink?

Now you are in a better position to ask about the negative side. This will cover dependency criteria of *salience* of drug-seeking behaviour as well as *continued use despite harm*.

### Salience (neglect of normal activities)

- It sounds like alcohol has become one of the most important things in your life . . .
- Anything you feel you miss out on because of it?
- How would life have been different if you hadn't used it?

### Continued use despite harm

- Has alcohol caused you any problems or difficulties?
- Does it affect your health?/Have you had to see a doctor because of it?
- Has it affected your mood/memory?
- How does it affect your work/studies/relationships?
- Has it got you into any trouble? Or debt?

## Past use and other history

### Current substance

- When did you first try it?
- How has your use changed since then? (tolerance)
- Have there been times you've used more than this?
- Have you ever tried to stop or get help in the past?
  - What happened? (withdrawal/reinstatement after abstinence)
  - What was the longest time you were able to stop? What helped the most?
  - When you started drinking again, how quickly did you return to your usual levels?

### Other substances

- What else have you tried in the past?
- How old were you? (each substance)
- Do you still use this now? If not, what happened?

## Future use

- Do you think your drinking is a problem?
- What are you most *worried* about, if you keep drinking?
- It's helped you through the hard times, but it sounds like it's making things worse for you now. What do you think about that?

Drug-using patients are often treated with disdain, anger, and sometimes even cruelty because they are seen as 'bad' patients who cause their own problems. Nevertheless, the snowboarder who breaks their leg on the slopes is usually dealt with compassionately. Of all the people this patient could meet, they're going to meet *you*—make that a good thing for them and set the example for your colleagues.

> **BOX 10.9** The CAGE screening questionnaire
>
> This only relates to alcohol, where two positive answers indicate that you should take a further alcohol history since your patient may have problems with their drinking. In alcohol OSCEs it's best to include it—there are usually points available.
>
> **C** Have you ever felt that you should *cut down* on your drinking?
>
> **A** Have people *annoyed* you by criticizing your drinking?
>
> **G** Have you ever felt *guilty* about your drinking?
>
> **E** Have you ever had a drink first thing in the morning, to steady your nerves or get rid of a hangover? (*eye-opener/early-morning drink*)

## 1. Alcohol misuse history (15 minutes)

### Candidate's instructions

John Darwin is a 40-year-old builder who has been told to see the GP by his manager. You are a medical student attached to the GP surgery.

Please take a history of alcohol use.

### Patient's brief

*Key characteristics*

- I'm restless and my hands are shaky.
- I want a drink, having not had one this morning.
- I'm cooperative, but annoyed about being 'made' to come in.

My boss will sack me if I don't deal with my 'drinking problem'. He wouldn't even have noticed if he hadn't confused our water bottles—he took a sip of mine and found I wasn't drinking water. I don't operate heavy machinery at work but he's afraid I'll fall off the scaffolding.

Mum and Dad were both alcoholics. She left us when I was little and Dad took his anger out on me, beating me 'til I left home at fifteen. I stayed with friends and found I'd forget everything with a few beers. I needed to drink more to forget as the years passed but gave up five years ago after breaking both arms while drink driving. After drying out in hospital I joined Alcoholics Anonymous and didn't drink again until two years ago when I heard Dad had died and the old memories flooded back. I was soon drinking as much as I had before the crash. I no longer drive.

Each day's the same now. I wake feeling shaky and sick each morning until I drink the can of Stella (500mL, 5.2% lager) that I keep by my bed. That first drink is like medicine for my body and I've had fits when I've missed it. I get through a small (350mL) bottle of vodka at work, which I hide in a water bottle. I'm desperate for beer by the end of the day and always go down the pub for a drink. I can't stop at one drink, though—it always ends up as four or five pints of Stella. I pick up another four cans on my way home and usually get another small bottle of vodka to finish off my evening. I drink 'til I fall asleep around 1am. There isn't room in my life for anything but drinking and working to pay for my drinking. I've lost my close friends, haven't had a girlfriend in years, and have been banned from most pubs for fighting. I get blackouts, so I can't remember most of the fights.

My workmates keep telling me I drink too much but it just annoys me—they've got no right to judge me. Why should I feel guilty? My Dad's to blame for my drinking. I don't want to cut down, but I know I must and the idea fills me with dread.

*Other history*

- Apart from indigestion, I was fit until I vomited a few days ago and saw blood in it.
- My GP gave me antidepressants for depression 6 months ago but they made me feel sick so I stopped them. I feel no better since then.

- I take vitamin tablets because I eat mostly microwave meals, and take indigestion tablets
- I smoke 40 cigarettes a day. I've never tried other drugs
- I feel depressed and I don't enjoy anything anymore. I'm tired and feel like I'm dragging myself about at work. I'm not suicidal but can't see a future beyond drinking.

*Questions*

Can I get a detox?

*Worries*

I'm worried I've done myself permanent damage and the blood I vomited is a sign of cancer.

## 2. Opiate use history (15 minutes)

### Candidate's instructions

Elaine Smith is a 23-year-old woman with a history of IV heroin use. She was admitted with a groin abscess. She is pre-operative and wants a doctor to prescribe methadone. The surgical team are in theatre.

You are a medical student attached to the surgical team. The SHO has asked you to take a substance misuse history so that he can address the situation quickly once out of theatre.

### Patient's brief

*Key characteristics*

- I'm tense and irritable. I just want methadone, the operation, and to get home.
- I don't want to be 'fobbed off' with a medical student, but can be calmed down. A judgemental/unkind student will make me angry and sullen.
- I'm *not* in much pain from my abscess at present.
- I talk openly once calm, though am edgy when discussing funding my habit.

I first smoked smack (heroin) when I was seventeen. I got a modelling contract at sixteen and drugs were everywhere. It made me happier and calmer than I'd ever felt before, but after a while I couldn't get the hit I wanted no matter how much I smoked. My boyfriend, Mark, convinced me to inject. The high was *amazing*, like falling in love. I vomited that time, but didn't care, I just wanted the hit again. It quickly stopped being about the high and became more about stopping the withdrawal. You feel sick and shivery, like you've got flu—then there's diarrhoea, vomiting, goosebumps, and cramps.

I spend £60 on 1g of smack everyday. I inject three times a day to feel normal, and use sleepers to get me through the night (2 × 10mg diazepam). I've used up my arms (veins) and inject in my groin. Using smack becomes a full-time job: heroin's the most important thing in my life and I've done stuff I'm not proud of to get it. *(If pushed)* After I lost my modelling contract, Mark put me on the game (prostitution). He takes most of what I earn and gives me back my wages in smack. I know it doesn't sound fair, but he looks out for me. Sometimes I steal stuff to sell but I haven't been caught.

I know it's wrecked my life. I lost my family and friends; I had a leg blood clot last year and I've accidentally over-dosed twice. I share needles when desperate and I'm Hep B positive. Smack controls me now—I lost control of *it* years ago. I detoxed two years ago and though it was hard I felt great afterwards. Problem was, Mark wouldn't give up and I was soon back on the smack. I went to the community drugs team a couple of times for methadone, but they wanted meetings and urine samples and it was just easier to carry on. I want a detox (but not yet) but they won't arrange it.

*Other history*

- I've tried most things (E, coke, crack, weed, speed) but smack and sleepers are all I use now. I drink a glass or two of wine at weekends. I smoke twenty fags a day.
- Mum and my brother were both drinkers. My childhood was great until I was twelve when my Mum got a new boyfriend. He was horrible—that's all I'm saying.
- I'm not depressed or suicidal now, but I took a paracetamol overdose a few years ago.
- I use inhalers for asthma.

*Questions*

Can I have methadone now?
When will I see the doctor?

*Worries*

I won't make it through the night without methadone.

# NEXT STEPS

## Aggression: 72 hours after a road traffic accident

You are the junior doctor on an orthopaedic team. A nurse calls you, requesting help with Terry Harrison, a 28-year-old man who was admitted three days ago. He suffered multiple fractures in a road traffic accident while drink-driving. He has undergone open reduction and internal fixation of his right ankle and has his right arm in a plaster cast.

The nurse tells you that he has become acutely confused this morning and he is aggressively swinging his plastered arm at anyone who comes too near.

1. What could be happening (differential diagnosis)?
2. How will you assess Terry?
3. How will you manage him?

### Issues

- Risk assessment
- Diagnosis
- Management: immediate and longer-term

While on the phone, advise the nurse to safeguard other patients and staff and contact security, letting her know how soon you will attend.

### Differential diagnosis

1. Alcohol-related problems:
   (a) acute intoxication
   (b) severe withdrawal/delirium tremens
   (c) Wernicke's encephalopathy.
2. Other causes for delirium.
3. Missed head injury.
4. Other psychiatric disorder, e.g. psychosis.
5. A non-medical explanation—has he become distressed and angry about something?

### Assessment

On arrival, don't leap straight into prescribing sedative medication without first assessing this man's condition —the assessment will be much harder if you've knocked him out with heroic doses of medication! Spend a few minutes reviewing the medical notes and talking to the staff, looking for evidence of substance misuse and past psychiatric history. Review his admission physical examination and observations (temperature, pulse, and blood pressure). For example: Was there a head injury? What was his Glasgow Coma Scale score on admission? Reviewing his investigations, look for evidence of substance misuse (macrocytosis, raised γGT, deranged LFTs, positive UDS). You should also consider the management so far, particularly whether he received benzodiazepines or parenteral thiamine as a means of alcohol detoxification. He is at risk of seizures but could *already* be in a post-ictal state without anyone noticing his seizure.

Swiftly move on to assess the patient, taking security staff with you if required and using de-escalation techniques to defuse the situation (see p.18) so that you can proceed safely. Find out what is happening from Mr Harrison's perspective. Then:

- Assess his orientation to time, place and person.
- Observe for signs of alcohol withdrawal (e.g. sweating, tremor) and delirium tremens (clouding of consciousness, hallucinations).
- Perform a physical examination (as far as practically possible) to identify evidence of head injuries and other causes of delirium.

### Management

If there is evidence of a treatable cause for delirium this should be managed as quickly as possible, e.g. antibiotics for pneumonia. Alcohol withdrawal and delirium tremens should be treated with benzodiazepines. In addition, you should have a low threshold for treating Wernicke's encephalopathy. The classic triad (confusion, ataxia, and ophthalmoplegia) rarely present altogether, so even if you observe only one of these and it is unexplained, give high-potency B vitamins either IM or IV (e.g. Pabrinex) for 2–5 days.

Acute psychotic symptoms may require antipsychotics (ideally check for past history and use medication that has been tolerated and effective before); give at low dose and titrate upwards as necessary. Benzodiazepines can also be used on a PRN basis as rapid tranquillization for associated agitation.

Terry should be nursed 1:1 in a well-lit side room, with security present as necessary. He will remain in hospital, receiving treatment in the short term under the Mental Capacity Act, as the physical causes for the acute change in mental state are assessed and treated. If Terry remains disturbed and resistant to care beyond 48 hours, the Mental Health Act may need to be considered.

Once the situation is under control there is an opportunity for some psycho-education for Mr Harrison to seriously address his alcohol problem *and* for the admitting doctor to seriously address their reluctance to prescribe sedatives and parenteral vitamins when admitting patients with alcohol problems. This situation could be avoided in the majority of cases!

### Film list

**Alcohol**
*Withnail & I* (1987)

**Opiates**
*Pure* (2002)
*Trainspotting* (1996)
*The Basketball Diaries* (1995)

**Stimulants**
*Walk the Line* (2005)
*Human Traffic* (1999)

**Other**
*A Scanner Darkly* (2006)

### Books

**Alcohol**
Doyle, R. (1998) *The Woman Who Walked Into Doors*. London: Vintage. Novel exploring alcoholism in the context of domestic violence.

Johnstone, N. (2002) *A Head Full of Blue*. London: Bloomsbury. Frank account of alcoholism, particularly resonant in examining the development of addiction in adolescence.

**Opiates**
Burgess, M. (1997) *Junk*. London: Penguin. Novel aimed at adolescent readers exploring heroin addiction in teenagers, including the descent into prostitution to fund a habit.

Burroughs, W.S. (1953) *Junky*. London: Penguin. Autobiographical account of drug addiction, with graphic scenes of withdrawals.

De Quincey, T. (1822) *Confessions of an English Opium-Eater*. London: Wordsworth, 1994. Historical text examining addiction to opiates in the nineteenth century, when addiction was one of a long list of 'moral' sicknesses.

Welsh, I. (1999) *Trainspotting*. London: Vintage. Also a film, this has become a cult classic, examining the bleak reality of heroin addiction.

**Stimulants**
Burroughs, W.S. (1993) *Naked Lunch*. London: Flamingo. A rollercoaster ride of drug-induced hallucinations—written while Burroughs himself was under the influence of opiates and stimulants.

Wurtzel, E. (2003) *More, Now, Again*. London: Virago. Wurtzel's follow-up to *Prozac Nation* sees her descend into stimulant addiction, including cocaine and Ritalin.

### Quotes

The addict regards his body impersonally as an instrument to absorb the medium in which he lives, evaluates his tissue with the cold hands of a horse trader.
**William S. Burroughs,** *Naked Lunch*

The doctor never saw me. He studied parts of me but he never saw all of me. He never looked at my eyes. Drink, he said to himself. I could see his nose moving, taking in the smell, deciding.
**Roddy Doyle,** *The Woman Who Walked Into Doors*

There is no pain, you are receding.
A distant ship's smoke on the horizon.
You are only coming through in waves.
Your lips move but I can't hear what you're sayin' . . .
The child is grown, the dream is gone.
I have become comfortably numb.
*Comfortably Numb*—Pink Floyd

Whiskey river take my mind don't let her memory torture me
Whiskey river don't run dry you're all I've got take care of me.
*Whiskey River*—Willie Nelson

## Note

1. Conan Doyle, A. (1890) *The Sign of Four*. London: Penguin, 1982.

## References/Further reading

Babor, T.F. *et al.* (2001) *AUDIT (Alcohol Use Disorders Identification Test)* (2nd edn). Geneva: World Health Organization. Available online at: http://whqlibdoc.who.int/hq/2001/WHO_MSD_MSB_01.6a.pdf

Crome, I.B. (1997) Gender differences in substance misuse and psychiatric comorbidity. *Current Opinion in Psychiatry*, **10**, 194–8.

Edwards, G. and Gross, M.M. (1976) Alcohol dependence: provisional description of a clinical syndrome. *British Medical Journal*, i,1058–61.

Faggiano, F., Vigna-Taglianti, F., Versino, E., and Lemma, P. (2003) Methadone maintenance at different dosages for opioid dependence. *Cochrane Database of Systematic Reviews* **3**: CD002208.

Farrell, M. and Marsden, J. (2008) Acute risk of drug-related death among newly released prisoners in England and Wales. *Addiction*, **103**, 251–5.

Gossop, M., Marsden, J., Stewart, D., and Kidd, T. (2003) The National Treatment Outcome Research Study (NTORS): 4–5 year follow-up results. *Addiction*, **98**, 291–303.

Kessler, R.C., Berglund, P.A., Demler, O., *et al.* (2005a) Lifetime prevalence and age-of-onset distributions of DSM-IV disorders in the National Comorbidity Survey Replication (NCS-R). *Archives of General Psychiatry*, **62**, 593–602.

Kessler, R.C., Chiu, W.T., Demler, O., and Walters, E.E. (2005b) Prevalence, severity, and comorbidity of twelve-month DSM-IV disorders in the National Comorbidity Survey Replication (NCS-R). *Archives of General Psychiatry*, **62**, 617–27.

Matheson, C., Bond, C.M., and Hickey, F. (1999) Prescribing and dispensing for drug users in primary care: current practice in Scotland. *Family Practice*, **16**, 375–9.

Miller, W.R. and Rollnick, S. (2002) *Motivational Interviewing* (2nd edn). New York: Guilford Press.

Orford, J. and Keddie, A. (1986) Abstinence or controlled drinking in clinical practice: a test of the dependence and persuasion hypotheses. *British Journal of Addiction*, **81**, 495–504.

Prochaska, J.O. and DiClemente, C.C. (1982) Transtheoretical therapy: toward a more integrative model of change. *Psychotherapy: Theory, Research and Practice*, **19**, 276–88.

Robins, L.N. (1993) Vietnam veterans' rapid recovery from heroin addiction: a fluke or normal expectation? *Addiction*, **88**, 1041–54.

West, R. (2006) *Theory of Addiction*. Oxford: Blackwell.

WHO (1992) *International Classification of Diseases, 10th Revision (ICD-10)*. Geneva: World Health Organization.

 Go to www.oxfordtextbooks/orc/stringer for an array of additional references, including indicative mark sheets for OSCEs, self-assessment questions, guidance, and exercises.

# 11 Organic psychiatry

*Juliet D. Hurn*

## True or False? Test your existing knowledge—answers in the chapter and online

1. Lesions to the left frontal lobe result in expressive dysphasia in right handed people.

2. A two-day history of confusion can diagnose dementia following a severe stroke.

3. Pick's disease is characterised by rounded collections of hyperphosphorylated tau protein, known as Pick's bodies.

4. Normal pressure hydrocephalus is characterised by the triad of dementia, tremor, and urinary incontinence.

5. Patients with sporadic CJD tend to have an earlier onset and more prominent psychiatric symptoms than those with variant CJD.

6. Amnesic syndrome is characterised by a profound retrograde amnesia.

7. Approximately 50% of patients with epilepsy or multiple sclerosis suffer with depression.

8. Depression in patients who have had a stroke should be treated as for primary depression.

9. Assessing verbal fluency gives an indication of temporal lobe function.

10. If a patient who is medically unfit to drive refuses to inform the driving authorities of their continued driving, it is legal to override their confidentiality and inform the authorities.

## Contents

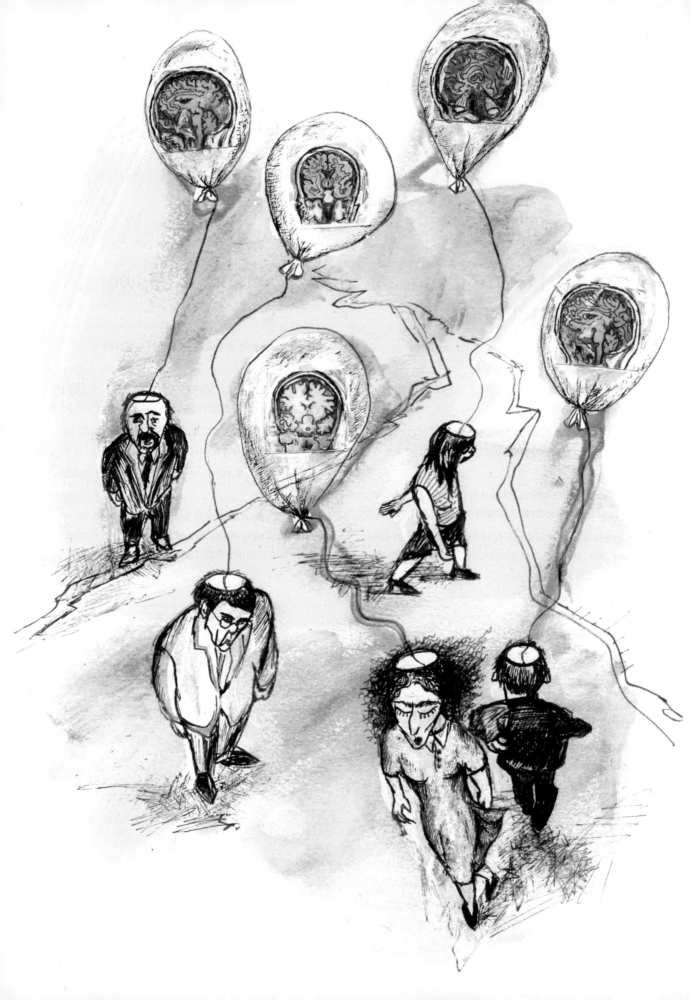

# PRINCIPLES

It was odd, I reflected, that my one remaining protection against the uncertainties of waking life was itself an uncertainty: I had amnesia. All my movements through memories and locations still hadn't told me who I was. I didn't have a surname, or parents with faces, or even a good idea of my age. And now the means to end that uncertainty was in my hands. The papers in the briefcase would tell me what I had been doing and thinking about in the very last hour before the attack. At the very least, they would reveal my profession, and I felt sure that from that basic piece of information, the remaining secrets of my history would fall quite naturally into place.

*The Coma*—Alex Garland[1]

## Introduction

*Organic* psychiatric disorders are those caused directly by a demonstrable physical problem (e.g. brain tumour, hypothyroidism). *Functional* illnesses are those traditionally viewed as having no organic basis (e.g. schizophrenia), although it is becoming clear that many of these *do* have some underlying physical pathology. Philosophers may argue about whether we are dealing with the mind or the body but, pragmatically, doctors focus on the most helpful way of dealing with a patient's problem.

## Basic neuroanatomy: lobes and lesions

Knowing the roles of different parts of the brain will give you clues to the areas affected by local disease or damage, long before your patient has a CT or MRI scan. More generalized involvement (e.g. delirium) can produce a wide variety of symptoms due to the whole-brain effect. Figure 11.1 and Table 11.1 briefly review anatomy, function, and the results of lesions.

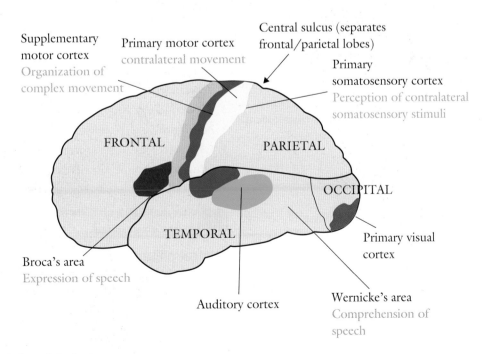

FIGURE 11.1 Lobes of the brain

**TABLE 11.1** Lobes, functions, and lesions

| Lobe | Functions | Symptoms of dysfunction |
|------|-----------|-------------------------|
| Frontal | Executive function | Poor judgement/planning |
| | Personality/social behaviour | Inappropriate behaviour/impulsivity |
| | Initiative/motivation | Apathy/decline in self-care |
| | Speech production | Expressive dysphasia: problems producing language |
| | Broca's area: dominant lobe | Telegraphic speech: short words and sentences, e.g. 'Want cake' (I want some cake). |
| | | Normal comprehension |
| | Motor cortex | Contralateral spastic hemiparesis |
| | Suppression of primitive reflexes | Primitive reflexes re-emerge (e.g. sucking, rooting) |
| Temporal | Auditory, olfactory, gustatory perception | Auditory impairment/agnosia |
| | | Auditory, olfactory, gustatory hallucinations (e.g. in temporal lobe epilepsy) |
| | Understanding of speech | Receptive dysphasia: problems comprehending speech |
| | Wernicke's area: dominant lobe | Speech is fluent, but nonsensical with mistakes, additional sounds/words/neologisms, e.g. 'I filly iver want a gar some cakes' |
| | Memory | Amnesic syndrome (see text) |
| | Emotional regulation | Lability |
| Parietal | Somatosensory perception | Contralateral sensory impairment |
| | Integration of sensory perception allowing awareness and movement of body | Apraxias = inability to carry out skilled tasks despite intact sensory and motor function, e.g. drawing, dressing |
| | | Agnosias = inability to recognize a sensory stimulus despite normal peripheral sensation |
| | | Contralateral sensory neglect = inattention to information presented to one side of the body, despite normal peripheral sensation |
| | Communication between Broca's and Wernicke's areas (dominant lobe) | Receptive dysphasia |
| | Calculation | Dyscalculia = inability to calculate |
| Occipital | Visual perception and interpretation | Contralateral visual defects |
| | | Visual agnosia |
| | | Cortical blindness |

NB Language is dealt with by the 'dominant' lobe which is the left hemisphere in right-handers *and* the majority of left-handers.

# Delirium ('acute confusional state')

Delirium is an acute and transient state of global brain dysfunction with *clouding of consciousness*: the patient is not fully aware of (or 'in touch with') their environment. It is common (Burns *et al*. 2004), occurring in up to:

- 20% of medical inpatients
- ~50% of post-operative patients
- 70% of elderly ITU patients.

Delirium is a sign that something is physically wrong, so always search for the underlying cause. Risk factors for delirium include old age, pre-existing physical or mental illness (especially dementia), substance misuse, polypharmacy, and malnutrition. Remember that relatively minor problems, such as urinary tract infections, can tip vulnerable people into delirium. Causes include:

- Trauma: e.g. head injury, burns.
- Hypoxia: cardiovascular/respiratory.

- Infective: intracranial (e.g. encephalitis) and systemic (e.g. septicaemia).
- Metabolic: e.g. liver failure, renal failure, electrolyte imbalance.
- Endocrine: e.g. hypoglycaemia.
- Nutritional: e.g. Wernicke's encephalopathy.
- CNS pathology: e.g. raised intracranial pressure.
- Drugs and alcohol: intoxication/withdrawal.
- Medication: e.g. anticholinergics, opiates.

 **Rule out delirium if there is *any* change in an elderly person's mental state.**

## Clinical picture

Onset is sudden (hours to days) and symptoms fluctuate throughout the day, often worsening in the evening or at night. The patient is usually disorientated with poor attention and short-term memory. Mood changes may be prominent—don't mistake them for depression or mania. Illusions and hallucinations are common (usually visual), and transient muddled delusions may be present. It can be difficult for patients to communicate these experiences because of disorganized thinking and impoverished, pressured, or rambling speech. Sleep is commonly disturbed, with insomnia or reversal of the sleep–wake cycle. Behavioural change usually takes one of two forms:

---

**BOX 11.1** Delirium mental state examination

- **Appearance and behaviour** Agitated 82-year-old woman in a hospital gown. Plucking at cubicle curtains. Fearful expression. Hitting out with her stick. Smells of urine.
- **Speech** Screaming; incoherent mumbling.
- **Mood**

  (S) Refused to comment

  (O) Frightened, irritable, suspicious.
- **Thought** Persecutory delusions: 'They're experimenting on me!'
- **Perception** Visual hallucinations: insects on her bed. Illusions: misinterpreting curtains as 'ghosts'.
- **Cognition** Unable to engage in MMSE. Disorientated to time, place, and person. Poor attention and concentration. Unable to retain simple facts.
- **Insight** Refusing all interventions; does not believe she is ill.

---

**TABLE 11.2** Comparison of delirium and dementia

| Feature | Delirium | Dementia |
| --- | --- | --- |
| Onset | Sudden (days–weeks) | Gradual (weeks–months)[a] |
| Course | Fluctuating | Slowly progressive[a] |
| Duration | Short (days–weeks) Officially <6 months | Lifelong Officially >6 months |
| Consciousness | Impaired | Normal |
| Attention | Poor | Normal |
| Thinking | Disorganized[b] | Impoverished |
| Delusions | Common, fragmented | Sometimes later in illness |
| Hallucinations | Common | Sometimes later in illness[c] |
| Prognosis | Recovery once underlying cause resolves, but often residual deficits | Deterioration likely |

[a]Except vascular dementia which progresses 'stepwise' or may have sudden onset.
[b]Impoverished in 'quiet' delirium.
[c]But a central feature of Lewy body dementia.

- **Hyper**activity, agitation, aggression.
  - Wandering, climbing into other patients' beds, pulling out catheters.
  - Easily spotted!
- **Hypo**activity, lethargy, stupor, drowsiness, withdrawal.
  - *Quiet delirium*, e.g. silently lying in bed.
  - Easily missed: these patients appear 'well-behaved' to busy staff!

 A two-day history of confusion does *not* diagnose dementia!

## Investigations

1. Physical examination.
2. Collateral history (especially: Is this patient usually forgetful?).
3. Check the drug chart for recently added drugs.
4. Essential: FBC, U&Es, G, $Ca^{2+}$, MSU, $SaO_2$, ECG, CXR, septic screen.
5. Consider: LFTs, blood cultures, CT head, CSF, EEG.

## Management

1. **Treat the cause** and manage aggravating factors like dehydration, pain, and constipation. Stop unnecessary medications.

2. **Behavioural management** Work with nursing staff to ensure:
   - Frequent reorientation, e.g. clocks, calendars, verbal reminders.
   - Good lighting—gloomy conditions increase hallucinations and illusions. At night, ensure enough light for the patient to recognize where they are without being kept awake.
   - Address sensory problems, e.g. hearing aids, spectacles.
   - Avoid over- or understimulation. If the main ward is disruptive, a side room may be calming, although isolated side rooms can increase disorientation.
   - Minimize change:
     - Don't keep moving the patient.
     - One staff member to engage the patient each shift.
     - Establish a routine, including regular toileting and sleep hygiene.
   - Remove things that can be thrown or tripped over.
   - Silence unnecessary noises, e.g. beeping alarms.
   - Allow safe or supervised wandering if possible (restraining people increases accidents).

3. **Medication** A small nocturnal dose of a benzodiazepine may promote sleep and help correct the

sleep–wake cycle. If sedation short-term is absolutely necessary, use *low-dose* typical antipsychotics or benzodiazepines. Beware the increased risk of falls.

4. **Consider referral** on recovery to an old age physician or psychiatrist to manage ongoing physical or psychiatric problems.

5. Help to **prevent delirium** through:
   - Good sleep hygiene without medication.
   - Minimal moves around the hospital.
   - Encouraging mobility.
   - Proactive management: minimize dehydration, pain, constipation, urinary retention, and sensory problems.

➡ Confused patients become frightened if you suddenly 'appear' beside them. Give warning by approaching from the front and catching their attention from a distance.

## Prognosis

Delirium is associated with increased mortality, longer admissions, and higher readmission rates, as well as subsequent nursing home placement (Inouye *et al*. 1998). It may take days or weeks (rarely, months) to completely resolve after treatment of the underlying cause. Some patients never fully recover to their premorbid level.

➡ The brain is like a jelly being 'poked' by a physical problem; delirium is the resultant 'wobble'. When the poking stops, the jelly will wobble for a while afterwards. Don't expect delirium to resolve as soon as the physical cause has been treated.

## Dementia

Alzheimer's disease, vascular dementia, and dementia with Lewy bodies (DLB) are covered under old age psychiatry (Chapter 12); in this section we review the *rarer* dementias more often found in *younger* patients

---

**BOX 11.2** Cortical and subcortical dementias

Dementias can be divided into cortical and subcortical types, although features often overlap.

- *Cortical* (e.g. Alzheimer's disease):
  - Affects *cortical* functions, e.g. memory, language.
- *Subcortical* (e.g. Huntington's disease):
  - Affects functions controlled by *subcortical structures* like the thalamus and basal ganglia. Problems include bradyphrenia (mental slowing), bradykinesia, depression, movement disorders, and executive dysfunction (due to connections between basal ganglia and frontal lobes).

---

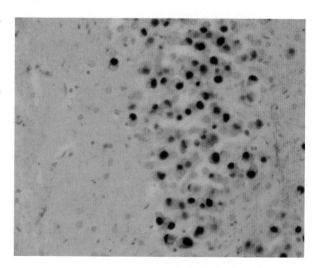

FIGURE 11.2 Pick bodies stained with antibodies to hyperphosphorylated tau (by kind permission of Dr Andrew King)

(under 65). Management is similar to that outlined in Chapter 12.

## Frontotemporal lobar degenerations

This term describes the pathology of asymmetrical frontal and/or anterior temporal lobe atrophy (Snowden and Neary 2002). It causes three clinical syndromes which usually begin between the ages of 40 and 60. Most cases are sporadic, although up to 40% show autosomal inheritance. There is no clear-cut correlation between the pathological and clinical forms.

### Pathology

Cortical atrophy unites these disorders. In the Pick's disease subtype (Figure 11.2), neurons contain 'Pick bodies' (rounded collections of hyperphosphorylated tau protein). In FTLD-U (frontotemporal lobar degeneration with tau-negative ubiquinated inclusions), tau-negative inclusions are found, similar to those in motor neuron disease.

### Clinical forms

- *Frontotemporal dementia*: this causes frontal lobe syndrome with prominent disinhibition and social/personality changes (Figure 11.3).
- *Semantic dementia*: progressive loss of understanding of verbal and visual meaning.
- *Progressive non-fluent aphasia*: this begins with naming difficulties and progresses to mutism.

Death usually occurs within 5–10 years.

## Huntington's disease (Huntington's chorea)

This autosomal dominant disease causes dementia and chorea. The mutation is a trinucleotide CAG repeat in

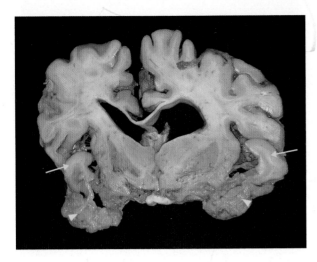

**FIGURE 11.3** Coronal slice through the cerebral hemispheres of a patient with a frontotemporal lobar degeneration. Note the degeneration of medial/temporal structures (arrowheads) and the relative preservation of the superior temporal gyri (arrows) (by kind permission of Dr Andrew King)

the Huntingtin gene on chromosome 4. Onset is usually in early middle age, although longer CAG repeats cause earlier and more severe presentations; lengthening occurs with each inheritance, so that onset is younger in subsequent generations ('anticipation').

Deposits of abnormal *Huntingtin* protein cause atrophy of the basal ganglia and thalamus, as well as some cortical neuron loss, mostly frontal. CT/MRI may show caudate nucleus atrophy (Figure 11.4) and the EEG may be flat.

Clinically, there are personality and behavioural changes, sometimes with aggression. Depression, irritability, or euphoria are common, and a subcortical dementia emerges later. Chorea affects limbs, trunk, face, and speech muscles, and produces a wide-based lurching gait. Genetic testing is available, although there is currently no cure and death usually occurs within 15 years.

> ➡ Chorea may be due to a relative excess of dopamine in the atrophied basal ganglia, and as such, can be thought of as the 'opposite' of parkinsonism. Antipsychotics may help.

## HIV dementia (HIV encephalopathy)

HIV dementia is due to the direct effect of the virus on the brain. Incidence has halved since the introduction of HAART (highly active anti-retroviral therapy), but prevalence has risen due to increased survival rates. It affects 10% of HIV patients (Manji and Miller 2004). Early apathy and withdrawal progress to a subcortical dementia, with neurological features such as ataxia, tremor, seizures, and myoclonus. MRI may show atrophy and diffuse white matter signal changes.

> ⊙ Depression, mania, psychosis, and other psychiatric problems are more common in people with HIV.

## Normal pressure hydrocephalus

This is a relatively rare, but potentially reversible, cause of dementia, usually affecting older adults. Causes include meningitis and head injury; although up to 50% of cases are idiopathic. Cerebrospinal fluid (CSF) absorption is impaired in the subarachnoid space, with normal

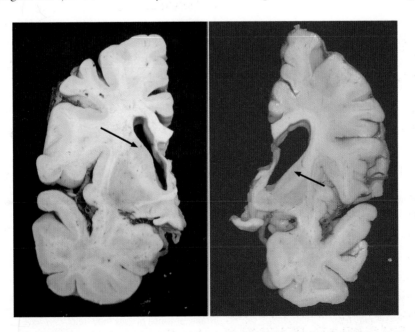

**FIGURE 11.4** Coronal slices from cerebral hemispheres comparing a control case (left) with a case of Huntington's disease (right). Note the significantly flatter caudate nucleus in the Huntington's case (arrows) (by kind permission of Dr Andrew King)

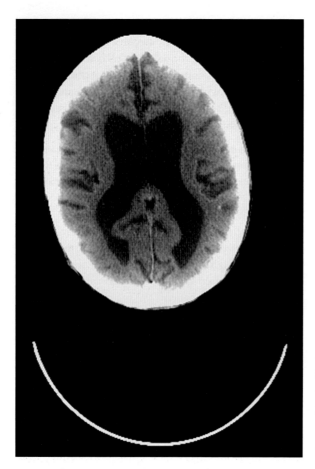

FIGURE 11.5 Normal pressure hydrocephalus: CT shows dilated ventricles out of proportion to the degree of involutional changes or cortical atrophy (by kind permission of Dr Mona Sriharan)

communication between here and the ventricles. CSF accumulates in the ventricles (*hydrocephalus*), although CSF pressure remains fairly *normal* as CSF production adjusts. Distortion of periventricular white matter tracts produces the classic symptom triad:

- dementia (subcortical)
- unsteady gait
- urinary incontinence.

A ventriculo-atrial shunt may allow CSF drainage from the brain ventricles to the heart. Prognosis is worse in those where the cause is unknown.

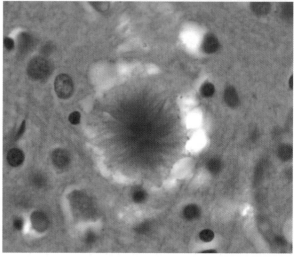

FIGURE 11.6 Florid plaque from the brain of a 27-year-old woman with vCJD (by kind permission of Dr Andrew King)

TABLE 11.3 Comparison of sporadic and variant CJD

|  | Sporadic CJD | Variant CJD (vCJD) |
|---|---|---|
| Cause | Unknown | Eating BSE-infected beef |
| Onset | Older: 40–60 years | Younger: mostly in twenties |
| Clinically | Various neurological signs: extra-pyramidal, pyramidal, cerebellar, myoclonus<br>Dementia | Prominent psychiatric symptoms: dementia, depression, irritability, psychosis, behavioural changes<br>Ataxia and sensory symptoms |
| EEG | Typically, triphasic sharp wave complexes | Less typical changes |
| MRI | May be high signal in *anterior* basal ganglia | The pulvinar sign: high signal in *posterior thalamus* (sometimes) |
| Other | CSF: raised 14-3-3 protein.<br>Brain biopsy[a] may help | CSF: raised 14-3-3 protein less common<br>Brain[a] or tonsil biopsy may help |
| Death | 6–12 months | May be over a year |

[a]Brain biopsy is risky and only used if diagnosis is uncertain

## Prion diseases (transmissible spongiform encephalopathies)

These rare disorders often cause rapidly progressive neurological and psychiatric symptoms. The main human form is Creutzfeldt–Jakob disease (CJD), of which the most common is sporadic CJD. Other human types include variant CJD (vCJD), iatrogenic CJD, kuru, and various familial prion diseases. Animal forms include scrapie in sheep and bovine spongiform encephalopathy (BSE) in cattle.

In prion diseases, the normal prion protein changes into an abnormal insoluble form which appears to act as a template for further transformation of normal to abnormal prion. This positive feedback mechanism is the 'protein-only hypothesis'. Accumulations of abnormal prion protein are linked to spongiform and amyloid changes in the cerebrum, basal ganglia, and cerebellum. Although occasional cases are genetic and the protein can also undergo change from 'infection' or 'transmission' via another affected individual, the cause of the conversion from normal to abnormal protein is not well understood in most patients. There is currently no specific treatment.

## Amnesic syndrome (amnestic syndrome)

The amnesic syndrome is characterized by a profound anterograde memory loss—an inability to lay down new memories from the time of brain damage onwards. Although there can be some retrograde loss (of memories before the damage), other brain functions are relatively intact. Damage affects the limbic structures dealing with explicit memory (hippocampus, mamillary bodies, parts of the thalamus, and surrounding cortex). Causes include hypoxia, encephalitis, and carbon monoxide poisoning. *Korsakoff's syndrome* is the most common type of amnesic syndrome and is due to thiamine (B$_1$) deficiency, usually secondary to alcohol abuse. Wernicke's encephalopathy (acute confusion, ataxia, and ophthalmoplegia) precedes the onset of Korsakoff's syndrome (see p.97).

---

**BOX 11.3** A theoretical patient with amnesic syndrome

Your patient could hold a normal conversation and score full marks for immediate recall on the MMSE, but would be disorientated with impaired delayed recall. At the next meeting, they would not remember you, but might relate nostalgic stories of your holiday together in Spain. If you arranged classes, they could learn to salsa, despite having no recollection of the lessons.

---

The main problem is anterograde amnesia, despite intact short-term ('working') memory; information is lost once it is no longer being actively used. Some patients *confabulate*, talking about things they 'remember' but which never happened; they are not deliberately lying, but trying to make sense of confusing memory gaps, using any memories that come to mind. Since the cortex, basal ganglia, and cerebellum are undamaged, procedural memory (remembering *how* to do things) is intact.

Although prompt parenteral thiamine may prevent further damage in Korsakoff's syndrome, nothing reverses the amnesic syndrome once the damage has been done.

## Transient global amnesia

This is an acute global memory loss, lasting from one to 24 hours. It may be due to transient ischaemia affecting memory structures and is sometimes precipitated by physical or emotional stress. Patients are usually over 50 and otherwise healthy. Anterograde memory is particularly affected, but there may also be retrograde loss. Patients are often bewildered, repeatedly asking 'Where am I?' In contrast with psychogenic amnesia, the patient does *not* forget their identity. Consciousness and cognition are otherwise normal, with no signs of neurological disease (it is important to exclude intoxication, head injury, stroke, and epilepsy). Although episodes sometimes recur, prognosis is good.

## Frontal lobe syndrome

Frontal lobes are the *brakes* of the brain—the part that shouts 'Stop! Do you *really* want to do that?' Rather than letting you react to situations with basic impulses (e.g. *eat it, fight it, have sex with it*), frontal lobes weigh all the available information to produce a more reasoned plan of action, which they then motivate you to follow. Anything that damages this area (e.g. head injury, dementia, or stroke) can cause *frontal lobe syndrome*. The syndrome consists of symptoms from the following domains:

- **Executive dysfunction**
  - Poor judgement
  - Poor reasoning and problem-solving
  - Poor planning and decision-making
- **Social behaviour and personality change**
  - Loss of social awareness: irresponsible/disinhibited/inappropriate behaviour
  - Impulsivity
  - Euphoric or 'fatuous' mood; lability
  - Repetitive or compulsive behaviours

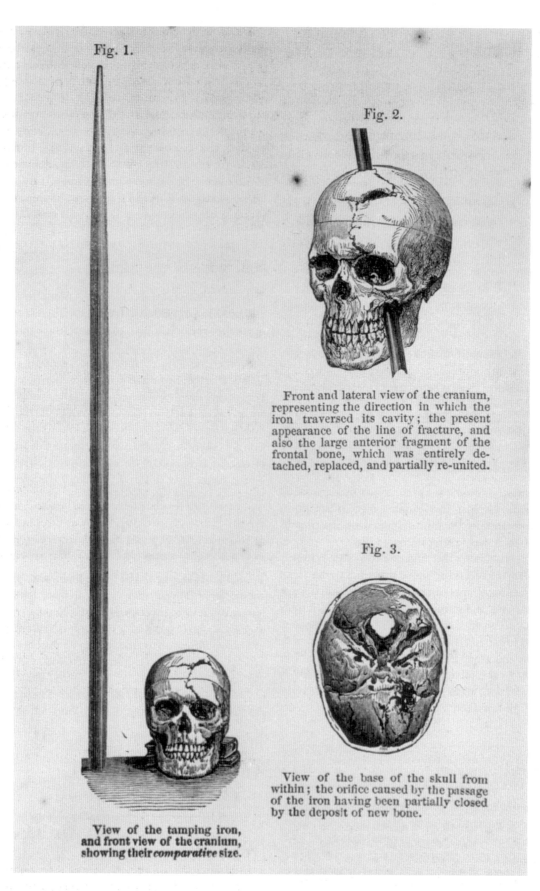

Fig. 1.

Fig. 2.

Front and lateral view of the cranium, representing the direction in which the iron traversed its cavity; the present appearance of the line of fracture, and also the large anterior fragment of the frontal bone, which was entirely detached, replaced, and partially re-united.

Fig. 3.

View of the base of the skull from within; the orifice caused by the passage of the iron having been partially closed by the deposit of new bone.

View of the tamping iron, and front view of the cranium, showing their *comparative* size.

FIGURE 11.7  Phineas Gage's skull (from Harlow, J.M. (1848) Passage of an iron rod through the head. *Boston Medical and Surgical Journal*, **39**, 389–93, courtesy of the National Library of Medicine)

- **Apathy**
  - Lack of motivation and initiative
  - Decline in self-care.

Depending on the part of the lobes most affected, people tend to be either apathetic *or* disinhibited, impulsive, aggressive, and socially inappropriate.

MRI brain may be helpful (e.g. atrophy, space occupying lesion) but formal occupational therapy and neuropsychological testing will give insight into functional impairment. Unless the cause can be treated, management is usually through rehabilitation and supporting the family.

>> *Bedside frontal lobe tests are included in Reality (p.128).*

---

**BOX 11.4** Phineas Gage's frontal lobes

Phineas Gage was a railway worker in Vermont in 1848, whose job involved packing sand over gunpowder with a tamping iron (3ft long metal rod). One day the gunpowder exploded unexpectedly and shot the iron through his left cheek, his frontal lobes, and out of the top of his head (Figure 11.7). He survived the accident *and* the subsequent wound infections. His employers had viewed him as their most capable and conscientious worker, but were unable to re-employ him because of a drastic personality change following the accident. Phineas became impatient, impulsive, rude, bad-tempered, and stubborn. He was notably distractible and unable to finish tasks. Friends described him as being 'no longer Gage' (Harlow 1848).

---

## Head injury

Head injuries are either *open* (where the skull is penetrated, causing local cerebral damage) or *closed* (no penetration, but brain damage is caused by acceleration/deceleration and shearing forces). Severity is graded as mild, moderate, or severe, according to the Glasgow Coma Scale score, duration of coma, and duration of post-traumatic amnesia (PTA).

Immediately after a head injury, consciousness may be impaired to the point of delirium or coma. This is more common in closed injuries. Once consciousness is regained, memory impairments often occur.

- *Post-traumatic amnesia* (PTA) lasts from the time of injury until recovery of normal memory. The longer it lasts, the greater the risk of complications.

- *Retrograde amnesia* (RA) is memory loss *before* the injury (from the last clear memory until the injury occurred). It is not a good predictor of outcome.

Longer term, *cognitive impairment* ranges from mild deficits to severe dementia. It is more likely to be *focal* (e.g. frontal, parietal) in open head injuries and *global* in closed head injuries. Typical problems affect attention/concentration, memory, speed of processing, and problem-solving. *Personality change* can occur after any trauma, but is particularly associated with frontal damage. Previous personality traits may be exaggerated. *Depression* and *anxiety* occur in up to 50% of head injury survivors and can persist. Suicide risk may be increased.

*Post-concussional syndrome* may follow a head injury with loss of consciousness. Symptoms occur in at least 50% of those with mild head injury, and a significant proportion persist for at least a year. People become preoccupied with their symptoms:

- mood, e.g. depression, anxiety, irritability
- cognitive, e.g. poor concentration and memory
- somatic, e.g. headache, dizziness, fatigue, insomnia, noise sensitivity.

Organic and psychological factors are probably involved, since microscopic axonal injury can be found in even mild head injury. The syndrome is influenced by premorbid personality and highly comorbid with anxiety and depression.

### Management

Specialist head injury services provide rehabilitation, as well as support for the family. Psychotropic drugs may be needed but are used with care, partly because of the increased risk of seizures. Education and reassurance in mild head injury may help to prevent post-concussional syndrome.

## Parkinson's disease

Parkinson's disease (PD) is an idiopathic movement disorder. Degeneration of dopaminergic cells in the substantia nigra causes depletion of dopaminergic tracts, leading to the basal ganglia. The classic triad of extrapyramidal symptoms is:

---

**BOX 11.5** Secondary forms of parkinsonism

- Drug-induced e.g. antipsychotics.
- Multiple cerebral infarcts.
- Repeated head injury ('boxing encephalopathy'/ 'punch-drunk syndrome').
- '*Parkinson plus* syndromes' (a group of neurodegenerative disorders), e.g. progressive supranuclear palsy, corticobasal degeneration, multiple system atrophy.

---

- *tremor* (pill-rolling type)
- *rigidity* (experienced as stiffness)
- *bradykinesia* (slowed movement).

Other signs and symptoms include a stooped posture and shuffling gait, 'mask-like' facies, recurrent falls, constipation, and urinary problems.

## Depression

Ask about depression, since it occurs in up to 45% of patients. It can be difficult to diagnose since PD and depression symptoms can overlap, e.g. lack of smiling and psychomotor slowing. Treatment is as for primary depression.

> When physical illnesses resemble depression, focus on cognitions (e.g. hopelessness, guilt) and the *experience* of depression (e.g. sadness, anhedonia). This helps separate out a diagnosis of depression.

## Parkinson's disease dementia

Up to 80% of Parkinson's patients eventually develop dementia (Aarsland *et al.* 2003). It is linked to increased mortality, carer stress, and nursing home admission. An early symptom is bradyphrenia, which progresses to more profound dementia. This is distinguished from dementia with Lewy bodies (DLB) by the presence of PD *before* cognitive impairment; in DLB, the pattern is the other way round (see p.138). Acetylcholinesterase inhibitors can help in both cases.

## Psychotic symptoms

These affect up to 40% of patients and are the strongest predictor of nursing home placement. PD dementia is a risk factor. Visual hallucinations, often of animals or people, are common. Symptoms sometimes result from the use of dopaminergic anti-Parkinson's drugs. Management involves trying to gain a balance between too much dopamine (psychotic symptoms) and too little (parkinsonism). Dopaminergic drugs can be slowly withdrawn or cautious doses of atypical antipsychotics tried, though both options may exacerbate parkinsonism. If the patient and family are coping, it may be best not to change anything.

## Multiple sclerosis

Multiple sclerosis (MS) is characterized by episodes of inflammation and demyelination occurring at different sites, and at different times, within the white matter tracts of the CNS. The disease may run a relapsing–remitting course and then become progressive; or less commonly may be progressive from the start.

---

### BOX 11.6 Wilson's disease

- Autosomal recessive disorder of copper metabolism.
- Copper deposition leads to pathology of the liver, brain, cornea, and other organs.
- Kayser–Fleischer rings can be seen in the eyes.
- Motor disturbance, e.g. tremor, dysarthria.
- Psychiatric symptoms in a young person may be the first sign, e.g. depression, psychosis, personality change.
- Treat with chelating agents.

## Depression

Up to 50% of patients suffer depression, and the risk of suicide is substantially increased. Depression may relate to disability and pain, or to MS medication (e.g. steroids, anti-spasticity drugs or interferon). As with Parkinson's disease, diagnostic difficulties arise when symptoms are common to both MS and depression; additionally, brief mood changes (e.g. emotional lability, pathological crying) can occur as part of MS (Jefferies 2006). Treatment is as for primary depression. Mania is also common (see Next steps).

## Cognitive impairment/dementia

Patients commonly have memory and concentration problems, and dementia affects up to 60% of those in the late stages of MS.

## Stroke

Strokes, whether ischaemic or haemorrhagic, are a major cause of mortality and morbidity. Mortality rates are 30% within the first year, and up to 70% within 3 years. A third of survivors return to independent living, often with ongoing disability.

## Cognitive/neurological symptoms

These relate to the pattern of brain damage, e.g. frontal lobe syndrome, dysphasia, dyspraxia, dementia.

---

### BOX 11.7 Tertiary neurosyphilis

Neurosyphilis can occur if primary syphilis is not adequately treated. Prevalence may rise as syphilis rates increase.

- *General paralysis of the insane* was one of the most common reasons for admission to asylums before penicillin. It is characterized by grandiose delusions, cognitive decline, and neurological deficits.
- *Meningovascular syphilis* usually presents as delirium.

## Depression

Depression affects up to a third of stroke patients, and impairs rehabilitation. It may relate to the consequences of the stroke or to adverse life events *before* the stroke occurred. Additionally, depression can be related to the site of the lesion. Treat as for primary depression while addressing rehabilitation needs.

## Epilepsy

Epilepsy is defined as recurrent (two or more) seizures, unprovoked by an immediate identifiable cause. There is an increased risk of psychiatric disorder in those with epilepsy, particularly in treatment-resistant epilepsy or in temporal lobe epilepsy. This may relate to the psychosocial burden and stigma of the illness, the physiological effects of epilepsy, or underlying brain abnormalities. Problems include cognitive impairment, psychotic symptoms, and learning disabilities. Depression is common (50%), and suicide rates are four times higher than in the general population (Gaitatzis *et al.* 2004).

## Systemic conditions and psychiatric symptoms

Many systemic conditions can present with psychiatric symptoms—Table 11.4 is not exhaustive!

**TABLE 11.4** Systemic conditions causing psychiatric symptoms

| | Systemic illnesses to consider |
|---|---|
| Depression | Addison's disease (hypoadrenalism)<br>B$_{12}$ deficiency<br>Corticosteroids<br>Cushing's syndrome (hyperadrenalism)<br>Hypo/hyperparathyroidism<br>Hypothyroidism<br>Systemic lupus erythematosus (SLE) |
| Mania | Corticosteroids<br>Cushing's syndrome<br>Hypothyroidism (rarely, 'myxoedema madness') |
| Anxiety | Hypoglycaemia<br>Hyperthyroidism<br>Phaeochromocytoma |
| Psychosis | Acute porphyria<br>Corticosteroids<br>Cushing's syndrome<br>Hypothyroidism (rare)<br>SLE |
| Dementia | Addison's disease<br>B$_{12}$ deficiency<br>Cushing's syndrome.<br>Folate deficiency<br>Hypo/hyperparathyroidism<br>Hypothyroidism |

# REALITY

## General approach: tips, tricks, and cautionary tales

This section focuses on working with *delirious* patients.

### 1. Behaviour is communication

When people can't express themselves verbally, they communicate *non-verbally*. On meeting a confused person with behavioural problems, ask yourself: *What are they trying to tell me?* Identify the underlying message, and engage your patient on *that* level. For example, rather than wrestling with a stick-wielding elderly man, you may realize that he feels threatened and ask: *What's scaring you?* This is more likely to stop the aggression than confiscating his stick.

> Wandering may communicate pain, boredom, a full bladder, a search for relatives, etc.

### 2. Cut out the competition

Delirium makes it hard to focus: information can't be filtered out or held onto easily, making the ever-changing environment overwhelming and distracting. You need to cut out the competing stimuli (e.g. the television) to let your patient focus on *you* and retain *your* message. Make the environment stable, calm and quiet, and then take centre stage.

### 3. Give them a clue

Repeatedly reorientate your patient to time, place, and person. Introduce yourself and remind them who you are every time you meet them; ensure that they wear their watch, glasses, and hearing aid if they have them; tell them the date and remind them they are in hospital. If visitors are due at certain times, leave messages to remind your patient of this, e.g. *Henry will visit at 2pm* (make sure that they have a clock nearby to check the time).

## 4. Comfort always

Being confused is frightening. Gently but firmly reassure your patient of their safety and your wish to help them feel better. Explain their situation and your actions, speaking clearly and simply, with a single idea in each sentence. Ensure they know how to get help: a working call button may stop someone screaming by reassuring them that staff can be contacted.

## 5. Recruit experts

Family and friends are comforting and can provide essential assistance on a busy ward. Explain the situation and what they can do, for example with calming and reorientation. They may also make sense of the patient's behaviour; for example, knowing that your patient was recently widowed may explain their wandering as a search for their lost partner.

## 6. Delirium's left hook

Confused and agitated patients may lash out. Seemingly frail elderly women can give you a lovely black eye, so be careful!

> Delirious patients are temporarily not 'themselves'. You need to protect them, their values, and their dignity until they recover and can do this for themselves again.

---

## 1. Frontal lobe testing (7 minutes)

### Candidate's instructions

Mr Bekir Kassim is a 35-year-old chemist who suffered a frontal subdural haematoma in a road traffic accident, five weeks ago. His wife now says he is a 'changed man'.

His consultant has asked you to perform bedside frontal lobe testing, before considering referral to a neuropsychologist.

### Patient's brief

*Key characteristics*

- I'm cheerful, flirtatious, and keen to follow instructions, but I am not aware of my mistakes.
- Hand movements: I repeat the first movement, over and over.
- Finger pointing test: I *copy* the examiner's movements.
- Word testing: I manage two or three different words or animals, and then keep returning to them.
- With proverbs, I give very uncreative, straightforward interpretations, e.g. 'Birds of a feather flock together': '*Birds with the same feathers stay together*'. I don't understand the metaphor.
- When asked to 'guess' amounts, I am *very* wrong! For example, a racehorse runs at 300 miles an hour.
- When the examiner strokes my:
  – palm, I grasp their hand;
  – lip, I purse my lips;
  – cheek, I turn my head towards their hand.

### Guidance for candidate: frontal lobe testing

There are many versions of these *screening* tests and only a few are given here. Record exactly what your patient does, since there are a number of ways of getting them wrong; this explains more than writing *failed*. Remember, formal testing is useful, but a collateral history and observation on the ward are *essential*.

*Set-shifting*

The Luria test assesses the ability to shift from one action or idea to another—a key component of sequencing and monitoring behaviour.

- Can you do this? Watch me . . .

  *Place one hand flat, palm upwards. With your other hand, make a sequence of three movements onto it: a fist, a slice ('karate chop'), and a slap.*

- Now do it with me . . . keep going until I say stop.

Once the patient has mastered it, they should manage three perfect cycles by themselves.

## Go–no-go task

This primarily assesses the ability to inhibit an inappropriate response (i.e. here the patient has the urge to copy you, but has to inhibit this and do the opposite). It also assesses set-shifting, as above.

- When I touch my nose, you raise your finger, like this.

  *Show patient: point to the ceiling with your right index finger.*

- And when I raise my finger, you touch your nose, like this.

  *Show patient: touch your nose with your right index finger.*

- It can be tricky. Can you explain what I just said?

  *Check your patient understands.*

- OK. Let's go . . .

Start with either move and see what your patient does. Leave your finger in place while waiting for a response. Make a sequence of a few moves before stopping.

## Verbal fluency

This primarily tests the ability to initiate the retrieval of words held in semantic memory. Normal ranges vary with age and premorbid ability, but as a rule of thumb, scoring less than 15 should raise concerns.

### 1. FAS testing

- I'm going to ask you to give me all the words you can, beginning with a certain letter. I can't accept people's names or place names, so if we were doing the letter B, I couldn't count Bob or Berlin. The words need to be different from each other, so I couldn't accept brave *and* braver or bravest. Keep going until I say stop. Does that make sense?

  *Check patient understands*

- OK, please give me words beginning with *F*. Go.

  *Time for a minute. Repeat for A and S.*

### 2. Animals in a minute

This is the one-minute alternative to FAS testing.

- Name all the animals you can think of, starting now.

## Abstract reasoning

These test reasoning and abstract thinking. Concrete interpretation of proverbs suggests frontal lobe pathology. In cognitive estimates, the patient needs to make *reasonable guesses* for things that they are unlikely to know, using relevant information in their knowledge (e.g. how fast a car can move compared with a racehorse). Frontal impairment produces extreme answers.

### 1. Proverbs

- Some phrases have a hidden meaning. For example, *too many cooks spoil the broth* isn't actually about cooks—it means that jobs aren't done well when too many people are involved. Does that make sense to you? *(Check)* Can you think of a hidden meaning for these . . . ?
- Birds of a feather flock together.
- A stitch in time saves nine.
- People in glass houses shouldn't throw stones.

➜ **Many proverbs don't translate across cultures, and some aren't understood by healthy people anyway! Concrete interpretation also occurs in people with schizophrenia, autism, and learning disability.**

### 2. Cognitive estimates

Please give me your best guesses to these questions . . .

- How fast can a racehorse run?
- What is the best paid job in this country?
- How many camels are there in Holland?
- How many eyelashes are on your lower eyelid? (Out of interest, the actual answer is 60.)

## Primitive reflexes

Frontal lobes inhibit the primitive reflexes we all had as babies; if damaged, these reflexes may re-emerge.

- Could you hold your hands out, please?

  *Stroke across the patient's palm towards their thumb.* (Grasp reflex)

- Could I touch your face, please?

  *Lightly tap the patient's lips or stroke down their philtrum.* (Suck/pout reflex)

  *Stroke the patient's cheek with your finger.* (Rooting reflex)

# NEXT STEPS

## Fitness to drive and multiple sclerosis

You are a junior doctor in the neurology outpatient clinic. Mrs Sharma is a 38-year-old teacher who was diagnosed last year with multiple sclerosis. She recently relapsed, so her GP started high-dose oral steroids and arranged for her to be urgently reviewed in clinic.

Mrs Sharma is ushered in, ahead of two patients who were due to be seen before her, as she was becoming disruptive in the waiting room. She explains that she has been taking steroids for five days and now feels 'great'. She is restless, talkative, and giggly, referring to you by your first name. She mentions that she thought she was going to be late but managed to 'put her foot down' on the main road and hence arrived on time.

1. What could be happening in this situation and what will you do?
2. What are your duties regarding Mrs Sharma's driving?

### Issues

- Assessment of current physical and mental state
- Diagnosis
- Risk assessment
- Management

### Immediate assessment and management

You need to perform a psychiatric history, mental state examination, and physical examination to gain clues to the cause of her presentation. The steroids treating her relapse may now be precipitating a manic episode. Other possible causes for elated mood could be the MS itself, other organic causes (e.g. substance misuse), or a *functional* illness (i.e. mania without an organic cause). Look for clinical features and risks associated with a manic episode, in particular considering whether Mrs Sharma is able to manage at home with the support of her family or whether she needs a brief admission to a psychiatric or medical bed. The decision to admit will be based on the risk assessment and in consultation with Mr and Mrs Sharma.

The most likely diagnosis is that of an organic mood disorder. She is currently *hypomanic* since there is elated mood without marked loss of function. You should seek advice from your consultant as well as a liaison psychiatrist regarding Mrs Sharma's management. If the acute MS relapse has been treated adequately and underlying causes (e.g. infection) excluded, her steroids should be stopped and a mood stabilizer considered (see p.43). The psychiatrist will advise on mood stabilizers and can arrange a psychiatric admission or involve community psychiatric services if it is agreed that Mrs Sharma can return home today.

Longer term, there should be careful discussion between neurologists, psychiatrists, and her GP because of the high risk of relapse in her mental state; she will be very susceptible to steroids in future, and this drug reaction must be documented clearly in medical notes, letters, and drug charts. Additionally, CBT should be provided to address her hypomanic episode, e.g. awareness of relapse indicators. Psychological support would be beneficial regarding two recent life events: diagnoses of both mental illness *and* a chronic progressive neurological condition.

### Driving

The subject of driving often arises. Doctors who don't think to ask or give advice about driving remain blissfully unaware of this minefield, but are negligent in their duties to their patients and society at large. You should find out how Mrs Sharma and her husband understand the law regarding her driving status and what action she has taken so far. She should have already contacted the Driver and Vehicle Licensing Agency (DVLA)[2] in the UK (or appropriate body in your country) to notify them of her MS. If you believe that she has been driving when she was not safe, for physical or mental health reasons, you have a duty to inform her of this and encourage her to contact the DVLA herself. If she continues to drive, you must contact the DVLA on her behalf, letting her know of your responsibility to do this. In extreme cases a doctor may have to call the police to prevent their patient from driving while grossly unfit to do so.

Mrs Sharma's hypomania prevents her from driving safely and she should be informed of this. You must ensure that she makes arrangements to return home safely (e.g. by taxi) and advise her not to drive until she has been well and stable for at least three months.

> Your patient may be fit to drive when they leave your clinic, until they take the tablets you have just prescribed! Always advise patients not to drive if they feel affected by medication side effects (particularly sedation and coordination problems). Many psychotropic medications are sedative.

### Film list

*Memento* (2000): amnesic syndrome following head injury.

*Hilary and Jackie* (1998): cellist Jacqueline du Pre's increasingly erratic behaviour may be explained as frontal lobe syndrome secondary to MS.

*The Madness of King George* (1994): mental illness, possibly due to acute porphyria.

*Regarding Henry* (1991): personality change following head injury.

*Awakenings* (1990): catatonia and parkinsonism following encephalitis lethargica.

### Books

Amis, M. (2003) *Yellow Dog*. London: Jonathan Cape. Post-head injury personality changes—in particular, the destruction of previously held ethical values.

Dostoevsky, F. (1868) *The Idiot*. Translated and edited by A. Myers. New York: Oxford University Press. The life of a man with epilepsy, with a particularly good description of prodromal symptoms.

Garland, A. (2004) *The Coma*. London: Faber & Faber. Novel exploring post-head-injury consciousness, examining existential themes around what differentiates the mind from the brain.

McEwan, I. *Saturday* (2005) Describes the near-fatal encounter between a neurosurgeon and a man with Huntington's disease.

Sacks, O. (1985) *The Man Who Mistook His Wife for a Hat, and Other Clinical Tales*. Summit Books. Precise but patient-centred accounts of neuro-psychiatric conditions.

### Quotes

We know the human brain is a device to keep the ears from grating on one another.
**Comfort Me with Apples**, Peter de Vries

I like nonsense; it wakes up the brain cells.
**Dr Seuss**

The surgeon knows all the parts of the brain but he does not know his patient's dreams.
**Mortal Lessons**, Richard Selzer

## Notes

1. Garland, A. (2004). *The Coma*. London: Faber & Faber.
2. Driver and Vehicle Licensing Agency. For guidance refer to their *Guide to the Current Medical Standards of Fitness to Drive*'. http://www.dvla.gov.uk/medical/ataglance.aspx

## References/Further reading

Aarsland, D., Andersen K., Larsen, J.P., *et al.* (2003) Prevalence and characteristics of dementia in Parkinson disease: an 8-year prospective study. *Archives of Neurology*, **60**, 387–92.

Burns, A., Gallagley, A., and Byrne, J. (2004) Delirium. *Journal of Neurology, Neurosurgery, and Psychiatry*, **75**, 362–7.

Cummings, J.L. and Trimble, M.R. (2002) *Neuropsychiatry and Behavioural Neurology* (2nd edn). Washington, DC: American Psychiatric Publishing.

Dilley, M. and Fleminger, S. (2006) Advances in neuropsychiatry: clinical implications. *Advances in Psychiatric Treatment*, **12**, 23–34.

Eisenberg, L. (1986) Mindlessness and brainlessness in psychiatry. *British Journal of Psychiatry*, **148**, 497–508.

Gaitatzis, A., Trimble, M.R., and Sander, J.W. (2004) The psychiatric comorbidity of epilepsy. *Acta Neurologica Scandinavica*, **110**, 207–20.

Harlow, J.M. (1848) Passage of an iron rod through the head. *Boston Medical and Surgical Journal*, **39**, 389–93.

Harlow, J.M. (1868) Recovery from the passage of an iron bar through the head. *Publications of the Massachusetts Medical Society*, **2**, 327–47.

Hodges, J.R. (1994) *Cognitive Assessment for Clinicians*. Oxford; Oxford Medical Publications.

Inouye, S.K., Rushing, J.T., Foreman, M.D., *et al.* (1998) Does delirium contribute to poor hospital outcomes? A three-site epidemiologic study. *Journal of General Internal Medicine*, **13**, 234–42.

Jefferies, K. (2006) The neuropsychiatry of multiple sclerosis. *Advances in Psychiatric Treatment*, **12**, 214–20.

Korsakoff, S.S. (1889) Psychic disorder in conjunction with multiple neuritis (English translation with commentary). *Neurology* **5**, 394–406, 1955.

Manji, H. and Miller, R. (2004) The neurology of HIV infection. *Journal of Neurology, Neurosurgery, and Psychiatry*, **75** (Suppl 1), i29–35.

Price, B., Adams, R., and Coyle, J. (2000) Neurology and psychiatry; closing the great divide. *Neurology*, **54**, 8–14.

Slater, E. (1963) The schizophrenia-like psychoses of epilepsy. *British Journal of Psychiatry*, **109**, 95–112.

Snowden, J. and Neary, D. (2002) Frontotemporal dementia. *British Journal of Psychiatry*, **180**, 140–3.

Will, R.G., Ironside, J.W., Zeidler, M., *et al.* (1996) A new variant of Creutzfeldt–Jakob disease in the UK. *Lancet*, **347**, 921–5.

Young, L.J. and George, J. (2003) Do guidelines improve the process and outcomes of care in delirium? *Age and Ageing*, **32**, 525–8.

 Go to www.oxfordtextbooks/orc/stringer for an array of additional references, including indicative mark sheets for OSCEs, self-assessment questions, guidance, and exercises.

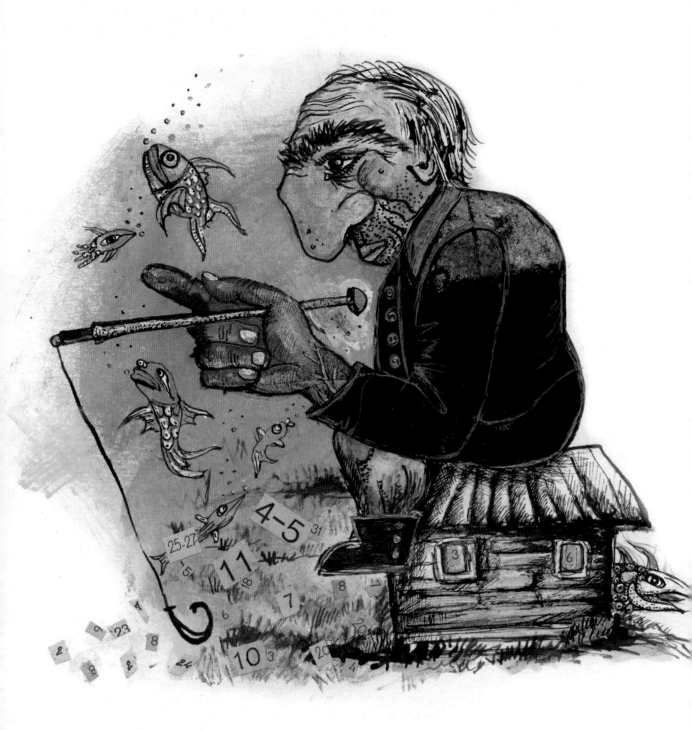

# 12 Old age psychi

*Sarah Stringer and Alice M. Roberts*

## True or False? Test your existing knowledge—answers in the chapter and online

1. Dementia with Lewy bodies is characterised by stable cognitive impairment with parkinsonism and psychotic symptoms.

2. Cognitive behavioural therapy is of limited value in depressed people over the age of 75.

3. Female sex, poor hearing, and social isolation all increase the risk of developing late onset schizophrenia.

4. Amyloid plaques and neurofibrillary tangles are implicated in the pathology of Alzheimer's disease.

5. Dysphasia is more indicative of dementia with Lewy bodies than of vascular dementia.

6. Low doses of antipsychotics are useful in the management of dementia with Lewy bodies.

7. Trazodone is an acetylcholinesterase inhibitor used to slow the progression of Alzheimer's disease.

8. Social isolation, physical disability, and male sex are all characteristics which increase a person's risk of being a victim of elder abuse.

9. The majority of patients over 80 years of age will require you to speak in very simple, short sentences.

10. A 78 year old woman has fallen for the fourth time at home. She accepts that she often falls but maintains that she wants to go home. A Mini Mental State Examination will ultimately decide whether or not she lacks capacity to make this decision.

## Contents

'That's not Mother. She still knows who she is. She may not talk correctly, but she's still able to take part in a conversation. She still has her social skills.'

The doctor is good-naturedly persistent. 'Her prosodic variation is still intact.'

It's the word 'still' that bothers me. 'You keep telling me what has been lost, and I keep telling you something remains.'

*Scar Tissue*—Michael Ignatieff[1]

## Introduction

The mental health of older adults (MHOA) has arisen as a separate speciality because of the particular needs and vulnerabilities of elderly people (65+ years). MHOA teams are experts in dementia and skilled in managing cases with a complex interplay of social, physical, and mental health problems. The crux of old age psychiatry is not the symptoms *per se*, but how these symptoms affect a person's everyday life and ability to function. MHOA teams usually assess older people at home, since this gives a realistic view of how they are managing in their own environment. Teams then utilize the skills of social workers, specialist nurses, psychologists, occupational therapists, and psychiatrists—in conjunction with carers—to keep people in their own homes for as long as possible. Their emphasis is on quality of life.

---

**BOX 12.1  To optimize your reading**

Old Age Psychiatry deals with *any* mental illness in old age. Problems such as depression, anxiety, and psychosis are covered only briefly, but are comprehensively discussed in their own chapters. Read *with* this one for best effect! You will also benefit from referring to the chapter dedicated to organic psychiatry as you explore old age psychiatry.

---

## Depression

Fifteen per cent of older people in the community are depressed at any time, but this rises to 30% in hospitals. Problems such as multiple bereavements, social isolation, poverty, physical illness, and chronic pain are more common in older adults, playing an important aetiological role in depression. The presentation is similar to that of younger people, although there may be more obvious:

- physical symptoms (e.g. constipation)
- agitation or retardation
- memory problems (and pseudodementia).

There is a high risk of completed suicide, particularly in men; always take suicidal ideation seriously. Risks of self-neglect and poor food and fluid intake are extremely important in older depressed people. It's important to follow-up people who suffer pseudodementia, since they are at higher risk of developing actual dementia.

Management is similar to that of younger patients.

1. Problem-solving, increasing socialization and daytime activities.
2. Psychological therapies, e.g. cognitive behavioural therapy (CBT), psychodynamic, group, family or couple therapy.
3. Antidepressants: selective serotonin reuptake inhibitors (SSRIs) are usually first line (e.g. citalopram).
4. Electroconvulsive therapy (ECT) is sometimes used for psychotic or life-threatening depression.

See p.32 for depression, and p.59 for suicide and self-harm.

> SSRIs may cause hyponatraemia in the elderly, so remember to check sodium levels.

## Anxiety disorders

The prevalence and incidence of anxiety disorders fall with age, possibly because of under-reporting. They remain more common in women and in those who are isolated or have suffered adverse life events. Management is usually psychological (CBT), although SSRIs can be useful.

## Psychosis

Psychotic symptoms can occur in many conditions in older people (e.g. delirium, dementia) or secondary to sensory impairment.

**Late-onset schizophrenia** (late-onset psychosis/ paraphrenia) is more common in women—especially isolated, single, widowed, or childless. Sensory deficits are a risk factor. Positive symptoms (delusions and hallucinations) are more prominent than negative symptoms.

Management involves reduction of sensory impairment, exclusion of an organic cause or Lewy body dementia (see later), and then low-dose antipsychotics. See p.73 for more on schizophrenia.

 Charles Bonnet syndrome: complex visual hallucinations, secondary to visual impairment alone.

## Dementia

Dementia is not a normal part of ageing. It is an acquired, chronic, and progressive cognitive impairment, sufficient to impair activities of daily living (ADLs) (Box 12.2). The effect of dementia on ADLs is an important part of the assessment since a low Mini Mental State Examination (MMSE) score alone does not diagnose dementia (Box 12.3). For a confident diagnosis, problems should have been present in *clear consciousness* for at least six months.

---

**BOX 12.2 Activities of daily living**

- Financial management
- Using the toilet
- Washing
- Dressing
- Grooming
- Shopping
- Cooking
- Housework
- Mobilizing/transfers/stairs

---

**BOX 12.3 Causes of a low MMSE score**

- Dementia
- Delirium
- Most psychiatric illnesses, e.g. depression, anxiety, psychosis
- Learning disability
- Sensory impairment
- Language barrier
- Feeling unwell, tired, irritable

---

 See the ORC for an MMSE role-play, score sheet, and guidelines for asking the questions.

### Epidemiology

The risk of dementia increases with age and the prevalence is:

- 5% over 65 years
- 20% over 80 years.

Alzheimer's disease (AD) is the most common type, accounting for around two-thirds of cases. Next most common is vascular dementia (VD), and then dementia with Lewy bodies (DLB).

>> *Early onset (<65 years) dementias are discussed in Chapter 11.*

### Clinical features

Dementia often begins with forgetfulness, principally for recent events. There may be mild mistakes in day-to-day activities (e.g. muddling up appointments, mislaying items). Initial problems are often attributed to normal ageing or absent-mindedness. Anxiety or depression may occur early, especially when insight is intact. Forgetfulness worsens over time and new information becomes harder to retain. Disorientation sets in—for time, then place, and finally person. People with dementia may confuse day and night, become lost easily, or fail to recognize family and friends. Increasingly, people become less independent, needing more help with ADLs. Thinking and language become impoverished; mood and personality are also affected.

Subjectively, dementia can make the world incomprehensible; this is very distressing when someone was previously independent.

Eventually, behavioural or psychiatric problems may arise, making management at home difficult. Problems include:

- wandering
- sleep disturbance/day-night reversal
- delusions
- hallucinations
- calling out, shouting, screaming, swearing
- inappropriate behaviour, including sexual disinhibition
- aggression.

### Alzheimer's disease (AD)

#### Aetiology

1. **Age** is the main risk factor for AD. It is marginally more common in women.

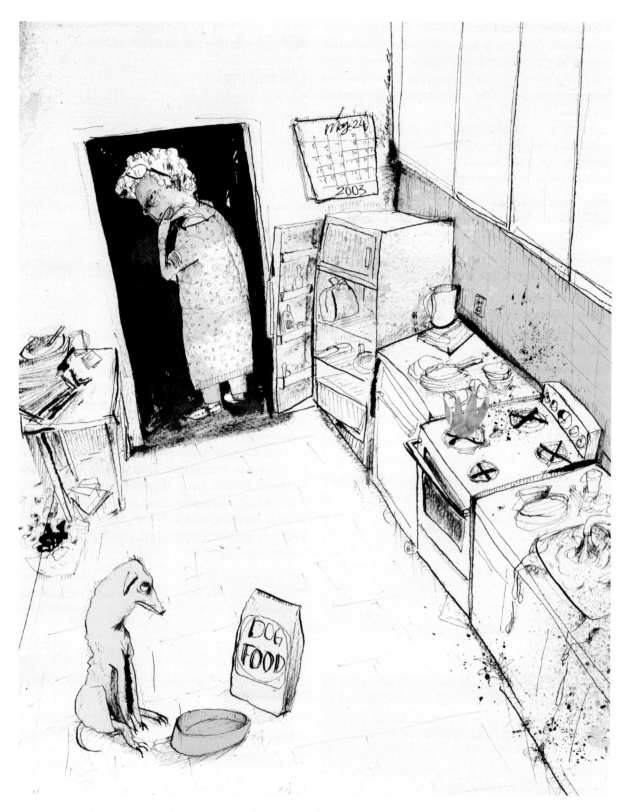

**FIGURE 12.1** If you were carrying out a home visit, what risks would you identify from viewing this woman's kitchen? How would you manage them?

2. **Genetics** Familial early-onset AD is usually due to rare autosomal dominant gene mutations causing increased β-amyloid. Mutations include:

- Presenilin 1 gene (chromosome 14)
- Presenilin 2 gene (chromosome 1)
- Beta-amyloid precursor protein (APP) gene (chromosome 21).

Late-onset (>65 years) AD is associated with the Apolipoprotein E4 allele (chromosome 19). The exact mechanism is yet unknown, though E4 increases early arteriosclerosis.

3. **Vascular risk factors**, e.g. hypertension
4. **Low IQ/poor educational level**
5. **Head injury**

➜ Children of people with dementia should know that *late onset* is less worrying than *early onset* in terms of inherited risk.

🔑 People with Down syndrome are at high risk of AD by middle age, probably because of the extra copy of the APP gene in trisomy 21.

## Pathology

The key elements are:

1. **Atrophy** due to neuronal loss. The hippocampus, essential for new learning and visuospatial skills, is affected early; temporal and parietal lobes later. On CT scans the natural spaces of the brain (sulci and ventricles) may be enlarged, although this occurs in normal ageing and so is not diagnostic.

2. **Plaque formation** APP can be abnormally cleaved into β-amyloid, which aggregates into insoluble lumps. These form the core of the plaques and are surrounded by dystrophic neurites that are filled with hyperphosphorylated tau protein.

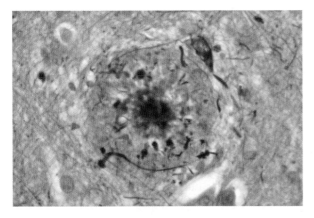

**FIGURE 12.2** AD plaque (silver stain) (by kind permission of Dr Andrew King)

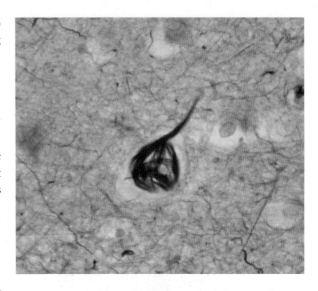

**FIGURE 12.3** AD neurofibrillary tangle (silver stain) (by kind permission of Dr Andrew King)

3. Intracellular **neurofibrillary tangles** (NFTs). These are made of abnormal (hyperphosphorylated) tau protein. Tau usually holds microtubules together within a neuron, but when phosphorylated it cannot attach to microtubules and so accumulates in the cell as insoluble paired helical filaments. These become tangles, which fill up the neuron and kill it. The severity of dementia is most closely associated with the number of NFTs.

4. **Cholinergic loss** Cholinergic pathways are most affected in AD.

## Clinical presentation: the four A's

- **A**mnesia: recent memories are lost first, disorientation occurs early.
- **A**phasia: word-finding problems occur; speech can become muddled and disjointed.
- **A**gnosia: recognition problems, e.g. faces (prosopagnosia)
- **A**praxia: inability to carry out skilled tasks despite normal motor function, e.g. dressing.

The personality may erode as these features progress.

## Vascular dementia (VD)

VD is due to infarcts caused by thrombo-embolus or arteriosclerosis ('stroke-related dementia'). Risk factors are the same as stroke disease (e.g. older age, male sex, smoking, hypertension, diabetes, hypercholesterolaemia, atrial fibrillation). The history may reveal other signs of arteriosclerosis, e.g. heart attacks or transient ischaemic attacks.

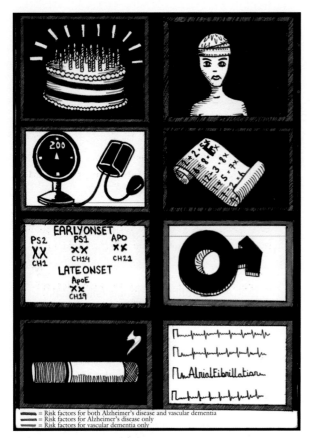

FIGURE 12.4 Risk factors for dementia

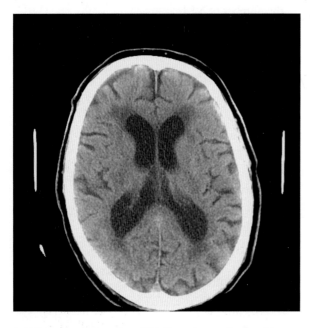

FIGURE 12.5 CT head multi-infarct dementia: on this non-contrast scan there are areas of lower density adjacent to the anterior and posterior horns of the lateral ventricles, which are due to chronic ischaemia (by kind permission of Dr Mona Sriharan)

### Pathology

Arteriosclerosis, cortical ischaemia, and infarction are the key points. The latter appear on CT scans as multiple lucencies.

### Clinical presentation

Classically, VD has a stepwise progression, with each 'step' representing a sudden deterioration as an infarct occurs (Figure 12.6). Many tiny infarcts cause a smoother, more subtle deterioration. Sometimes, one strategically located stroke can cause dementia (strategic infarct dementia). Symptoms reflect the sites of lesions and therefore the presentation may be 'patchy' with personality and some areas of cognition being spared. Neurological signs such as hemiparesis or aphasia may be present, and there may be episodes of confusion (especially at night).

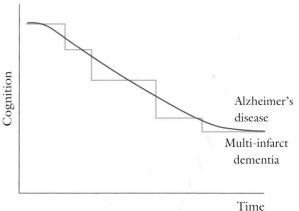

FIGURE 12.6 Gradual (AD) and stepwise (VD) cognitive decline

## Dementia with Lewy bodies (DLB)

This is probably greatly underdiagnosed. Risk factors are unknown.

### Pathology

Lewy bodies are eosinophilic intracytoplasmic neuronal structures. They are composed of α-synuclein with ubiquitin. In Parkinson's disease (PD) they are found in the brainstem, but in DLB they are also seen in the cyngulate gyrus and neocortex. DLB is therefore one end of the spectrum of Lewy body diseases which includes PD (see p.125).

### Clinical presentation

Two of the following three symptoms should alert you to the possibility of DLB (McKeith *et al.* 2005):

• fluctuating confusion with marked variation in levels of alertness

• vivid visual hallucinations (often of people or animals)

• spontaneous (new) parkinsonian signs.

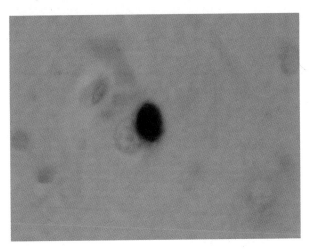

FIGURE 12.7 A cortical Lewy body from the temporal lobe of a patient with DLB. The immunohistochemistry is for α-synuclein (by kind permission of Dr Andrew King)

It can be hard to diagnose, especially if parkinsonian signs are late to present. Other suggestive features include repeated falls, syncope, and transient losses of consciousness. Short-term memory is less affected. DLB can resemble delirium (due to fluctuating cognition with visual hallucinations), but you *must not* prescribe antipsychotics (e.g. haloperidol). Extreme antipsychotic (neuroleptic) sensitivity in DLB can result in death!

 The 'mirror sign' is sometimes seen in dementia. Sufferers no longer recognize their own reflection (autoprosopagnosia).

*Sun-downing*: confusion in dementia often worsens as evening draws in. The exact cause is unknown, but may relate to the increased risk of illusions in poor light and when tired.

Memorize this book at the gym—being educated and physically active protect against AD.

TABLE 12.1 Summary of Alzheimer's disease, vascular dementia, and dementia with Lewy bodies

|  | Alzheimer's disease | Vascular dementia | DLB |
|---|---|---|---|
| Risk factors | Age<br>Vascular risk factors<br>Low IQ/poorly educated<br>Head injury<br>FHx *early* onset (Presenilin 1 and 2; APP)<br>Late onset (ApoE E4 allele) | Age<br>Vascular risk factors | Age<br>Largely unknown |
| Histopathology | Plaques and tangles<br>Neuronal loss, especially cholinergic | Multiple cortical infarcts<br>Arteriosclerosis | Lewy bodies |
| Onset | Insidious | Sudden | Varies |
| Course | Gradual decline | Stepwise decline | Gradual decline |
| Main features | The 4 As:<br>Amnesia<br>Aphasia<br>Agnosia<br>Apraxia | Patchy cognitive impairment | Fluctuating cognition<br>Visual hallucinations<br>Parkinsonian symptoms |
| Affect | Depression or anxiety (early)<br>Flattened affect (later) | Depression<br>Lability | Depression |
| Personality | Eroded: 'It's just not Mum anymore'<br>Socially withdrawn | Relatively preserved | More apathetic |
| Other suggestive features | *Absence* of physical signs | Focal neurology | Neuroleptic sensitivity<br>Autonomic instability<br>Recurrent falls<br>Syncope |
| CT changes | Generalized atrophy, especially medial temporal and parietal | Multiple lucencies<br>Atrophy | Mild atrophy (less than AD) |

## Differential diagnosis

1. **Delirium**: presents *suddenly* with altered or 'clouded' consciousness—losing touch with surroundings (poor attention is a good marker of this). The presentation usually fluctuates and there may be evidence of underlying physical problems; symptoms resolve once the underlying cause is treated (see p.117).

2. **'Reversible' dementias**: present with cognitive impairment that may resolve if treated. For example:
   - Brain: subdural haematoma, space-occupying lesion, normal pressure hydrocephalus.
   - Endocrine: hypothyroidism, hyperparathyroidism, Addison's disease, Cushing's syndrome.
   - Vitamin deficiency: $B_{12}$, folate, thiamine, niacin.

3. **Pseudodementia**: memory problems in severe depression can resemble dementia. In depression, low mood usually *precedes* cognitive problems; there may be a past history of depression. Depressed people lack motivation to answer questions, commonly saying, 'I don't know'. People with dementia are often keen but make mistakes.

> If someone presents for the first time in later life with *any* psychiatric illness, rule-out an underlying organic cause.

## Investigations

1. Basic observations and physical examination.
2. Blood tests:
   - FBC (infection/anaemia)
   - U&Es (dehydration/renal failure/hyponatraemia)
   - Glucose
   - TFTs (hypothyroidism can mimic dementia)
   - LFTs (abnormalities may suggest alcohol misuse —a risk factor for falls and subdural haematomas, alcohol-related dementia, or Korsakoff's syndrome)
   - $B_{12}$ and folate (deficiencies can cause reversible dementias)
   - Calcium levels
   - VDRL (neurosyphilis can cause cognitive impairment).
3. MMSE.
4. Collateral history.
5. Septic screen: MSU (exclude UTI); chest X-ray, blood cultures, wound swabs, sputum/stool samples as suggested by symptoms.
6. CT or MRI head if:
   - unusual presentation/neurological signs

- first onset of psychotic symptoms later in life (especially olfactory/visual hallucinations)
- planning to start anti-dementia medication.

## Management

Although dementia cannot be cured, management focuses on quality of life and preservation of independence and dignity. The MHOA team works closely with GPs, social services, voluntary groups, and carers, providing a multidisciplinary approach to management.

1. **Adaptations for patients**
   - Always carry ID, address, and contact number in case of getting lost.
   - Dossett boxes/blister packs to aid medication compliance.
   - Change gas to electricity (to decrease risks of the gas being accidentally left on).
   - Reality orientation: visible clocks, calendars, etc.
   - Environmental modifications, e.g. patterned carpets can predispose to visual hallucinations.
   - Assistive technology, e.g. door mat buzzers alert relatives to wandering.

2. **Social support**
   - Personal care, meal preparation, or medication prompting.
   - Day centres provide enjoyable daytime activities and social contact.
   - Day hospitals enable daily psychiatric care for more complex patients.

3. **Support carers**
   - *Emotional* support.
   - *Educate* about dementia.
   - *Train* to manage common problems.
   - *Provide respite care*, e.g. sitting services/temporary placements.

> Partners often soldier on, in very difficult circumstances, as they do not consider themselves 'a carer'; a carer's assessment should be a routine part of your work.

4. **Optimize physical health**
   - Treat sensory impairment (hearing aids, glasses).
   - Exclude superimposed delirium.
   - Treat underlying risk factors, e.g. with antihypertensives, statins.
   - Review all medication, prescribed and non-prescribed: some non-psychotropic medications can impair cognition in dementia patients because of anticholinergic effects.

## 5. Psychological therapies

- *Behavioural approaches*: identify and modify underlying triggers for difficult or risky behaviours, e.g.:
  - Wandering may be due to disorientation, boredom, anxiety, pain, hunger, or needing the toilet. Providing regular food or a calm environment may resolve it.
- *Reminiscence therapy*: talking about 'the old days' enhances a sense of belonging, reinforces identity, and builds confidence.
- *Validation therapy*: reassure and validate the emotion behind what is said, e.g. if your patient is looking for their mother, recognize the possible underlying need for reassurance.
- *Multisensory therapy*: as dementia advances and speech is lost, it may be easier to respond to touch, music, etc.
- *Cognitive stimulation therapy*: memory training and relearning.

## 6. Psychotropic medications:

The golden rule for prescribing in older adults is: *start low, go slow*. Remember, older people are often very sensitive to drug side effects.

- Treat comorbid psychiatric illness, e.g. antidepressants if depressed.
- Acetylcholinesterase inhibitors (ACIs), e.g. donepezil, rivastigmine. These drugs prevent acetylcholinesterase destroying the acetylcholine, increasing neurotransmitter levels in the synapse and compensating for the overall cholinergic loss. They don't cure dementia, but are used as 'brakes' in AD and DLB (Courtney *et al.* 2004).

- Drugs are a last resort in the management of behavioural disturbance, e.g. trazodone (sedative antidepressant), sodium valproate, low dose antipsychotics or benzodiazepines (Howard 2003).

> It's hard to be concordant with medication if you don't *remember* you need tablets, can't *read* the instructions, and can't *open* the bottles. Ask to *see* the patient's medications—this may be very revealing!

> Avoid using risperidone or olanzapine to treat behavioural symptoms in dementia—they increase the risk of stroke.

## Prognosis

Two-thirds of people with dementia live in their own home or with a carer. As dementia progresses, increasing levels of help may be needed. People should be supported to stay in their own homes for as long as possible. Placement in a nursing home is never the first solution to problems, but should be considered as part of a stepwise approach to increased levels of need; GP and MHOA in-reach support is extremely important in care homes. Elderly mentally infirm (EMI) placements care for the small proportion of people with otherwise unmanageable behavioural problems.

> Elder abuse in the form of neglect or psychological, financial, physical, or sexual abuse is more likely to occur in victims who are female, living alone with the abuser, and depending on them for physical and mental health needs. Look for signs of bruising, neglect of diet and personal care, and changes in behaviour. Carers are more likely to abuse if they are socially isolated, unsupported, mentally ill (e.g. depressed, substance misuse), or have a personal history of childhood abuse. Concerns should be reported to social services. Support should be offered to the carer, who may be overwhelmed. You should also be alert to elder abuse within care homes: poor supervision and training of staff working in isolation can be risk factors for abuse in institutions.

# REALITY

## General approach: tips, tricks, and cautionary tales

### 1. Basics

Home visits are the gold standard to see how someone copes in their own environment. If you can't do a home visit, ask as much as possible about their home situation. Speak with a collateral historian (with permission), e.g. family, day care centre staff. Always check that your patient can hear and see you (provide them with their hearing aids and glasses if needed). Before starting, remove distractions, e.g. turn off the television.

### 2. Hearing problems

Don't shout! Many people lip-read to some extent, so don't cover your mouth. Speak clearly and slightly slowly, sitting on the side of their better ear. When speaking to carers, keep your face in view of your *patient* or they won't follow the conversation. Presbyacusis affects high-pitched noises most, so speaking in a slightly deeper voice can help. If still no luck, try writing down short questions.

### 3. Visual problems

Don't sneak up on patients; sit close with good lighting.

### 4. Speech problems

Ask relatives and carers to help if you can't understand someone. Dentures aid clarity; see if they have any teeth! Ask *them* to slow down. Dysphasias are tricky for both of you: use short sentences and repeat what they say back to them to ensure you understood correctly.

### 5. Extra considerations in cognitive impairment

Remember that 80% of the over-eighties are *not* suffering from dementia—it seems patronising if you use this as an approach to *all* elderly people. For the 20% with cognitive problems, keep your message simple, and speak slowly and clearly. If you are not understood the first time, repeat yourself exactly—people with dementia take time to process information and different phrasing can further confuse. If this doesn't work, use simpler closed and clarifying questions.

**You:** What did you do for a living?

**Molly:** ?

**Y:** What did you do for a living?

**M:** ?

**Y:** Did you work?

**M:** Yes.

**Y:** What did you do?

**M:** I was a ballet dancer.

Be encouraging. If your patient becomes distressed over their poor memory, try exploring areas of the history that are easier (e.g. childhood/early adulthood memories).

### 6. No sweethearts

More often than with younger patients, elderly people prefer to be addressed formally (e.g. Mr Smith)—how they would have been addressed throughout their life. The idea of being addressed by first name or a 'sweet' term, such as *Honey*, *Dear*, *Poppet*, or *Love*, by a complete stranger is rude and patronising.

➤ Accept a cup of tea if offered. It builds rapport and tells you a lot about functioning! If it's served cold with the kitchen plug instead of a teabag, your host needs help around the house (or wants you to leave).

## 1. History of memory loss (10 minutes)

### Candidate instructions

Thomas Locke is the 66-year-old deputy manager of a sports shop. He has come to see the GP at the request of his manager, who is worried about his memory. You are a third-year medical student at the practice.
   Please take a history of memory loss.

### Patient instructions
*Key characteristics*

- I don't remember exact details and need to be asked directly about most symptoms to remember that they have been a problem.
- I feel frustrated when I can't remember things.
- I have problems finding the right word sometimes.
- I'm fairly happy otherwise—just worried.

My manager called me in for a chat two weeks ago. He'd noticed I'd been making mistakes for a few months, like not setting the alarm each evening and forgetting to re-order stock. He wasn't angry but wanted to know if there was anything on my mind. When I couldn't think of anything, he said I should see the GP. I'm one of the best employees he's ever had and the firm doesn't want me to retire!

When I told my partner (Geoffrey), he admitted he'd also been worried for about 6 months. He's noticed I go shopping and come home with completely random things, forgetting the important items I'd gone out for. He said I kept losing my keys and reminded me I'd locked myself out a few times (unusual for me). We attended a party last week and Geoffrey said I couldn't remember much about the conversations afterwards.

I've started writing things down so that I don't forget them, like the names of Saturday staff and a 'to do' list at work. I've even started taking notes on *EastEnders*, because I can't follow the storylines. I've only got lost once, when Geoffrey and I drove to Guildford a few weeks ago. We split up to shop and agreed to meet at the car park but I couldn't find my way back and had to call him to find me.

I don't have any problems with the names of people I've known for years, and can remember old memories as clearly as if they'd happened yesterday. I'm not depressed —life is good . . . as far as I can remember! My energy levels are good and I really enjoy my time with Geoffrey— especially gardening together. I look after myself, but Geoffrey is taking over the cooking and shopping because I make mistakes. He hasn't mentioned a change in my mood or personality.

*Other history:*

- My older brother, Jack, got Alzheimer's in his late fifties. He died in a nursing home at 63.
- Nobody in my family, including me, has suffered any mental illness.
- I have high blood pressure and take tablets for this.
- I smoke 20 cigarettes a day and drink 2 pints of beer a week, but don't use drugs.

*Questions*

What happens next?

*Worries*

I'm losing my memory like my brother.
I'll end up in a home.

## 2. Collateral history of memory loss (10 minutes)

### Candidate's instructions

Naomi Walters is a 21-year-old bank clerk who lives with her grandmother. She has brought her grandmother to the GP because she is worried about her memory. You are a medical student working with the GP.

You will see Naomi while the GP examines her grandmother. Please take a collateral history of memory impairment.

### Patient's brief

*Key characteristics*

- I'm worried about how much Gran's gone downhill and whether I can cope with her.
- I'm tired and need help.
- I'm tearful at times.
- I feel like I'm letting Gran down.

I moved in with Gran about eight months ago as she'd been finding it difficult on her own. I remember she locked herself out after shopping in December and got really distressed. She's always been a great cook and entertained the whole family for Christmas dinner every year for as long as I can remember. This year she couldn't get the timings right and all we had was roast potatoes. That wasn't like her. We had a family meeting and we decided I'd move in with her to help out. Her memory seems to have taken sharp drops downhill. It was perfect until about nine months ago, when there was a sudden drop about November. She suddenly got a lot worse in March, but she's stayed at that level since then.

I have to wash and dress her. It's not that she can't physically do it, but she can't organize herself and wouldn't remember it needed doing. I do all the cooking and shopping. She comes shopping with me but I keep a close eye on her because she gets lost easily, even though she's lived here her whole life. Gran sometimes confuses me with my mum and calls me Julia.

She has too much energy—she's always pacing around the house. She's not been trying to get out, but I keep finding her in the kitchen, trying to cook a meal in the middle of the night. We've got a gas stove and I worry she'll try to cook on it (she hasn't, so far). She's wet herself a couple of times and it's really upset her. Sometimes she gets really scared and says she sees 'spirits' but I can't see anything. Otherwise, she seems fairly happy and enjoys pottering about the house.

*Other history*

- Gran's never had any mental health problems before this.

- She had two 'mini strokes' last autumn: one side went limp and her speech was slurred. She got better each time within a few hours. Gran's had high blood pressure and diabetes for years.
- She takes aspirin, a water tablet, and insulin injections.
- My great-grandmother died of a heart attack.
- She's never smoked or drunk alcohol.

*Questions*

Will social services help us?
Does she have Alzheimer's?

*Worries*

I can't keep taking time off work, but I'm worried about what she'll do if she's left alone.

# NEXT STEPS

## Capacity and a dangerous discharge

You are a Care of the Elderly doctor. Miss Lily Watson is a 78-year-old retired librarian who was admitted under your team's care following her fourth fall at home in six months. She has a three year history of multi-infarct dementia and has been reluctantly under the care of the MHOA community team recently.

Miss Watson has a good relationship with her niece, who phones daily and visits monthly despite living 50 miles away. She receives Meals on Wheels and twice-daily carers. She has always maintained that she will live at home until her death and is described by her niece as 'fiercely independent'.

The physiotherapist has concerns that Miss Watson will not be safe at home. He tried to discuss this with her today and she told him she would manage 'perfectly well' once home, and would have 'no problems whatsoever' using the stairs to reach her bedroom and bathroom. Miss Watson then crossly packed her bags and demanded that the nurses call her a taxi to go home.

1. You have been called to the ward to 'sort the situation out'.
2. How will you assess and manage this situation?

### Issues
- Immediate containment
- Capacity assessment
- Discharge planning

### Immediate containment

While on the telephone, ask the staff to let Miss Watson know that you are coming to see her and how soon this will be. Don't call any taxis just yet! Courtesy and a cup of tea should suffice in the short term, but if Miss Watson makes active attempts to leave the ward, staff will need to know that they can keep her there until your arrival because of the concerns raised about her *capacity* to make such a decision. You should attend as soon as you can.

### Capacity assessment

You need to assess Miss Watson's ability to make decisions regarding going home. To do this, you gather information from her notes, the MHOA community team, the GP, and ward staff involved in her care; with her permission, you also speak with her niece and any other close contacts. You ensure that you understand:

- The concerns about her ability to manage at home, especially with regard to safety, e.g. falls, leaving gas taps on, not eating, wandering, letting strangers into the house.
- Any objective evidence of problems both before and during this admission, e.g. falls.
- Whether there is the opportunity for an increase in her care package and if this would be likely to help her to live independently and safely at home.
- Whether she has made any provision such as Lasting Power of Attorney (LPA) or any advance directives regarding her medical care.

Armed with this information, you interview Miss Watson, taking a focused psychiatric history and performing a mental state examination. In particular:

- Look for evidence of disorientation, poor memory or concentration, low mood, delusional ideas, and hallucinations.
- Perform formal cognitive testing, e.g. MMSE and frontal lobe testing.

- Decide if you agree with the diagnosis of multi-infarct dementia, and estimate how severely she is actually impaired.
- Check if Miss Watson understands the risk to herself of the current situation. For example:
  - How does she plan to manage at home?
  - Does she think she will need any help? If so, what?
  - Is she aware of anyone being concerned about her?
- Give her feedback regarding the concerns of the medical team. For example:
  - She forgets to use her Zimmer frame and thus falls; at home, she has repeatedly left the gas on, unlit.
- Consider whether Miss Watson is able to:
  - **Understand** the information you give her
  - **Retain** the information long enough to . . .
  - **Weigh** the decision (pros and cons) to come to a conclusion, *and then*
  - **Communicate** her decision?

If you think she has the capacity to make this decision, document this clearly, inform all relevant parties, and ensure she receives urgent follow-up with social services and the MHOA team. She can go home.

If you suspect that there is a reversible problem affecting Miss Watson's capacity to make this decision, you deal with this. For example:

- If you suspect delirium, you treat the underlying cause and allow time for this to resolve.
- If Miss Watson is deaf/doesn't speak English etc., you have to make every effort to overcome these problems (with hearing aids, interpreters, etc.), or she will be unfairly prevented from understanding the information given to her

You then reassess her capacity.

## Discharge planning

Miss Watson optimistically maintains that she has been using the stairs safely all week on the ward, which is not true. She refuses to consider moving into a residential home and does not believe that she is at risk at home. You document clearly in the notes that Miss Watson currently lacks capacity to make informed decisions regarding her ongoing care, explaining which aspect(s) of capacity she lacks and why. You inform the nursing staff that it is in her *best interests* that she be prevented from leaving the ward because she is at risk. Fortunately, Miss Watson now appears to be much calmer and accepts your recommendation that she should remain in hospital until there has been a meeting to plan her care and discharge.

You arrange such a meeting, involving the multi-disciplinary team and Miss Watson's niece. It is agreed that Miss Watson would be at high risk of potentially life-threatening falls as she continues to lack insight and understanding into her lack of safety using the stairs. However, it is very clear that she wants to go home and her niece insists that she has always wanted to be at home. For this reason, every effort is made to facilitate her safe discharge home, and it is decided that her risks can be minimized to a satisfactory level by:

- Arranging a limited microenvironment with a bed and commode on the ground floor of her house, and preventing access to the stairs with safety gates.
- Increasing her care package to four home care visits a day.
- Arranging a personal alarm so that she can gain help in case of falls.
- Leaving notes to remind her to use her Zimmer frame.
- Turning off the gas to her stove.
- MHOA team follow-up.

Two weeks later, Miss Watson is re-admitted after falling when trying to climb over the safety gates on her stairs. The risk can no longer be managed safely at home, and placement in a residential home *in her best interests* is agreed. Should this decision be challenged (e.g. by another family member), a referral to the IMCA (Independent Mental Capacity Advocates) Service for an independent assessment is required.

### Film list
*Away From Her* (2006)
*The Notebook* (2004)
*Iris* (2001)
*Harold and Maude* (1971)

### Books
Bayley, J. (1998) *Iris: A Memoir of Iris Murdoch*. London: Abacus. Memoir written by Iris Murdoch's husband John Bayley—provides a poignant examination of life before and after the onset of Iris's dementia, reminding readers of the wealth of talent and experience lost to her.

Boylan, C. (1999) *Beloved Stranger*. London: Abacus. Beautifully written novel examining late-onset mania—useful in reminding readers of the impact of mental illness upon carers (daughter) and also on long-married couples through the wife's deterioration following her husband's hospitalization.

Grant, L. (1998) *Remind Me Who I Am, Again*. London: Granta Books. Memoir which factually explores multi-infarct dementia, notions of loss and guilt, and additional distress caused by bureaucratic interventions.

Ignatieff, M. (1993) *Scar Tissue*. London: Chatto & Windus. Novel exploring Alzheimer's from the perspective of a son—useful for examining the vast gap between scientific explanation and personal experience.

Rule, J. (1987) *Memory Board*. Tallahassee, FL: Naiad Press. This novel won praise for its frank and illuminating expressions of sexuality and also the inclusion of older adults as central rather than marginalized characters.

### Quotes

Old age is no place for sissies.

**Bette Davis**

All would live long, but none would be old.

**Benjamin Franklin**

Beautiful young people are accidents of nature, but beautiful old people are works of art.

**Eleanor Roosevelt**

## Note

1. Michael Ignatieff (2004) *Scar Tissue*. Copyright © Penguin Group (Canada).

## References/Further reading

Bovee, B.F. (2005) Clinical, diagnostic, genetic, and management issues in dementia with Lewy bodies. *Clinical Science*, **109**, 343–54.

Courtney, C., Farrell, D., Gray, R., *et al.* (2004) Long-term donepezil treatment in 565 patients with Alzheimer's disease (AD2000): randomised double-blind trial. *Lancet*, **363**, 2105–15.

Folstein, M., Folstein, S., and McHugh, P. (1975) Mini-Mental State: a practical method for grading the cognitive state of patients for the clinician. *Journal of Psychiatric Research*, **12**, 189–98.

Howard, R. (2003) Management of behavioural problems in patients with dementia. *Progress in Neurology and Psychiatry*, 7(5).

Knapp, M. and Prince, M. (2007) *Dementia UK—The Full Report*. London: Alzheimer's Society.

McKeith, I.G., Dickson, D.W., Lowe, J., *et al.* (2005) Diagnosis and management of dementia with Lewy bodies: third report of the DLB consortium. *Neurology*, **65**, 1863–72.

Murphy, E. (1982) Social origins of depression in old age. *British Journal of Psychiatry*, **141**, 135–42.

Perry, E.K., Tomlinson, B.E., Blessed, G., *et al.* (1978) Correlation of cholinergic abnormalities with senile plaques and mental test scores in senile dementia. *British Medical Journal*, **ii**, 1457–9.

Richards, D., Clark, T., and Clarke, C. (2007) *The Human Brain and its Disorders*. Oxford University Press.

Walker, L.C. and Rosen, R.F. (2006) Alzheimer therapeutics —what after the cholinesterase inhibitors? *Age and Ageing*, **35**, 332–5.

 Go to www.oxfordtextbooks/orc/stringer for an array of additional references, including indicative mark sheets for OSCEs, self-assessment questions, guidance, and exercises.

# 13 Anxiety, obsessions, and reactions to stress

*Anna Streeruwitz, Matthew Hagger, Sheena Webb, Debbie Walker, and Noreen Jakeman*

## True or False? Test your existing knowledge—answers in the chapter and online

1. GABA receptor agonists reduce anxiety.

2. Negative reinforcement allows habituation to a fearful stimulus.

3. The onset of agoraphobia is bimodal, peaking in the 20s and mid 30s.

4. Social phobia is equally common in males and females.

5. Needle phobic patients characteristically become tachycardic during blood tests.

6. During a panic attack, paraesthesia may be experienced, secondary to hypocalcaemia.

7. Streptococcal throat infections are a risk factor for obsessive compulsive disorder.

8. Following a catastrophic event, formal psychological debriefing helps prevent the development of post traumatic stress disorder.

9. An anxious patient experiencing difficulties exhaling should be helped to rebreathe $CO_2$ with the use of a paper bag.

10. A medical student in your teaching group confides in you that she is prescribed beta blockers by her GP for anxiety during exam times. You have a duty to report this matter to the clinical tutor if she refuses to see them herself.

## Contents

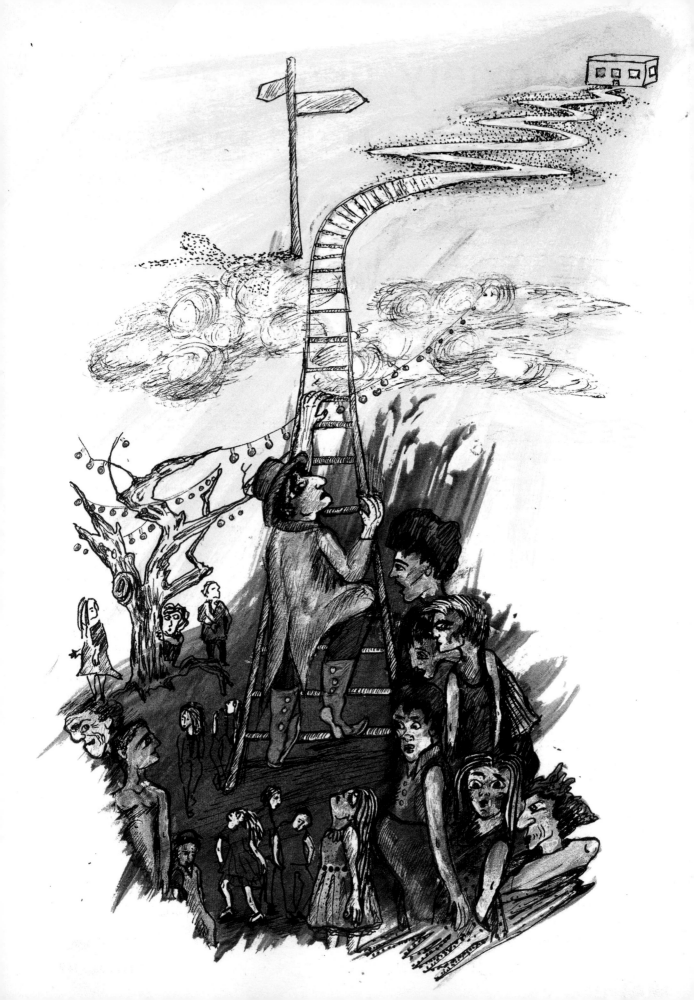

# PRINCIPLES

*'You asked me once', said O'Brien, 'what was in Room 101. I told you that you knew the answer already. Everyone knows it. The thing that is in Room 101 is the worst thing in the world. [ . . . ] The worst thing in the world', said O'Brien, 'varies from individual to individual. It may be burial alive, or death by fire, or by drowning, or by impalement, or fifty other deaths. There are cases where it is some quite trivial thing, not even fatal.' [ . . . ] 'In your case,' said O'Brien, 'the worst thing in the world happens to be rats.'*

*Nineteen Eighty-Four*—George Orwell[1]

## Introduction

Anxiety is a normal and necessary human emotion, for which we should be grateful. Over the years, it has surely protected the human race from multiple nonchalant extinctions, inspired us to develop bungee-jumping, and given medical students the extra 'push' they needed to pass exams. Useful, if a little unpleasant at times. Exaggerated anxiety to trivial or absent threat is unpleasant or even disabling.

Anxiety is often first recognized by its physical symptoms (Table 13.1). Anxiety disorders include generalized anxiety disorder (GAD), phobias, and panic disorder. This chapter will also cover obsessive–compulsive disorder (OCD) and post traumatic stress disorder (PTSD) because anxiety is a strong feature of both.

In some cultures, there is no directly equivalent word for anxiety. Patients might describe their bodily experience or a specific aspect of their anxiety, e.g. 'my heart is not at rest' (West African language Yoruba) or 'thinking too much' (Cambodia).

## Epidemiology

Anxiety disorders are very common, and affect women roughly twice as commonly as men (Table 13.2).

## Aetiology

### Genetics

Relatives of people with anxiety disorders have higher rates of these disorders than the general population, although specific genes have yet to be identified. This heritable vulnerability may be partly expressed through the personality trait of *neuroticism* (Fullerton *et al.* 2003). People with high neuroticism scores are more likely to experience anxiety, guilt, depression, and anger,

**TABLE 13.1** Symptoms of anxiety

| Symptom group | Examples |
|---|---|
| Psychological | Fears/worries<br>Poor concentration<br>Irritability<br>Feelings of unreality (depersonalization, derealization)<br>Insomnia: difficulties *falling* asleep<br>Night terrors |
| Motor symptoms | Restlessness, fidgeting<br>Feeling 'on edge'/unable to relax |
| Neuromuscular | Trembling/tremor<br>Headache (tension headache = a 'tight band' around the head)<br>Muscle aches (especially neck and back)<br>Feeling dizzy, light-headed, or unsteady<br>Tinnitus |
| Gastrointestinal | Dry mouth<br>Difficulty swallowing or a 'lump in the throat'<br>Nausea<br>Indigestion or stomach pains<br>'Butterflies' (abdominal churning)<br>Flatulence<br>Frequent or loose motions |
| Cardiovascular | Chest discomfort<br>Palpitations, feeling the heart 'pound' or 'miss beats' |
| Respiratory | Difficulty inhaling<br>'Tight'/constricted chest |
| Genitourinary | Urinary frequency<br>Erectile dysfunction<br>Amenorrhoea |

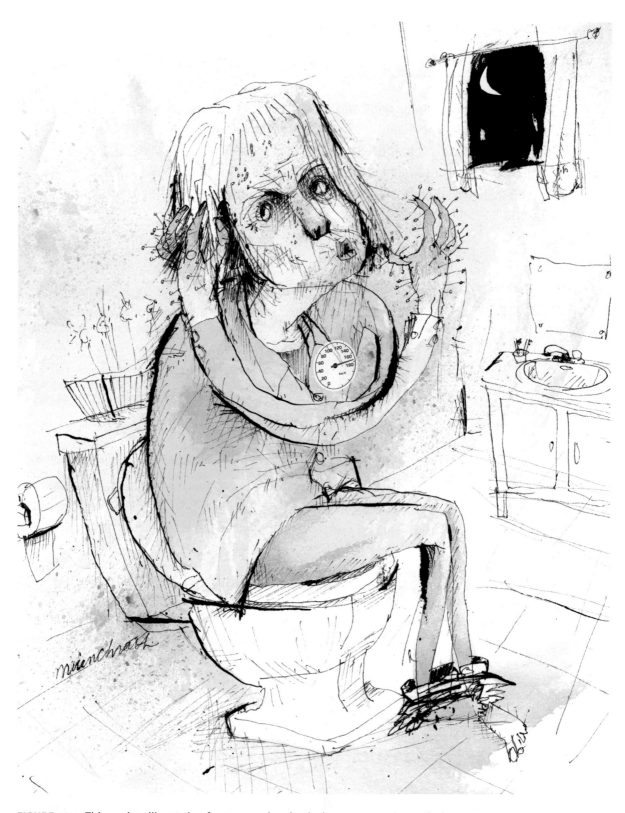

**FIGURE 13.1** This anxiety illustration focuses on the physical symptoms—in much the same way as an anxious patient does. Which symptoms can you see? What might this person be thinking?

**TABLE 13.2** Prevalence of anxiety disorders, OCD, and PTSD

| Disorder | 12-month prevalence[a] | Lifetime prevalence[b] | Predominantly Female | Predominantly Male |
|---|---|---|---|---|
| Specific phobia | 8.7% | 12.5% | ✓ | |
| Social phobia | 6.8% | 12.1% | – | – |
| GAD | 3.1% | 5.7% | ✓ | |
| Panic disorder | 2.7% | 4.7% | ✓ | |
| Agoraphobia (without panic disorder) | 0.8% | 1.4% | ✓ | |
| Obsessive–compulsive disorder | 1.0% | 1.6% | | ✓ |
| PTSD | 3.5% | 6.8% | ✓ | |
| Total: any anxiety disorder | 18.1% | 28.8% | ✓ | |

[a]Kessler *et al.* 2005b
[b]Kessler *et al.* 2005a

and feel easily overwhelmed by minor frustrations. Twin studies have shown genetic overlap between depression and GAD (Kendler 1996).

## Early experiences and life events

Childhood adversity predisposes to anxiety disorders (Brown and Harris 1993). Life events can trigger anxiety disorders, especially if they are experienced as threatening (e.g. possible redundancy).

## Neurochemical theories

It is thought that the central neurotransmitters serotonin, noradrenaline, and gamma-aminobutyric acid (GABA) are dysregulated in anxiety disorders. Evidence for their involvement is complex, but includes the fact that they are the target of drugs that can successfully combat anxiety symptoms:

- serotonin—selective serotonin reuptake inhibitors (SSRIs)
- noradrenaline—tricyclic antidepressants (TCAs)
- GABA—benzodiazepines (GABA agonists).

## Behavioural and cognitive theories

- **Classical conditioning** The repeated pairing of a neutral stimulus with a frightening one results in a fear reaction to the neutral stimulus (Box 13.1).
- **Negative reinforcement** Behaviours that relieve anxiety (e.g. running away) are repeated. This prevents habituation (getting used to the stimulus and calming down), so escaping from a fearful stimulus maintains the fear response.

> **BOX 13.1** Little Albert and the rat
>
> Little Albert, an 11-month-old boy, played happily with a white rat until scientists made loud clanging noises whenever the rat appeared. Being very little, Albert was naturally frightened of loud noises. However, through pairing of the rat with the noises, Albert became terrified of the rat itself (and anything resembling the rat, including a white beard).
>
> Watson and Rayner 1920

- **Cognitive theories** Worrying thoughts are repeated in an automatic way which both induces and maintains the anxiety response (see Management section).
- **Attachment theory** The quality of attachment between children and their parents affects their confidence as adults: insecurely attached children become anxious adults.

## Clinical picture

### Generalized anxiety disorder (GAD)

In GAD, anxiety is not triggered by a specific stimulus, but instead is continuous and generalized ('free-floating'). Life is a worry—past mistakes and future imagined catastrophes occupy the mind ceaselessly. Symptoms listed in Table 13.1 can occur at any time; severe cases have panic attacks as well. To diagnose GAD, symptoms must be present for at least six months, although the intensity may fluctuate.

## Differential diagnosis

- **Hyperthyroidism**: look for goitre, tremor, tachycardia, weight loss, arrhythmia, exophthalmos.
- **Substance misuse**:
  - intoxication (e.g. amphetamines)
  - withdrawal (e.g. benzodiazepines, alcohol).
- **Excess caffeine**.
- **Depression**: anxiety is a common feature of depression —and depression complicates anxiety. Which came first and which is currently most prominent are useful clues. If full-blown depression *and* GAD are present, diagnose them both. Diagnose *mixed anxiety and depressive disorder* if there are low-level depressive and anxiety symptoms present equally together, neither of which justifies diagnosis alone.
- **Anxious (avoidant) personality disorder**: from late adolescence onwards, the patient describes themselves as 'an anxious person', with no recent major increase in anxiety levels.
- **Dementia**: anxiety may be an early feature of this.
- **Schizophrenia**: in early schizophrenia, anxiety may occur before delusions and hallucinations are evident (delusional mood describes an unnerving sense that something is 'wrong').

> Anyone would appear to have 'GAD' if they drank 20 espressos a day.

## Phobic anxiety disorders

In these disorders, intermittent anxiety occurs in specific but quite ordinary circumstances. Patients characteristically avoid feared situations and the seriousness of the phobia depends on the resultant disability, for example, a pilot with a fear of flying would have a severe disorder.

### Agoraphobia

The uniting fear in agoraphobia is of being unable to easily escape to a safe place (usually home). Agoraphobia includes fear of open places *and* fear of situations that are confined and difficult to leave without attracting attention. Common problem situations include:

- travelling on trains, planes, or buses
- queuing
- supermarkets
- large crowds
- parks
- sitting in the middle row of a cinema.

Onset is commonly in the twenties or mid-thirties and may be gradual or precipitated by a sudden panic attack. The overwhelming urge is to return home to safety. The prospect of leaving home generates anxiety, the severity increasing with distance from home or difficulty returning. The presence of a dependable companion (or sometimes a car) increases range and makes otherwise avoided situations bearable. Those worst affected become housebound, dependent on a small circle of family or friends. Unsurprisingly, depression is common.

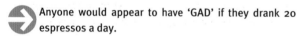 If the patient is successfully avoidant of all triggers, they might currently experience little or no anxiety. Ask about the past.

### Differential diagnoses

1. **Depression** can cause social withdrawal and is commonly comorbid with agoraphobia.
2. **Social phobia**: the fear here is of scrutiny or humiliation.
3. **Obsessive–compulsive disorder**: time-consuming rituals can confine people to their home.
4. **Schizophrenia**: patients may stay at home because of social withdrawal or as a way of avoiding perceived persecutors.

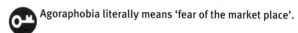 Agoraphobia literally means 'fear of the market place'.

>> *See Reality for Agoraphobia OSCE (p.163).*

### Social phobia

Onset is normally in the late teens, with *men and women equally affected*. The core fear in social phobia is of being scrutinized or criticized by other people, and patients often worry that they will embarrass themselves in public. They tolerate an anonymous crowd, unlike agoraphobic patients, but small groups (e.g. dinner parties, board meetings) feel very intimidating. There are sometimes specific worries, such as eating in public. Self-medication with alcohol or drugs perpetuates the problem as it offers psychological avoidance. Patients complain most about embarrassing symptoms, e.g. blushing, trembling, sweating, and urinary frequency.

### Differential diagnosis

1. **Shyness**: some people are naturally shy and feel uncomfortable in social situations. In social phobia, there is *overt fear*.
2. **Agoraphobia**: the need to get somewhere safe is more important than the fear of scrutiny.
3. **Anxious (avoidant) personality disorder**: there is a lifelong history of disabling shyness and anxiety.
4. **Poor social skills/autistic spectrum disorders** (e.g. Asperger's syndrome): people who are socially awkward will not show good social skills when relaxed—they remain awkward.
5. **Benign essential tremor**: this tremor is familial, worse in social situations, and responds to benzodiazepines and alcohol. There are no other features of anxiety.

6. **Schizophrenia/psychosis**: patients may avoid social situations because of paranoia or because they have delusions that they are being watched. Patients with social phobia recognize that their fears are exaggerated.

### Specific phobias

These phobias are restricted to a single, specific situation (e.g. spiders = arachnophobia). They often develop in childhood, although sometimes begin later, usually after a frightening experience. Phobias result in avoidance and, in severe cases, disability. Phobias are rarely confused with other diagnoses, but you should always exclude comorbid depression.

> Blood, injury, and needle phobias cause a strong vasovagal reaction, leading to bradycardia and low blood pressure. Although this may have an evolutionary advantage (fainting into the 'recovery position' once injured), it can cause problems for phlebotomists. Lay phobic patients flat before taking blood—or you may have to deal with a head injury after they collapse to the floor!

## Panic disorder

This disorder is also known as *episodic paroxysmal anxiety*. Anxiety is intermittent and without an obvious trigger—it comes 'out of the blue'. A panic attack is a sudden attack of extreme ('100%') anxiety with accompanying physical symptoms, such as:

- breathing difficulties/choking feelings
- chest discomfort/tightness
- palpitations
- tingling ('pins and needles') or numbness in hands, feet, or around the mouth
- depersonalization/derealization
- shaking
- dizziness/faints
- sweating.

The patient commonly fears that they will die, lose control, become incontinent, or go mad. These alarming thoughts provoke further panic until the patient gains reassurance or engages in *safety behaviours*. Safety behaviours are actions adopted to avert catastrophe, e.g.

---

**BOX 13.2** Calcium and pins and needles

Hyperventilation (rapid shallow breathing) blows off carbon dioxide ($CO_2$), resulting in lowered $P_{CO_2}$, raised pH, and hypocalcaemia. This in turn affects nerve conduction, causing paraesthesia (tingling and numbness) in hands, feet, and around the mouth. In extreme cases, carpopedal spasm (curling of fingers and toes) can occur.

---

calling an ambulance, taking aspirin. Panic attacks are self-limiting, lasting no more than 30 minutes, although this can feel never-ending.

> The mischievous Greek god, Pan, supposedly leapt out and surprised travellers in the woods, causing attacks of extreme anxiety—hence, *panic*.

For a diagnosis of panic *disorder*, there must be recurrent panic attacks (preferably several within a month). In between episodes, the person should be relatively free of anxiety.

### Differential diagnosis

1. **Other anxiety disorder:** especially GAD and agoraphobia.
2. **Depression**: if depressive symptoms preceded the panic attacks or the criteria for depressive disorder are fulfilled, the diagnosis of depression takes precedence.
3. **Alcohol or drug withdrawal** can cause severe anxiety that may be mistaken for panic attacks.
4. **Organic causes**: exclude cardiovascular and respiratory disease before diagnosing simple panic attacks. Disorders that mimic panic include the very, very rare phaeochromocytoma.

> Patients sometimes say 'panic' when they mean momentary shock and worry, rather than '100% anxiety'.

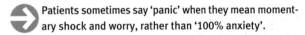

## Investigations

1. A good history and physical examination will establish whether an organic cause is likely and may prompt further investigations (Table 13.3).
2. Rating scales of anxiety include the Beck Anxiety Inventory and the HADS (Hospital Anxiety and Depression Scale). These can assess severity or provide baseline 'scores' against which to measure treatment response.
3. Social and occupational assessments for effect on quality of life.
4. Collateral history.

## Management

### Initial help

1. **Advice** and **reassurance** may be enough to prevent early or mild problems from worsening. Psycho-education (explaining the anxiety disorder) helps patients to understand their illness.
2. **Basic counselling** addresses the patient's worries.

**TABLE 13.3** Organic causes of anxiety: anxiety pattern and investigation

| Organic cause | Anxiety pattern | | Investigations |
|---|---|---|---|
| | Continuous | Episodic | |
| Hyperthyroidism | ✓ | | TFTs |
| Caffeine | ✓ | ✓ | – |
| Alcohol | ✓ | ✓ | LFTs/γGT/MCV |
| Drugs | | ✓ | Urine drug screen |
| Arrhythmia | | ✓ | ECG/24-hour ECG |
| Hypoglycaemia | | ✓ | Glucose (while anxious) |
| Phaeochromocytoma | | ✓ | 24-hour urine for VMA |

VMA, vanillylmandelic acid.

3. A **problem-solving** approach can help to identify and deal with stressors.

4. **Self-help** material is available, including CBT-based books and computer programs. Encourage people to rely on their natural supports: friends, family, faith groups, etc.

5. **Relaxation techniques** and **breathing exercises** taught in person or using manuals or tapes must be mastered while calm—it is too hard to employ them for the first time when panicking! The idea behind these is *reciprocal inhibition*: it is not possible to both panic *and* relax at the same time, so practised relaxation can negate panic.

## Cognitive behavioural therapy (CBT)

People with anxiety disorders often think and behave as if they are in imminent danger when they are not. Cognitive behavioural therapy aims to reduce the patient's

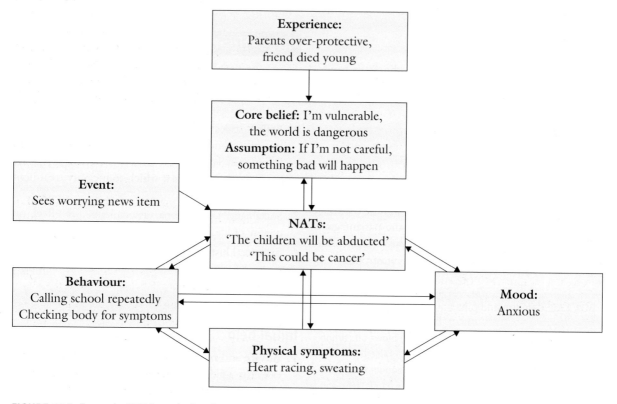

**FIGURE 13.2** Example CBT formulation for GAD. Negative automatic thoughts (NATs) occur in response to a trigger event set up a vicious cycle of worry

expectation of threat, and the behaviours that maintain threat-related beliefs.

Therapy often starts with education about the physiology of anxiety and techniques for managing arousal, such as relaxation and controlled breathing. Subsequent sessions explore the actual likelihood and impact of the anticipated catastrophe. Predictions such as 'I will go out of my mind' or 'I will embarrass myself' are discussed and behavioural experiments are set up to test them. These techniques gradually increase the patient's confidence in their capacity to cope with the feared situation. Over time, more adaptive coping mechanisms replace the unhelpful behaviours (e.g. avoidance and escape) that maintained anxiety.

- **GAD** The main feature of GAD is worry. Behavioural responses to worry include avoidance and reassurance seeking. Therapy involves testing predictions of worry with behavioural experiments and looking at errors in thinking.

- **Panic disorder** Panic may be triggered by misinterpretation of physical anxiety symptoms as signs of major catastrophe. As a result safety behaviours are adopted which merely reinforce beliefs: since no catastrophe then occurs, the conclusion is that the remedial behaviour prevented it, maintaining the problem. CBT educates the patient on the true meaning of their symptoms (panic, not perish). It helps them test whether their behaviours really keep them safe and whether their beliefs are true or misinterpretations.

## Exposure therapy

When there are strong elements of avoidance and escape —as with phobias—exposure therapy is used as part of the CBT approach. In the absence of actual harm, the body can only remain *extremely* anxious for a relatively short period (usually under 45 minutes) before *habituation* occurs and anxiety levels drop. Habituation is 'getting used to a fear', so that anxiety decreases until the fear dies out (extinction).

Exposure is usually through the gradual approach called *desensitization*. The therapist helps the patient to identify a goal and then construct a 'hierarchy' of feared situations, from the least to the most frightening. Table 13.4 shows an example dealing with the editor's cockroach phobia.

In this example there is no benefit to mastering fear over a locked room full of cockroaches, so the goal would be to catch and contain a live cockroach—this would be useful to remove cockroaches were they to enter the editor's clinic. The patient tackles each step as weekly homework, starting with the easiest and working upwards. The mission is to *stay* in the situation until the anxiety has subsided (habituated) in order to induce new learning and challenge existing thoughts. Repeated

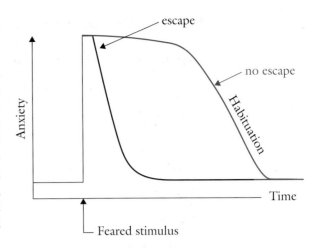

**FIGURE 13.3** Response to feared stimulus: fear and escape versus habituation

attempts at the same task cause the anxiety to decrease more quickly each time. This courageous tiptoeing can result in a complete cure.

**Agoraphobia** can be treated similarly. Tasks might include going shopping in a small, local shop, before progressing to a big supermarket, staying in the situation until the anxiety has abated. The first attempt at a task might be with a companion (e.g. spouse) and once successful, is repeated alone.

In **social phobia** the patient engages in safety behaviours and excessive self-monitoring to reduce the risk of embarrassment. These make things worse—focusing attention on one's own performance means not listening and responding properly to others. Therapy involves dropping these 'safety behaviours' whilst exposing the patient to social situations in order to challenge their assumptions. Video feedback and role-play may be helpful.

## Pharmacological

Remember that starting and *suddenly* stopping antidepressants can cause anxiety symptoms. Tell your patient beforehand to avoid further worry!

1. **Selective serotonin reuptake inhibitors (SSRIs)**, e.g. fluoxetine, paroxetine. These treat many anxiety disorders and may be combined with CBT. Therapeutic doses for anxiety disorders are generally higher than for depression, and response takes longer (6–8 weeks). For more details on SSRIs see p.39.

2. **Tricyclic antidepressants (TCAs)**, e.g. clomipramine, imipramine. TCAs can be used if patients don't tolerate or respond to SSRIs.

3. **Buspirone** is a serotonin partial agonist. Although it is non-dependency-forming, it is not very popular because of its delayed action and dysphoric side effects.

4. **Benzodiazepines**, e.g. diazepam. These can be useful *short-term* anxiety treatments (e.g. while waiting for

**TABLE 13.4** Hierarchy of fears

| Anxiety level[a] | Activity |
|---|---|
| 10 | Being in a locked room full of live, angry cockroaches |
| 9.5 | Catch a live cockroach in a container long enough to remove it from the room[b] |
| 9 | Holding a dead cockroach |
| 8 | Watching the therapist hold a live cockroach (this is called modelling) |
| 7 | Hold a glass jar containing a live cockroach |
| 6 | Hold the glass jar containing a dead cockroach |
| 5 | Look at a glass jar containing a dead cockroach |
| 4 | Look at a picture of a cockroach |

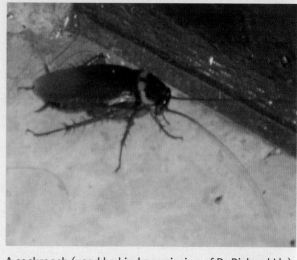

A cockroach (used by kind permission of Dr Richard Lin)

[a]A score of 10 = maximum anxiety, 0 = no anxiety.
[b]The phobic editor has heard that killing cockroaches releases millions of eggs which can then become new cockroaches—hence the wish to *remove* the cockroach.

SSRIs to take effect). Although they are very effective anxiolytics, tolerance builds rapidly and patients quickly become dependent. *Use must not exceed 2–4 weeks.* Benzodiazepines enhance GABA transmission in the brain by interacting with the GABA-A receptor, which is a ligand-gated chloride-ion channel. Side effects include amnesia, ataxia, and respiratory depression, especially in the elderly and patients with pre-existing respiratory disease.

5. **Beta-blockers**, e.g. atenolol. These are sometimes used to treat the adrenergic symptoms that social phobia patients find so disturbing, i.e. tremor and palpitations. However, take care in prescribing as there are many contraindications to beta blockade.

> Barbiturates are no longer used—they are highly addictive and fatal in overdose.

> Don't forget to treat comorbid depression/substance misuse.

> There is little use for medications in specific phobias—since these are usually intermittent problems.

## Prognosis

Anxiety disorders are common and often chronic. Overall, the rule of thirds applies:

- one-third recover completely
- one-third improve partially
- one-third fare poorly, suffering considerable disability and poor quality of life.

Early diagnosis and treatment are essential, as the shorter the duration of symptoms, the better the prognosis, e.g. if agoraphobia continues for a year, it is likely to go on for at least 5 years.

## Obsessive–compulsive disorder (OCD)

It is normal to experience unpleasant intrusive thoughts sometimes, although these are generally ignored and have no further impact. People with OCD cannot ignore these anxiety-producing thoughts and may try to relieve them with rituals (compulsions).

> People with OCD are often ashamed of their illness, which may delay presentation. Sometimes they present with symptoms resulting from the OCD, e.g. dermatitis following excessive hand-washing.

### Epidemiology

In any year, OCD affects 1% of the population, afflicting men and women equally.

### Aetiology

Relatives of patients with OCD are at a threefold increased risk of the disorder, but the means of transmission is unknown. A quarter of patients with OCD have premorbid anankastic personality traits (rigidity, orderliness). Stress may precipitate symptoms of OCD.

The basal ganglia are implicated, since they are affected by illnesses in which the risk of OCD is increased: Sydenham's chorea, encephalitis lethargica, and Tourette's syndrome. Anti-basal ganglial antibodies have been demonstrated in people who develop OCD following a streptococcal throat infection. (Note that streptococcal infection also causes Sydenham's chorea.) Neuro-imaging studies have linked OCD with a deficit in frontal-lobe inhibition, suggesting that intrusive or ritualistic thoughts might be harder to suppress in OCD.

## Clinical picture

**Obsessions** are recurrent unwanted intrusive thoughts, images, or impulses that enter the patient's mind, despite attempts to resist them. The thoughts are unpleasant but the patient recognizes them as both irrational and their own (unlike delusions or thought insertion). Themes of obsessions often concern:

- contamination
- aggression (thoughts of harming self or others)
- infection
- morality (commonly sex/religion).

Obsessions make the patient feel acutely uncomfortable or anxious. Sometimes they feel responsible for the damage that their thought *might* do, e.g. a violent thought might really harm someone.

This tension or discomfort is often 'undone' or neutralized by a *compulsion* (Salkovskis *et al.* 1997). Compulsions are repeated, stereotyped, and seemingly purposeful rituals that the patient feels compelled to carry out, even though they are irrational and may lack any obvious link to the obsession. Common examples include cleaning, counting, checking, and ordering objects. Compulsions can take hours and severely affect quality of life. Resistance to both obsessions and compulsions may decrease or disappear in chronic cases.

## Differential diagnosis

1. **Anxiety disorders**: obsessional symptoms are less prominent than other anxiety symptoms.
2. **Depression**: obsessions can occur within depression and up to 50% of patients with OCD experience depressive symptoms. If the episode meets the criteria for depression, this takes priority.
3. **Anankastic personality disorder**: a *lifelong* personality of rigidity, often with very high standards of orderliness, hygiene, etc. The pattern of obsessions and compulsions is absent unless OCD is superimposed.
4. **Schizophrenia**: beliefs are delusional not obsessional.
5. **Organic causes**: rarely, e.g. Sydenham's chorea.

## Management

As well as education and self-help as described for anxiety disorders, management may include the following.

1. **CBT: exposure and response prevention** Compulsions are in some ways analogous to escape in phobias, quickly reducing anxiety. CBT aims is to prevent compulsive behaviour, allowing the tolerated anxiety to habituate. For example, someone with obsessions about contamination is supported to touch something dirty (e.g. dustbin) and, instead of immediately washing their hands, they are encouraged to experience the anxiety and discuss it with the therapist. A hierarchy of feared situations is used, as in exposure therapy. This therapy is effective with well-motivated patients.
2. **SSRIs** are effective in OCD, as is clomipramine (a TCA).

## Prognosis

OCD tends to run a chronic course, with symptoms worsening at times of stress. It is often disabling and commonly comorbid with depression.

Patients describing obsessions might say, 'I know it's silly, but . . .' Delusional patients don't describe thoughts this way.

>> See Reality for an OCD OSCE (p.162).

## Reactions to extreme stress

Imagine witnessing your whole family die in a fire. What would be a *normal* reaction to that? With such a severely stressful event, you would expect to experience extreme emotions and behave accordingly. Following extreme stress, a wide variety of responses should be regarded as normal before considering someone to be 'ill'—and responses should be prolonged and disabling before being counted as an 'illness'.

## Acute stress reaction

Most people would regard the acute stress reaction as an understandable 'state of shock' that can follow traumatic events—the same events that can produce PTSD. The state is transient, starting within minutes of the trauma and resolving spontaneously within hours (1–3 days maximum). The person is usually anxious, but may seem to be dazed and in a 'dream world'; they may experience amnesia for the event as well as depersonalization and derealization. Often they are disoriented and agitated, but sometimes are irritable, panicky, or even aggressive.

Apart from excluding injury, support and reassurance are usually all that are required. Benzodiazepines can alleviate extreme short-term distress, but do not prevent later PTSD. More formal, immediate, psychological 'debriefing' (being required to describe the trauma and your emotional response to it) may *increase* the likelihood of later PTSD.

## Post-traumatic stress disorder (PTSD)

The disorder now called PTSD was initially recognized in military psychiatry, where the labels included 'shell shock', 'combat fatigue', and 'battle exhaustion'. PTSD follows a traumatic event that is often experienced as 'life-threatening'. The event suffered or witnessed by the patient must be 'an event of an exceptionally threatening or catastrophic nature likely to cause pervasive distress in anyone' (ICD-10 1992). Typical examples would include natural disasters, war, accidents, torture, terrorism, and rape.

### Epidemiology

PTSD has a one-year prevalence of 3.5% and a lifetime prevalence of 6.8%. In civilian life, women are at higher risk of developing PTSD than men.

### Aetiology

By definition, PTSD is caused by experiencing extreme trauma; aspects that increase the risk include the degree of exposure, proximity, and human design (e.g. torture victims). Only about 10% of people who experience an extreme trauma develop PTSD. Twin studies show that around a third of this variance in susceptibility is genetic. Risk factors include neurotic traits, a personal or family history of psychiatric problems, childhood abuse, and poor early attachment. 'Survivor guilt' and continual exposure to the trauma or other stressors can perpetuate symptoms (Fairbank *et al.* 2000).

Research in memory formation has suggested distortion in the processing and storage of traumatic events such that they are constantly 'relived' rather than 'remembered'. In PTSD, the amygdala (emotional processing) is hyperactive and the hippocampus (memory storage) is atrophied.

### Clinical picture

Although there is often a latency period following the trauma, PTSD usually begins within 6 months. Symptoms fall into the following groups.

### Re-experiencing

- Flashbacks: vividly reliving the trauma, feeling as though it is 'happening all over again'.
- Nightmares.
- Intrusive memories: being unable to keep the mind clear of memories of what happened.

Despite these often fragmented recollections, there may be difficulties in remembering the entire episode voluntarily.

### Avoidance

- Avoiding reminders of the event (these often trigger flashbacks and increased anxiety). People often try to avoiding thinking about the trauma.

### Hyperarousal

- Persistent inability to relax.
- Hypervigilance: the patient feels as though they are always on 'red alert'.
- Enhanced startle reflex (exaggerated reaction to the unexpected).
- Insomnia.
- Poor concentration.
- Irritability.

### Other changes

- Emotional detachment ('numbness').
- Decreased interest in activities.
- Powerful emotions including anger, loss of control, shame, and uncontrollable crying.

There is overlap with depression and other anxiety disorders, and many patients self-medicate with alcohol or drugs.

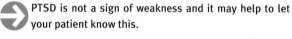 PTSD is not a sign of weakness and it may help to let your patient know this.

### Differential diagnosis

1. Depression or anxiety disorder—both common responses to severe stress.
2. Adjustment disorder (see Box 13.3).

### Management

It is important to be flexible and sensitive when working with PTSD patients; they can be 're-traumatized' in their interactions with services.

### Psychological treatments

. . . treatment sometimes consisted of simply encouraging the patient to abandon his hopeless attempt to forget, and advising him instead to spend some part of every day remembering. Neither brooding on the experience, nor trying to pretend it had never happened. Usually, within a week or two of his patients starting this treatment, the nightmares began to be less frequent and less terrifying.

*Regeneration*—Pat Barker[2]

- **Cognitive behavioural therapy** Following a traumatic event, people may find that their previous belief systems have been shattered, resulting in new belief patterns (Ehlers and Clark 2000), e.g.

– the world is unsafe and unpredictable

– I am vulnerable

– I can't cope.

These can be examined and tested in the same way as the anxiety disorders. *Exposure therapy* is an important aspect of the work, supporting the patient to work through their memories.

- **Eye movement desensitization and reprocessing (EMDR)** In this therapy, the original trauma is deliberately re-experienced in as much detail as possible, e.g. by the patient narrating or imagining every step that happened. While doing this, they fix their eyes on the therapist's finger as it quickly passes from side to side in front of them. Strange as this may seem, it is an effective treatment for PTSD! Eye movements can be replaced by any alternating left–right stimulus (e.g. tapping left then right hands). It is thought this aids memory processing.

### Pharmacological treatment

**SSRIs** are the first-line treatment, preferably in combination with psychological therapies (Baldwin *et al.* 2005).

*Prognosis*

The majority of patients recover, although some suffer for many years; chronicity can lead to enduring personality change. Symptoms can resurface at anniversaries associated with the trauma.

 See the ORC for a PTSD OSCE.

---

**BOX 13.3** Adjustment disorders

Life changes require adaptation to cope with new situations, tasks, roles, and responsibilities. Examples include going to university, breaking up with a partner, or moving house.

- Even for people who seem to take these changes 'in their stride' without too much distress, there are often fleeting symptoms of anxiety, low mood, irritability, or sleeplessness.
- In **adjustment disorders** the person's reaction is deemed greater than usually expected for the situation, but not severe enough to diagnose an anxiety or depressive disorder.
- Symptoms start within a month of the stressor and resolve within six months.
- Support, reassurance, and problem-solving are often all that are needed.

---

# REALITY

## General approach: tips, tricks, and cautionary tales

### 1. Ooze calm

Take a deep breath and relax. If you look frightened and jumpy, this will do nothing to calm a nervous person.

### 2. Read body language

Look for increased signs of nervousness in your patient, such as crossing arms and legs, trembling, or fidgeting. Think about *why* they are nervous and let this guide your interview. Remember that even discussing anxiety can make people feel anxious, and that the interview (or you) may be scaring them. Don't automatically change the subject, but be aware that your patient may need more time, encouragement, or reassurance to continue—ask how you can help them feel more comfortable.

### 3. Tough topics

Discussion can be a useful form of exposure therapy, but topics which have always been a secret, or provoke fear, guilt, shame, or embarrassment, can be extremely hard to discuss, so respectful and sensitive listening is essential. Do not push for details if they become very distressed—offer respite instead:

- 'This is hard to talk about. Are you OK to go on, or would you like to take a break?'

You can offer to return to a topic later in the interview or arrange a follow-up meeting, perhaps with a relative or friend for support. Remember, it can be harmful for patients to divulge sensitive information before they are ready.

### 4. Never dismiss fears

Few students actually laugh in the face of a fearful patient, but there are more subtle ways of being dismissive.

Jumping too readily to solutions and cures can leave your patient feeling that you regard their fear as a small, harmless obstacle that *you* could easily overcome. People sometimes apologize for their fear:

**Neil:** It's stupid. Cats terrify me!

**You:** Many people are scared of *something*. I think you're afraid I'll think it's silly and not see your courage in telling me.

If you join someone in calling a problem 'silly', embarrassment may prevent them seeking further treatment.

## 5. Paper bags and panic attacks

If your patient has a panic attack in front of you, it is not helpful if you join them in their panic. Speak calmly but firmly. Remove specific triggers (e.g. cockroaches) and get them to sit still. Explain that this is a panic attack and that, although frightening, it won't hurt them and will be over within a few minutes. Explain that they need to slow their breathing to undo the symptoms. One method is breathing in through the nose, slowly counting to three, then out for five through the mouth. Rebreathing $CO_2$ by holding a *paper* bag over the mouth and nose for ten or so breaths can help reduce symptoms by rebalancing respiratory gases. If a paper bag isn't available, cupped hands will do almost as well (avoid plastic bags). Successfully 'surviving' a panic attack without using safety behaviours will show your patient that their situation is not as serious as they fear it to be.

Panic attacks cause problems breathing *in*. If your patient is wheezing or having problems *exhaling*, fetch inhalers, not paper bags!

## The interview

There is a lot to remember when taking a focused history of anxiety and stress-related disorders, but remember, anxious people want to be SEDATED:

**S**ymptoms of anxiety

**E**pisodic or continuous

**D**rink and drugs

**A**voidance and escape

**T**iming and triggers

**E**ffect on life

**D**epression

This helps to diagnose the disorder *and* identify comorbid problems. The order of coverage is not important.

## Symptoms of anxiety

People may present with symptoms of anxiety (e.g. worries, palpitations) but if not, actively elicit them.

### Physical

- How does your body feel when you're nervous?
  - For example, choking feelings, breathing problems, palpitations, butterflies, shaking, . . .
  - \* What do you think is happening when you get these feelings?

### Psychological

- What worries do you have?/What worries you the most?
  - Do you find it hard to concentrate?
  - Can you relax and 'switch off'?
  - Have you felt as if you weren't real? (depersonalization)
  - Has the world around you felt unreal? (derealization)

## Episodic or continuous

The pattern of anxiety is important for diagnosis.

- Do you feel anxious *all* the time or just *some of the time*?
- \* Do you know what makes you anxious?
- \* What was happening or going through your mind when you last felt anxious?

If someone is anxious *all* the time, they probably have GAD. PTSD also leaves people feeling on edge all the time, although peaks in fear usually relate to re-experiencing or reminders of the trauma. If the anxiety is *some* of the time, establish any triggers. If the patient can't identify any but has recurrent spontaneous 10/10 anxiety, they have panic disorder. If there are triggers, they will have some form of phobia, OCD (obsessions causing anxiety), or PTSD.

## Drink and drugs

- Sometimes when they are stressed, people use alcohol or drugs to feel calmer. Is this something you do?

## Avoidance and escape

- Are there things you avoid because they'll make you too anxious?
- Does your fear ever get so bad that you have to leave a situation?
- \* How does this affect you? (work, relationships, personal freedom)

If your patient isn't sure what you mean, give examples. If they suffered a car crash and you're thinking about

PTSD, ask if they can still travel in cars, or if they have been able to walk past the site of the crash.

## Timing and triggers

- When did these problems start? Was anything stressful happening around then? Did you feel trapped?
- * What made you decide to talk about this *today*? (links to effect on life)
- * What triggers these feelings now?

## Effect on life

- How does this affect you?
- Have you missed out on anything because of it?

## Depression

Screen for low mood, anhedonia, and anergia. Always check for suicidal thoughts.

## Other relevant history

Briefly screen for relevant family, past psychiatric, past medical, and drug history. Remember to check the social history for social support.

## Specific disorders

### Generalized anxiety disorder

- How would friends have described you before you started feeling anxious all the time?

Consider anxious [avoidant] personality disorder if the anxiety really *has* been lifelong.

### Social phobia

Look for fears of being scrutinized, watched, or judged, fainting, or public embarrassment. Common symptoms include blushing, trembling, and sweating.

### Agoraphobia

This may have started with a panic attack, so check for this, as well as ongoing panic attacks. Look for a pattern of decreasing freedom and work out which places are 'safe' or 'unsafe'. Are they dependent on a close friend or relative?

### Panic attacks

Gain details of the attack and find out any known triggers as well as the frequency and duration of attacks.

- Take me through what happens when you have one of these episodes.

Ask specifically about panic attack symptoms. Look for interpretation of the attack as a medical emergency and ask about thoughts of death, madness, or loss of control during the attack.

- What do you think is happening to you?
- What thoughts go through your head when this happens?

Be vigilant for signs of developing agoraphobia.

 **Always find out what medical problems and investigations a patient with panic attacks has had.**

### OCD

*Obsessions* may be thoughts, impulses or images. Consider common themes: contamination, illness, aggression, sexual, religious, order, 'superstitions'.

- Do worrying thoughts or ideas bother you? Tell me about them . . .
- Are you quite superstitious? What kinds of things are you superstitious about?
- How do these thoughts make you feel?
- Do you try to block them out?
- Do they keep coming into your head even though you try to block them out?
- Where do the thoughts come from? Are they your own thoughts? (not thought insertion)
- How much truth is there in them, do you think?
- * How do you make the anxiety go away? (compulsions— 'undoing')

*Compulsions*

- Some people have rituals they have to do in a very exact way. Do you do anything like that?

Give examples if needed, e.g. counting, washing.

- Are there things you have to do, to put things right and feel better?
- Do they make you feel calmer for a while?
- What happens if you don't do them correctly?
- Do you think this is unreasonable or excessive?

Always find out how many times a day compulsions take place and how long they take. Consider cleaning, checking, ordering, and counting.

### PTSD

*Trauma*

- Did something awful happen?
- It's clearly hard to talk about . . . But could you tell me what happened? Take all the time you need.
- That's terrible . . . Did you think you were going to die?
- Were you badly hurt? Did anyone else get hurt?

Find out when it happened (usually in the six months before symptoms of PTSD started), and how things have worked out (police involvement, court cases, ongoing physical disability, etc).

## Re-experiencing

If your patient presents with re-experiencing phenomena (flashbacks, nightmares, intrusive thoughts, and memories about the trauma) it's often enough to ask,

- Does it remind you of something that's happened?

Questions that may uncover re-experiencing phenomena include:

- Do you ever feel like it's happening all over again?/Do you get 'flashbacks'?
  - What is that like?
  - \* What triggers this?
- Have you had bad dreams or nightmares?
- Do you find it hard to block out horrible memories of what happened?
- Do you find yourself thinking about it, even though you don't want to?

## Hyperarousal

- Have you been feeling on-edge or very jumpy, all the time?
- Do you feel as if you're almost waiting for something bad to happen again?
- \* How's your sleep?

## Avoidance of triggers

- Are there things you can't face, since this happened?
- Have you been able to visit the place where it happened?
- \* What happens if you can't avoid these things? Do they trigger flashbacks?

## Emotional changes

- Have you noticed changes in your feelings?
- Do you feel emotionally cut-off or numb?
- Do you feel more irritable than normal?

📖 For women who have been raped, questioning by a male student may feel intrusive and retraumatizing. A female colleague may be more appropriate.

# 1. OCD history (10 minutes)

## Candidate instructions

Jeremy Blaker is a 27-year-old bus driver. He has attended the GP surgery at the request of his employer, who is concerned about his fitness to drive.

You are a medical student attached to the GP surgery. The GP has asked you to take a psychiatric history.

## Patient's brief

### Key characteristics

- I'm embarrassed by the thoughts in my head.
- If the student makes me feel like I'm weird, I'll close down.
- I'm fairly calm but get anxious when talking about the worrying thoughts.

My manager's received complaints about me because my bus runs late. At first he said not to worry, but the complaints kept coming and he's losing patience. Last week I pulled in to a bus stop and just *couldn't* drive again. My passengers had to get off and another driver came out and drove me back to the depot.

It's embarrassing . . . About a year ago, I suddenly had this thought: 'The bus will crash and everyone will die!' I couldn't get it out of my head—it kept going round and round and really worried me. I got so distracted I went through a red light and nearly hit a car. I pulled over and tried to clear my head by counting all the people on the bus. When I finished I felt calm enough to drive again, but since then the thought's come more and more often. I feel the tension rising, my hands shake, and my heart pounds.

I can cope with the feelings until the next bus stop, when I have to count everyone again. It feels like counting puts everything right and keeps my passengers safe. It makes me feel calm again. If I think I've miscounted (especially if people are changing seats or crammed in), I have to count again until I'm sure. It makes me late. It's been getting worse over the months and now it's always in my head as I drive —no matter how hard I try to block it out, it comes back.

Last week I had a full bus and I couldn't get the count right so I couldn't leave the bus stop. People were shouting, getting off and on—it was too confusing. I couldn't drive unless I was sure it was safe, so I turned the engine off, took the keys out and sat down at the bus shelter. When I tried to explain it to my manager, he said I shouldn't work again until I saw the GP and got a brain scan.

Deep down, I know this is ridiculous. I don't honestly think that knowing the number of people on a bus will stop a crash happening! I just can't stop thinking, *what if?* What if the bus *does* crash and everyone dies? I can't take the risk of *not* counting, just in case. I can't tell my friends about this—they'd think I was crazy. I've always been the calm, practical one, not someone too superstitious to drive. I've stopped driving my car recently, because similar thoughts started happening there: 'I'll run someone over'. Fortunately, the thoughts only seem to happen while I'm driving, so otherwise I'm fine.

### Other history

- I'm not depressed and my energy's good. I'm too worried to enjoy my job. I am not suicidal.

- I'm physically fit. I had my tonsils taken out after lots of bouts of tonsillitis.
- I don't drink heavily or do drugs—it would be dangerous in my job.
- No-one in my family (including me) has ever suffered mental illness.
- I can't think of anything stressful around the time this started, although I did move house.

### Questions (if asked)

Am I going mad?

### Worries (if asked)

I won't be able to carry on driving.

## 2. Agoraphobia history (10 minutes)

### Candidate instructions

Mrs Grace Teaney is a 55-year-old solicitor who has been housebound for some time. Her son, Robert, has asked the GP to make a house call.

You are a medical student accompanying the GP. Take a history with a view to making a diagnosis.

### Patient's brief

*Key characteristics*

- I'm eloquent and personable.
- I try to make light of matters, but inwardly feel very sad.
- I'm embarrassed to need a house call (though I knew about it beforehand).
- I'm calm, but the memories of attacks make feel anxious when I have to talk about them.

Everything started about 9 months ago when I took the lift to my office on the eighteenth floor and it became stuck. I wasn't a great fan of enclosed spaces, but I thought I could cope. I calmly pressed the alarm button, but nothing happened other than a little bell noise. I called out—a little 'Hello?'—but no one replied. I banged on the doors and shouted, but to no avail. I realized I was trapped and panicked. There seemed so little space and the air seemed to be running out. My throat began to close up and I could feel my heart beating hard and fast, as if it would jump right out of my chest. Then my hands tingled and I thought I'd had a stroke! Just then, the engineer's voice came through the speaker, the lift shunted up, and the doors opened. I virtually fell out! I was dizzy, crying, and sweaty. Everything felt unreal—as if people were talking to me through water or thick glass. I was in such a state, I had to take the rest of the day off. I tried to tell myself that it was a one-off event but found that even thinking about lifts made me panicky. I preferred taking the stairs, though it was quite a workout climbing to the eighteenth floor each day!

Things didn't stop there. First, it was the trains. Going through tunnels triggered a similar sensation to that in the lift. One morning it was so bad that I got off a stop early and walked three miles to work. I haven't been on a train since. Buses became a problem a few weeks later . . . With the fear that it might happen again, my world shrank down to this house. It wasn't a deliberate decision, but there was always a reason to stay home: holding dinner parties for friends to visit me; giving Robert managerial experience at the firm by leaving him in charge . . . Eventually, I realized I'd given in to the fear. The further from home I am, the more frightened I am. For over six months, I've only been to the local mini-market with Robert. I trust him—and he understands I might need to run off. I really can't stand in a queue, so he queues while I wait in the car (which feels safe). We've told work that I have back problems and I work from home, e-mailing or sending work in via Robert.

Though I keep up the facade of coping and being the boss, I feel vulnerable, miserable, and lonely. The work Robert brings home is starting to feel overwhelming, and I don't enjoy it as I used to. It's become quite hard to concentrate on it. I wish I could get out and see my friends . . . I feel quite pathetic when I remember I can't leave home without pep talks and handholding.

*Other history*

- I've never seen a psychiatrist and no one in my family has had similar problems, though apparently my father was a nervous child.
- I'm not a big drinker but I do enjoy the occasional cognac. I've never smoked.
- I have high blood pressure, controlled with tablets.

## Questions

I want help, but I've heard it may mean facing my fears. Could this cause harm?

*Worries*

These 'incidents' could be mini strokes.

# NEXT STEPS

## An anxious colleague in need of help

Toby is a fellow medical student in your clinical firm. He is intelligent but rather quiet and shy. The group has had difficulty during paediatrics with the consultant, Dr Brand. During clinical teaching he picks on each student in turn and humiliates them. Toby has not been attending for the last few weeks, and Dr Brand has demanded that he present a case or will be failed.

Toby attends and is very different: he is calmer, but 'spaced out', performing poorly, despite well-prepared slides. You are surprised to see Toby in the university bar a few hours later, as he rarely socializes. He appears intoxicated, even on his first drink. He tells you in confidence that he took 10mg diazepam before his presentation because he was so nervous.

1. What issues need to be dealt with?
2. How can Toby's anxiety be treated?

### Issues

- **Dr Brand's behaviour** Teaching by bullying students is simply unacceptable. You should discuss this with your clinical tutor, either alone or as a firm.
- **The use of diazepam** Was Toby prescribed the diazepam? If not, he acted unprofessionally and possibly unlawfully. He needs to explain the situation to his clinical tutor so that it can be investigated and he can

be offered help. If Toby is unwilling to see the clinical tutor, then you should listen to his solution. You should not collude with a plan that allows the problem to continue. If he refuses to seek help, it is your professional responsibility to discuss matters with the clinical tutor yourself, even if this leads to disciplinary action. The effect that the diazepam had on Toby suggests that he has not developed tolerance to or dependence on the drug; however, the tutor should consider this. The help of an addictions specialist may be needed if Toby has an established problem with drugs or alcohol.

### Treatment

Toby may well have social phobia. The differential includes another anxiety disorder, anxious (avoidant) personality disorder, autistic spectrum disorder, depression, or psychosis. Toby should have a full psychiatric assessment, involving history, mental state examination, physical examination, risk assessment, and appropriate investigations. Social phobia would be managed primarily by psychological treatments (e.g. CBT), although SSRIs and beta-blockers may also help. Benzodiazepines should be avoided because of the risk of dependency in continued use. Toby may also benefit from self-help literature.

There are a variety of organizations that help doctors and medical students with psychological problems, e.g. Doctors Support Network (http://www.dsn.org.uk) or the British Medical Association 'Doctors for Doctors' scheme (www.bma.org.uk/doctorsfordoctors).

➜ Do you *really* need to involve the clinical tutor over a little diazepam? Yes, you do. If Toby needs diazepam now, how will he cope in the future? If drug abuse continues, it may be harder to detect and treat once he is a doctor, posing great risks to both him and his patients. This won't be comfortable for either of you, but Toby needs help *now*.

**Film list**

*The Aviator* (2004)—OCD

*As Good As It Gets* (1997)—OCD

*Copycat* (1995)—panic attacks, agoraphobia

*Apocalypse Now* (1979)—PTSD

*The Deer Hunter* (1979)—PTSD

**Books**

Barker, P. (1991) *Regeneration*. London: Penguin, 1992. Set in Craiglockhart Psychiatric Hospital during the First World War. Lots on shell shock (PTSD) and psychological treatments.

Haddon, M. (2006) *A Spot of Bother* London: Vintage, 2007. Touching and amusing novel focusing on a middle-aged retired man who becomes acutely anxious after finding a lesion on his leg which he believes to be cancerous.

Wilensky, A. (1999) *Passing for Normal*. London: Pocket Books, 2006. OCD in the context of Tourette's syndrome. It explores issues such as the use of medication, behavioural therapy, and support groups.

**Quotes**

Fear is the path to the dark side.

**Yoda**

For peace of mind, resign as general manager of the universe.

**Anonymous**

The brave man is not he who does not feel afraid, but he who conquers that fear.

**Nelson Mandela**

Worry often gives a small thing a big shadow.

**Swedish Proverb**

## Notes

1. Orwell, G. (1949) *Nineteen Eighty-Four*. London: Penguin, 1987.
2. Barker, P. (1991) *Regeneration*. London: Penguin, 1992.

## References/Further reading

Baldwin, D.S., Anderson, I.M., Nutt, D.J. *et al.* (2005) Evidence based guidelines for the pharmacological treatment of anxiety disorders; recommendations from the British association of psychopharmacology. *Journal of Psychopharmacology*, **19**, 567–96.

Bisson, J. ( 2002) Post-traumatic stress disorder. *Clinical Evidence*, 7, 913–19.

Brown, G.W. and Harris, T.O. (1993) Aetiology of anxiety and depressive disorders in an inner-city population. 1: Early adversity. *Psychological Medicine*, **23**, 143–54.

Ehlers, A. and Clark, D.M. (2000) A cognitive model of post traumatic stress disorder. *Behaviour Research and Therapy*, **38**, 319–45.

Fairbank, J.A., Elbert, L., and Costello, E.J. (2000) Epidemiology of traumatic events and post-traumatic stress disorder. In *Post-Traumatic Stress Disorder: Diagnosis, Management and Treatment* (ed D. Nutt, J.R.T. Davidson, and J. Zohar). London: Martin Dunitz, pp.17–27.

Fullerton, J., Cubin, M., Tiwari, H., *et al.* (2003) Linkage analysis of extremely discordant and concordant sibling pairs identifies QTL that influence variation in the human personality trait neuroticism. *American Journal of Human Genetics*, **72**, 879–90.

Heyman, I. (2006) Obsessive–compulsive disorder. *British Medical Journal*, **333**, 424–9.

Hull, A.M., Alexander, D.A., and Klein, S. (2002) Survivors of the Piper Alpha oil platform disaster: long-term follow-up study. *British Journal of Psychiatry*, **181**, 433–8.

ICD-10 (1992) *International Classification of Mental and Behavioural Disorders* (10th edn). Geneva: World Health Organization.

Kendler, K.S. (1996) Major depression and generalised anxiety disorder: same genes (partly) different environments—revisited. *British Journal of Psychiatry*, **168** (suppl 30), 68–75.

Kessler, R.C., Berglund, P.A., Demler, O., Jin, R., and Walters, E.E. (2005a) Lifetime prevalence and age-of-onset distributions of DSM-IV disorders in the National Comorbidity Survey Replication (NCS-R). *Archives of General Psychiatry*, **62**, 593–602.

Kessler, R.C., Chiu, W.T., Demler, O., and Walters, E.E. (2005b) Prevalence, severity, and comorbidity of twelve-month DSM-IV disorders in the National Comorbidity Survey Replication (NCS-R). *Archives of General Psychiatry*, **62**, 617–27.

Marks, I.M. (2005) *Living with Fear: Understanding and Coping with Anxiety* (2nd edn). New York: McGraw-Hill.

Salkovskis, P.M., Westbrook, D., Davis J., *et al.* (1997) Effects of neutralising on intrusive thoughts: an experiment investigating the aetiology of obsessive–compulsive disorder. *Behaviour Research and Therapy*, **35**, 211–19.

Shapiro, F. (2001) *Eye Movement Desensitization and Reprocessing: Basic Principles, Protocols and Procedures* (2nd edn). New York: Guilford Press.

Watson, J.B. and Rayner, R. (1920) Conditioned emotional reactions. *Journal of Experimental Psychology*, **3**, 1–14.

@ Go to www.oxfordtextbooks/orc/stringer for an array of additional references, including indicative mark sheets for OSCEs, self-assessment questions, guidance, and exercises.

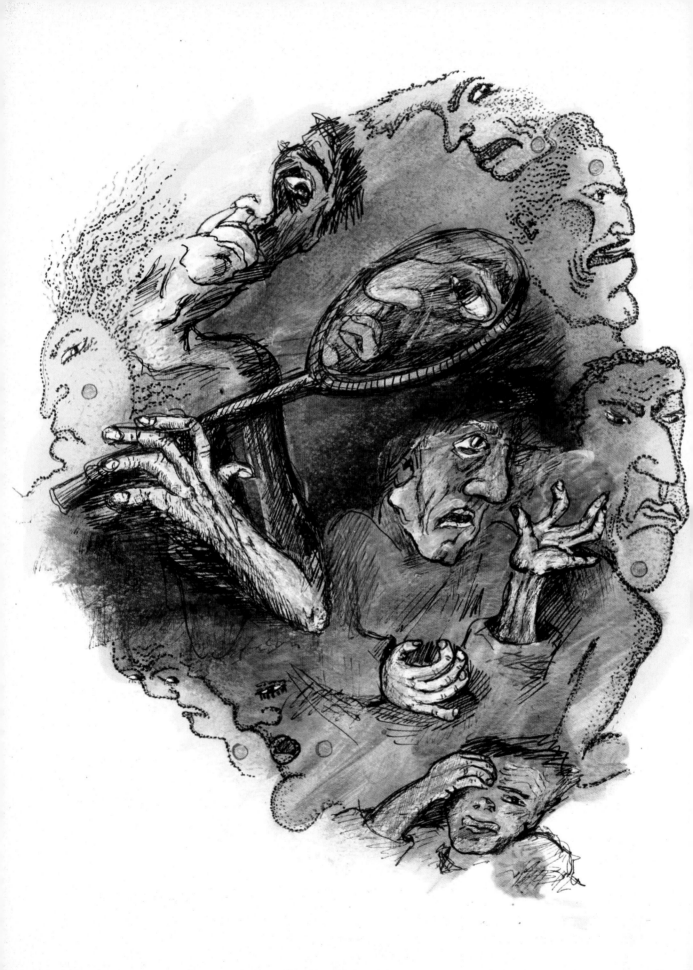

# 14 Medically unexplained symptoms

*Sarah Cader and Mark Haddah*

## True or False? Test your existing knowledge—answers in the chapter and online

1. Longer duration of formal education predisposes to the development of MUS.

2. Cognitive models of MUS show that the patient typically reduces their anxiety by taking their own pulse.

3. Chronic fatigue syndrome has been shown to be unrelated to previous viral infection.

4. People with chronic fatigue syndrome should be encouraged to exercise vigorously to break the cycle of fatigue.

5. In somatisation disorder, a patient's symptoms repeatedly focus on one particular part of the body.

6. Factitious disorder is the intentional production of physical or psychological symptoms to receive medical attention.

7. People presenting with conversion disorder may show a relative lack of concern despite very worrying symptoms.

8. Iatrogenic harm is one of the greatest risks to the health of people presenting with MUS.

9. The Reattribution Model consists of *contemplation, pre-attribution, reattribution*, and *maintenance*.

10. A patient with established irritable bowel syndrome should be referred for further investigation if they develop rectal bleeding – despite the potential for reinforcement of their anxiety.

## Contents

# PRINCIPLES

... often when I have been consulted in a Case, and found it to be what is commonly call'd Nervous, I have been in the utmost Difficulty, when desir'd to name the Distemper, for fear of affronting them ... If I call'd the case 'Glandular with nervous Symptoms', they concluded that I thought them pox'd, or had the King's Evil. If I said it was Vapours, Hysterick or Hypochondriackal Disorders, they thought that I call'd them Mad or Fantastickal ... I was in a Hazard of a Drubbing for seeming to impeach their Courage ... I myself was thought a Fool, a weak and ignorant Coxcomb, and perhaps dismiss'd in Scorn.

*The English Malady*—Dr George Cheyne[1]

## Introduction

Mind and body are *not* entirely separate, and teasing them apart is difficult and not always helpful. Medically unexplained symptoms (MUS) are physical complaints without evidence of an underlying organic cause. They are sometimes called *functional, psychosomatic, somatized,* or *somatoform* disorders. Most individuals with MUS are managed in medical outpatients and general practice; only a minority receive psychiatric referrals. Conflict, like that described by Dr Cheyne, arises when patients understandably attribute physical symptoms to physical pathology, while doctors conclude that 'non-organic' psychosocial factors are the cause. MUS can lead to frustration, excessive investigations, and chronic disability.

### Epidemiology

These disorders more commonly affect women. MUS affect around a quarter of general practice patients and a third of those seeing a neurologist. Over 50% of patients attending specialist medical outpatients at a London teaching hospital were found to have distressing medically unexplained symptoms (Nimnuan *et al.* 2001).

➡ Perhaps unexplained symptoms have 'no organic basis' because we haven't yet developed a test to find the underlying abnormality ...

### Aetiology

Genetics, a shorter duration of formal education, and childhood experiences (e.g. of parental illness) predispose to the development of MUS. Cultural and family attitudes to disease also play a role. Symptoms may be precipitated by stressful life events and maintained by unhelpful cognitive styles. The main underlying theories are as follows.

1. **Somatization** This is the unconscious expression of psychological distress through physical symptoms, e.g. rather than anger, a patient experiences abdominal pain.

2. **Psychiatric illness** Depression and anxiety symptoms can be psychological (e.g. sadness, fear) and physical (e.g. muscle aches, constipation, palpitations, headaches). Both disorders commonly present with physical symptoms in primary care.

3. **Cognitive models** An individual's interpretation of normal physiology can create anxiety and perpetuate MUS. Someone concerned about palpitations might *misinterpret* normal physiological experiences, such as a rapid heart beat while anxious, as a sign of a heart attack. *Selective attention* to the problem would lead to acute awareness of palpitations whenever they occurred. Behaviours such as *repeated checking* (e.g. of pulse rate) or constantly *seeking reassurance* would maintain anxiety long term; reassurance *reinforces* the importance of these behaviours whilst preventing patients from realizing that symptoms are benign (Salkovskis 1996).

### Clinical presentation

Symptoms are diverse with recognized syndromes, occurring in any system or specialty, e.g.

- rheumatology—fibromyalgia
- gastroenterology—irritable bowel syndrome, non-ulcer dyspepsia
- otolaryngology—dizziness, tinnitis.
- cardiology—non-cardiac chest pain, palpitations
- military medicine—Gulf War syndrome
- pain clinics—headache, pelvic pain, lower back pain.

- Also known as myalgic encephalomyelitis (ME).
- It may follow viral infection (e.g. glandular fever), but can also arise spontaneously.
- Extreme fatigue is the main complaint; patients are typically exhausted by mild exertion. This produces either an alternating pattern of activity and debilitating fatigue or complete exercise avoidance.
- Other symptoms are common, e.g. aches and pains.
- There is strong evidence for graded exercise; this is scheduled and gradually increasing activity (rather than rest).
- Pacing of activity is important: patients need realistic goals and should not do more activity than planned, even if they feel like it; otherwise they tend to exacerbate problems.
- Cognitive behavioural therapy (CBT) improves fatigue and physical functioning.

- Rare, disabling, and chronic condition.
- Ten times more common in women.
- *Multiple* medically unexplained symptoms affect any system of the body.
- Symptoms are difficult to treat, becoming a constantly moving target for clinicians.

Individuals may have very clear psychosocial stressors, but sometimes deny their relevance, either because they fear their symptoms will be dismissed as being 'all in the mind' or because they have been disappointed by previous doctors' responses to the lack of a physical cause. A patient's understanding of illness informs their symptoms, which may thus show unusual characteristics, e.g. pain of unvarying and maximal severity throughout the day, lacking usual relieving and exacerbating factors. This does *not* mean that they are making their symptoms up!

## Differential diagnosis

1. **Organic**: rule out any possible physical cause. Even if symptoms are multiple and changing, a multisystem physical illness may be responsible, e.g. sarcoidosis, occult malignancy, chronic infections (e.g. tuberculosis, HIV).

2. **Psychiatric illness**
   - **Anxiety** and **depression** can cause and exacerbate symptoms (e.g. depression lowers the pain threshold); they are commonly comorbid with MUS.
   - **Hypochondriasis**: an extreme form of health anxiety where patients believe that they have a

specific *illness* (e.g. cancer) ... with inexplicable *symptoms* ... to that of medically unex[plained] ... et al. 2002).

- **Schizophrenia, persistent** ... or affective psychosis sho[uld] ... hypochondriacal delusions ... tions may occur.

3. **Deliberate production of symptoms (rarely)**
   - **Factitious disorder**: the *deliberate* production of symptoms to receive medical treatment. Presentations include pyrexia of unknown origin, haematuria, and skin lesions. Extreme cases are termed Munchausen's syndrome.
   - **Malingering**: feigning symptoms to obtain external reward, e.g. escape military service, gain money or drugs.

The HADS (Hospital Anxiety and Depression Scale) focuses on the *cognitive* symptoms of anxiety and depression, and so helps to diagnose these disorders when physical symptoms (e.g. fatigue) are present.

## Management

1. **Therapeutic assessment** Engagement is crucial to resolution and progress. Take a full history and perform a brief physical examination.

2. **Explain and reassure** Many patients will be reassured by knowing that their symptoms are not serious, but common and familiar to you. Use the Reattribution Model (see Reality):
   - Ensure they feel understood.
   - Broaden the agenda from a physical cause to a physical *and* psychological explanation.
   - Make the link between symptoms and psychological factors.

3. **Avoid over-investigation, unnecessary specialist referrals or physical medications** These reinforce physical illness beliefs and may increase anxiety. Ensure *reasonable* investigation and review old notes and tests to prevent duplication.

4. **Emotional support** Encourage patients to discuss emotional difficulties; involve their social network and support them to deal with stress.

5. **Encourage normal function** Patients may avoid normal activities, thinking that they will exacerbate problems. Normal behaviour discourages disability!

6. **Antidepressants** may be useful, even without depression, e.g. tension headache, irritable bowel syndrome, fibromyalgia, and 'idiopathic pain' (Stahl 2003).

7. **Treat comorbid illness**, particularly anxiety or depression.

ssion, diaries, and behavioural experiments
...ents modify unhelpful cognitions, decreas-
...voidance and reassurance-seeking (Kroenke and
...indle 2000).

9. **Graded exercise** is very helpful in some disorders,
e.g. CFS and fibromyalgia.

⮕ The strength of patients' beliefs may encourage you to
order excessive investigations. Always ask yourself if
you would normally investigate *these* symptoms *this* way.

## Prognosis

Shorter duration of MUS and milder symptoms have a
better prognosis. Over a quarter of patients with problems
in primary care remain symptomatic after a year; this is
true for over half of those presenting to neurologists
with weakness or sensory symptoms. Chronic presentations fluctuate and stress can cause exacerbations. A few
patients with medically unexplained symptoms are subsequently diagnosed with organic pathology (Crimlisk
*et al.* 1998).

## Conversion (dissociative) disorders

Despite their separate classification, conversion disorders
represent a similar group of conditions. Internal conflict
is unconsciously 'converted' into neurological symptoms.
Presentations are *acute*, *specific*, and often dramatic,
following sudden stress or conflict (Aybek *et al.* 2008).
For example:

- paralysis
- blindness

- aphonia (inability to produce speech)
- seizures
- psychogenic amnesia (this is loss of *all* semantic
memories including own identity)
- multiple personality disorder (rare and controversial)
- fugue (patients lose their memory entirely and wander
away from home)
- stupor.

Again, the patient's own concept of illness informs
their symptoms, e.g. sudden anaesthesia might follow a
distribution that does not reflect dermatomes or other
sensory loss patterns. Again, this does not mean that it is
'deliberate'! Be aware that the acute stressor may not be
immediately obvious.

Exclude organic causes, before reassuring the patient
that their problem will resolve fully and quickly.
Encourage a return to normal activities and avoid reinforcing the symptoms or disability (e.g. by providing a
wheelchair). Patients should be supported to address
triggering stressors rather than focus on physical mani-
festations. The outcome tends to be better than for
other MUS.

⮕ Conversion disorder patients may show 'la belle indif-
ference'—a relative lack of concern despite obviously
worrying symptoms.

❗ A comorbid condition such as depression is associated
with particular risks (see p.41) and requires appropriate
treatment. If there is no underlying pathology, the greatest risk
to these patients is probably iatrogenic harm. Patient demands,
personal frustration, and a culture of defensive medical practice may encourage doctors to order unnecessary, invasive
investigations or provide speculative treatments. These prolong
symptoms and carry their own risks of harm.

# REALITY

## General approach: tips, tricks, and cautionary tales

### 1. A challenge

Be aware that unexplained symptoms often cause
strong feelings; negative labels are commonly applied,
e.g. 'heart-sink' or 'thick-folder' patients. These patients
have *unsolved*, rather than *unsolvable* problems. They
will challenge you to use your medical *and* psychiatric
knowledge.

### 2. Look before you leap!

Don't leap into explaining to your patient that they
are healthy; this will waste time and make them feel
that they need to correct you before discussing their
symptoms. Likewise, attempting to reassure your patient
before you've elicited *all* their fears will convince them
that you 'miss things'—both worries and deadly diseases.
Instead, be clear that their case is complex and may need
several appointments *just* to establish the history before
even considering management.

### 3. 'Feeling understood'

What do they think is wrong and why? Your history should include a 'typical day' of symptoms, including those of depression or anxiety. Explore their beliefs about the possible cause of symptoms (e.g. brain tumour). Elicit psychosocial factors which might have preceded symptoms and look at the impact of symptoms on the person's life. Note any personal or family history of medical mismanagement (e.g. undiagnosed meningitis).

### 4. 'Changing the agenda'

Your patient's agenda is physical. Your task is to bridge the gap to include a psychological *and* physical understanding. Feedback your (normal) examination/investigation findings while recognizing the reality of their symptoms, e.g.

> **You:** Your examination was normal, though your neck muscles are very tight. These headaches have been causing you a lot of pain, haven't they?
>
> **Kirsty:** Yeah—they're driving me mad.
>
> **Y:** Constant headaches are miserable! People can get headaches like this when under pressure. Other signs of being under pressure can include feeling shaky and tearful—a bit like you've been feeling since starting your new job. Do you think it's possible that this might be having an effect on your headaches?
>
> **K:** I guess . . .

This *reframes* your patient's symptoms in the context of life events and other symptoms identified during your assessment.

### 5. 'Making the link'

Make an explicit link between symptoms and your patient's emotional state, normalizing their experience. One way to is to draw a CBT-style diagram with them, e.g.

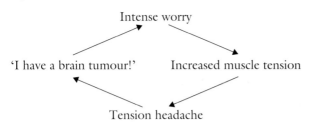

### 6. Real symptoms

Patients may feel disbelieved or accused of making up symptoms. Never say *nothing's wrong*; if that were true, they wouldn't keep consulting you! Symptoms are real: an itch is itchy, whether due to stress or scabies. By understanding this yourself, you legitimize it for your patient.

→ Talk in terms of biological *and* psychological models as early as possible, to prevent your patient feeling that they have been 'downgraded' to a psychological problem later on.

### 7. Negatives are positive

*Before* ordering tests, explain the meaning of a normal or negative result—you can both feel reassured that a frightening physical illness isn't causing their symptoms. Patients should know that you will still take their symptoms seriously if tests are negative; this is not the end of your management plan.

### 8. Believe in yourself

Patients may expect or demand specialist opinions, while *you* worry that you are missing something or feel that your expertise is being challenged. Listen to your patient, but trust your clinical judgement. If you are sure that you have excluded organic diagnoses, don't join your patient in their anxiety.

### 9. Boundaries

Offer regular scheduled appointments. One member of the team should see this patient; ten people will say ten very slightly different things—leading to ten different plans!

This opens the way for a shared understanding of the reality of symptoms, while recognizing psychosocial contributing factors.

---

**BOX 14.3** The Reattribution Model

..................................................................................

*Feeling understood*, *changing the agenda*, and *making the link* constitute Goldberg's Reattribution Model. See Goldberg *et al.* (1989) for more details.

---

# NEXT STEPS

## Suspected malignancy in a patient with a history of MUS

You are a junior doctor in a general surgical outpatient clinic, seeing Mrs Vanessa Ouade, a 52-year-old woman who has two large volumes of hospital notes. She has been seen and extensively investigated by a number of specialties within the hospital and her GP has now referred her for a year's history of irregular bowel habit and weight loss. The referral letter states that she has suffered 'largely hypochondriacal complaints' for many years. Mrs Ouade tells you: 'My GP said it was irritable bowel syndrome and there was no point seeing a specialist. I insisted, because I wasn't getting better'.

The history reveals further concerning symptoms, including PR bleeding. You state that you need to organize further tests immediately and she asks you anxiously if she has cancer. You reply that this is one possibility, but it is too early to know. Mrs Ouade tearfully asks, 'Has my GP been negligent? He kept on ignoring me and this should have been picked up sooner, right?'

1. How will you answer her question?
2. What other measures should you take?
3. How might Mrs Ouade's history of MUS affect her ongoing treatment?

### Issues
- Managing the immediate situation
- Management of a patient with previous MUS

### Your response

This is an uncomfortable situation and Mrs Ouade is aware of that. However, she does have the right to ask this question. Make sure that she understands the *facts*: she has worrying symptoms of weight loss, change in bowel habit, and rectal bleeding, but *you do not know what the diagnosis is yet*. Remain professional—neither leap to support your colleague unreservedly, nor criticize him openly, however tempting this may be. It is not *your* job to decide whether the GP was negligent, but Mrs Ouade has the right to complain which will lead to an investigation, providing an answer to her question. Explain the local complaints procedure and how she can make a complaint. Reassure her that this will *not* affect her medical management.

### Other measures

Document Mrs Ouade's symptoms in her own words, including her concerns about her treatment so far. Clearly detail the advice and explanations you have given her, remembering that your notes may be read in the event of a complaint. After the clinic, make your consultant aware of the situation. If there are concerns about the GP's fitness to practise, this should be taken up with the General Medical Council in the UK (or equivalent regulating body in other countries). Contact your medical indemnity provider to ensure that there is nothing more you can do.

### Effects on current treatment

Mrs Ouade may have had a long history of *unsatisfactory* consultations already; her confidence and trust in doctors may be very low, especially if a bowel cancer *has* been missed. This increases the complexity of her case: she may need extra time for explanations of her diagnosis and management, and to vent her feelings. She is at increased risk of depression and anxiety disorders, which may impact on management and prognosis. these must be identified and treated if present.

➜ Mrs Ouade may have *not* received the same basic history and examination from her GP because of her past consulting behaviour. Avoid over-investigation, but never dismiss new symptoms out of hand.

### Film list
*I Remember Me* (2001)—CFS
*Memento* (2000)—dissociative amnesia
*Joe Versus the Volcano* (1990)—hypochondriasis

### Books
Cardinal, M. (1975) *The Words to Say It*. London: The Women's Press, 1993 (translated by Pat Goodheart). Autobiographical account of Freudian analysis following a period of acute anxiety and depression, which manifests through medically unexplained vaginal bleeding.

Haddon, M. (2006) *A Spot of Bother*. London: Vintage, 2007. Depression and anxiety caused by a benign skin lesion and resultant belief of malignancy.

Strouse, J. (1981) *Biography of Alice James*. London: Jonathan Cape. A detailed biographical account of 'neurasthenia'—modern day CFS.

### Quotes
I told you I was ill.
**Spike Milligan, *epitaph***

The Doctor answered me quietly and calmly: 'Those are psychosomatic disorders. That doesn't interest me. Speak about something else.'
**Marie Cardinal, *The Words to Say It*.**

## Note

1. Cheyne, G. (1733) *The English Malady: or A Treatise of Nervous Diseases of all Kinds*. London: G. Strahan.

## References/Further reading

Aybek, S., Kanaan, R.A., and David, A.S. (2008) The neuropsychiatry of conversion disorder. *Current Opinion in Psychiatry*, **21**, 275–80.

Crimlisk, H., Bhatia, K., Cope, H., *et al.* (1998) Slater revisited: 6 year follow up of patients with medically unexplained motor symptoms. *British Medical Journal*, **316**, 582–6.

Fink, P., Rosendal, M., and Toft, T. (2002) Assessment and treatment of functional disorders in general practice: the extended reattribution and management model—an advanced educational program for nonpsychiatric doctors. *Psychosomatics*, **43**, 93–131.

Goldberg, D., Gask, L., and O'Dowd, T. (1989) The treatment of somatization: teaching techniques of reattribution. *Journal of Psychosomatic Research*, **33(6)**, 689–95.

Hatcher, S. and Arroll, B. (2008) Assessment and management of medically unexplained symptoms. *British Medical Journal*, **336**, 1124–8.

Kroenke, K. and Swindle, R. (2000) Cognitive-behavioral therapy for somatization and symptom syndromes: a critical review of controlled clinical trials. *Psychotherapy and Psychosomatics*, **69**, 205–15.

Lloyd, G. and Guthrie, E. (2007) *Handbook of Liaison Psychiatry*. Cambridge University Press.

Nimnuan, C., Hotopf, N., and Wessely, S. (2001) Medically unexplained symptoms: epidemiological studies in seven specialities. *Journal of Psychosomatic Research*, **51**, 361–7.

Salkovskis, P.M. (1996) The cognitive approach to anxiety: threat beliefs, safety-seeking behaviour and the special case of health anxiety and obsessions. In *Frontiers of Cognitive Therapy* (ed P.M. Salkovskis). New York: Guilford Press.

Stahl, S.M. (2003) Antidepressants and somatic symptoms: therapeutic actions are expanding beyond affective spectrum disorders to functional somatic syndromes. *Journal of Clinical Psychology*, **64**, 745–6.

Wessely, S., Nimnuan, C., and Sharpe, M. (1999) Functional somatic syndromes: one or many? *Lancet*, **354**, 936–9.

 Go to www.oxfordtextbooks/orc/stringer for an array of additional references, including indicative mark sheets for OSCEs, self-assessment questions, guidance, and exercises.

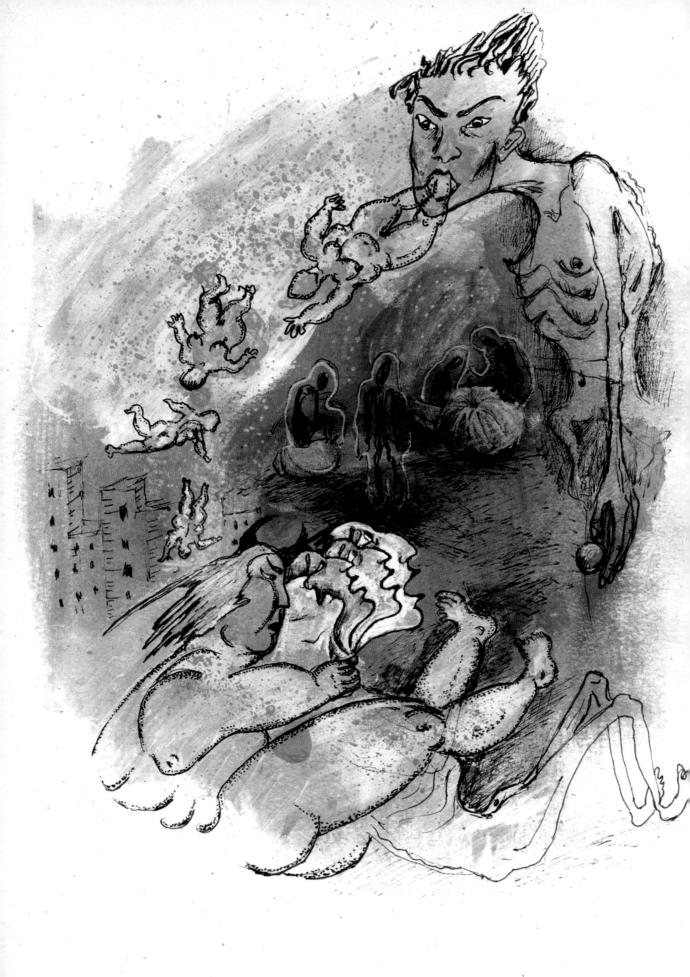

# 15 Eating disorders

*Sarah Cader and Janet Treasure*

## True or False? Test your existing knowledge—answers in the chapter and online

1. 5% of people with eating disorders are male.

2. Perfectionism and low self esteem are psychological traits strongly associated with anorexia nervosa but not bulimia nervosa.

3. Anorexia is a cause of pancytopenia.

4. Russell's sign is evidence of malnutrition in patients with eating disorders.

5. Most patients with a diagnosed eating disorder will require inpatient treatment, at least in the early stages of therapy.

6. Refeeding syndrome is characterised by low potassium and high magnesium and phosphate.

7. In anorexia nervosa, failure to complete the squat test is an indicator that inpatient treatment may be required.

8. High risk eating disorder patients invariably have a BMI <17.5.

9. Rather than building rapport, weight jokes are generally unhelpful when working with patients with eating disorders.

10. Patients with anorexia nervosa lose their right to confidentiality once their BMI falls below 17.0.

## Contents

# PRINCIPLES

Flesh is heretic.
My body is a witch.
I am burning it.

Yes I am torching
her curves and paps and wiles.
They scorch in my self denials.

*Anorexic*—Eavan Boland[1]

## Introduction

Eating disorders typically affect perfectionist, high-achieving young women with low self-esteem. In Western cultures the ideal of feminine beauty is to be slender, exemplified by abnormally thin fashion models. Dieting becomes an eating disorder when the pursuit of thinness becomes all-consuming: anorexia nervosa (AN) involves weight loss methods causing extreme emaciation, bulimia nervosa (BN) involves binge eating followed by vomiting, and binge eating disorder (BED) is BN without the purging. BED may result in obesity and is more usually seen by physicians, so will not be covered in this chapter.

## Epidemiology

Women are more commonly affected, although the incidence in men is increasingly recognized and accounts for 10% of cases. The lifetime prevalence of eating disorders is:

- anorexia nervosa—0.6%
- bulimia nervosa—1.0%
- binge eating disorder—2.8%.

AN mostly affects Westernized societies, where black and ethnic minority groups are at lower risk than white populations (Striegel-Moore *et al.* 2000). Onset is usually in girls aged 16–22, and affects all social classes.

BN is more common than AN, but is also probably largely undetected since patients are usually as secretive as in AN, but not as obviously emaciated. BN usually starts in mid-adolescence.

Eating disorders are commonly comorbid with other mental health disorders, especially depression and substance misuse.

## Aetiology

### Genetics

In AN, heritability is estimated at 58%, and the MZ:DZ twin concordance rates are 65:32. Genes are less salient in bulimia (Wade *et al.* 2007).

### Psychological theories

Perfectionism and low self-esteem are risk factors for both AN and BN. Theories for AN include the idea that successful weight loss enhances the patient's sense of achievement, autonomy, and perfectionism. When life feels uncontrollable, AN comforts by providing the ability to control *something* (weight). The disorder can also be seen as a way of avoiding separation from family or becoming an independent sexual being; it maintains dependency on close family *and* a peri-pubertal physique.

### Sociocultural

Social pressures to be thin and the promotion of dieting are important influences on the development of both AN and BN. High-risk groups include occupations where emphasis is on weight or body image, e.g. models, athletes, and dancers.

### Personal history

People with BN often have a history of obesity and up to 50% have previously suffered from AN (the reverse pattern occurs less frequently). Experiences of child abuse are commonly found in AN and BN, but no more so than in other psychiatric illnesses.

### Family

Parental overprotection and family enmeshment are associated with AN. Enmeshment describes relationships that are over-involved, with poor boundaries making it difficult for members to feel independent. BN is connected with disturbed family dynamics, parental weight concern, and high parental expectation. A family history of obesity, depression, or substance misuse are also risk factors.

## Anorexia nervosa

### Clinical presentation

There are four main diagnostic points in AN.

1. **Body mass index (BMI) <17.5** (or weight 15% less than expected).
2. **Deliberate weight loss** People with AN go to extraordinary lengths to lose weight, becoming extremely emaciated. They restrict calorie intake by avoiding 'fattening' foods (e.g. chocolate) and may also use laxatives, vomiting, or excessive exercise. Appetite suppressants, thyroxine, diuretics, and stimulants (e.g. cocaine) can all be used to lose weight. Diabetics may 'skip' insulin doses to prevent fat deposition.
3. **Distorted body image** Patients are preoccupied with body shape and a dread of weight gain. They hold overvalued ideas that they are fat, des[...] very thin.
4. **Endocrine dysfunction** The hypothalami[...] gonadal axis is affected, causing amen[...] women and impotence in men. Libido is lost in both sexes. If AN begins before puberty, menarche and breast development are delayed or arrested.

Weight loss sets up a vicious circle, as some of the symptoms of AN result from starvation. Preoccupation with food becomes constant, and people may cook elaborate meals for their families, concealing their avoidance of eating in a flurry of activity. A recent unhelpful development is online chat rooms where weight loss methods are swapped.

>> *See Reality for an AN role play (p.183).*

### Physical complications

Eating disorders may present with physical complications.

1. **General** Lethargy and cold intolerance are common. Pancytopenia occurs in severe anorexia where there is bone marrow hypoplasia; milder disorders may show anaemia, leucopenia, or thrombocytopenia. Infections may result from decreased immunity.

---

**BOX 15.1** Body mass index

$$BMI = weight\ (kg)/[height\ (m)]^2$$

---

**TABLE 15.1** Examination findings in anorexia nervosa

| System | Physical examination findings secondary to: | |
| --- | --- | --- |
| | **Malnutrition** | **Binge/purge/vomit** |
| General appearance | Emaciation<br>Dry skin, brittle hair/nails<br>Fine downy (lanugo) hair<br>Reduced sexual maturation<br>Blue/cold extremities<br>Oedema<br>Anaemia<br>Low $SaO_2$<br>Hypothermia | Russell's sign (calluses or cuts on the knuckles from self-induced vomiting)<br>Swollen salivary glands (puffy face)<br>Oedema |
| Cardiovascular | Bradycardia<br>Low BP/postural drop<br>Peripheral oedema | Arrhythmias |
| Gastrointestinal | Tender abdomen | Tender abdomen<br>Erosion of dental enamel<br>Caries |
| Musculoskeletal | Muscle wasting (general and proximal myopathy)<br>Short stature (early onset AN)<br>Previous or current fractures | |
| Metabolic | Hypercholesterolaemia<br>Hypercarotenaemia (yellow skin tinge, especially soles and palms) | Hypercholesterolaemia<br>Hypercarotenaemia |
| Neurological | Peripheral neuropathy | Peripheral neuropathy |

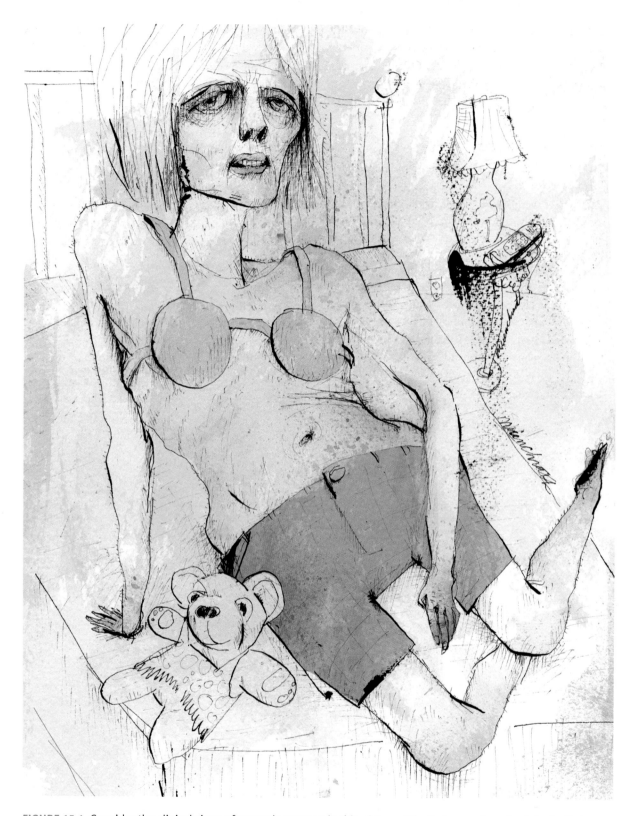

**FIGURE 15.1** Consider the clinical signs of anorexia nervosa in this picture. What's happening physiologically to account for this appearance?

2. **Cardiovascular** Over 80% of AN patients experience cardiac complications, risking sudden death. Problems include bradycardia, hypotension (postural drop), arrhythmias (usually secondary to hypokalaemia), mitral valve dysfunction, and cardiac failure.

3. **Gastrointestinal** These range from constipation and abdominal pain to ulcers, oesophageal tears, and gastric rupture due to vomiting. Delayed gastric emptying makes patients feel bloated after eating even small amounts. A nutritional hepatitis occurs in a third of patients, detected by a low serum protein, with raised bilirubin, lactate dehydrogenase, and alkaline phosphatase.

4. **Reproductive** In women, amenorrhoea is a diagnostic criterion, and infertility (due to atrophy of ovaries or testes) may also occur in both women and men. There is usually a loss of libido, and males may notice the loss of morning erections.

5. **Musculoskeletal** Osteoporosis leads to fractures and proximal myopathy is often severe.

6. **Neurological** Peripheral neuropathy, delirium, convulsions or even coma may occur.

🔑 Lanugo hair is the body's attempt to keep warm following body fat loss.

🔑 Swollen parotid and submandibular glands occur after bingeing.

## Differential diagnosis

1. **Medical causes of weight loss**, e.g. hyperthyroidism, malignancy, gastrointestinal disease, Addison's disease, chronic infection, inflammatory conditions, and AIDS.

2. **Depression**: weight loss can be severe in depression, but would not be denied. Low mood is common in AN, but weight gain would be resisted.

3. **Bulimia nervosa**: bingeing and vomiting can occur in anorexia nervosa, but BN should be diagnosed if this is the predominant behaviour and the patient is not underweight.

4. **Eating disorder not otherwise specified (EDNOS)**: the term for atypical presentations.

5. **Body dysmorphic disorder (BDD)**: BDD is a condition characterized by body image distortion (e.g. belief that the nose is misshapen). Deliberate weight loss in BDD would be unusual.

6. **Psychosis**: self-starvation might occur if food is believed to be poisoned.

## Investigations

1. Height, weight, and BMI.

2. Squat test: Ask the patient to squat down and rise to standing without using their arms (difficult with proximal myopathy).

3. Essential blood tests
   - ESR, TFTs—exclude most organic causes of weight loss, e.g. hyperthyroidism. ESR is normal or low in anorexia.
   - FBC, U&E, phosphate, albumin, LFT, creatinine kinase, glucose—evaluate nutritional state and risk.

4. ECG: Bradycardia, arrhythmias, and a prolonged QT interval.

5. Other tests as indicated, e.g. DEXA scans (low bone density).

**TABLE 15.2** Blood tests.

| | Abnormality | | Reason | |
|---|---|---|---|---|
| | **Low** | **High** | **Starvation** | **Binge/purge/vomit** |
| FBC | ✓ (Hb, WCC, platelets) | | ✓ | ✓ (WCC) |
| U&E | ✓ | | ✓ Urea | ✓ K⁺, Na⁺ |
| Phosphate | ✓ | | ✓ | ✓ |
| LFT | | ✓ (ALP, bilirubin) | ✓ | |
| Albumin | ✓ | | ✓ | |
| Creatine kinase | | ✓ | ✓ | |
| Glucose | ✓ | | ✓ | ✓ |
| TFT | ✓ (T₃) | | ✓ | |
| FSH, LH, oestrogen, progesterone | ✓ | | ✓ | |
| Calcium | ✓ | | ✓ | ✓ |
| Magnesium | ✓ | | ✓ | ✓ |
| Amylase | | ✓ | | ✓ |
| Chloride | ✓ | | | ✓ |
| Cortisol | | ✓ | ✓ | |
| Growth hormone | | ✓ | ✓ | |
| Cholesterol | | ✓ | ✓ | ✓ |

$T_3$ = tri-iodothyronine; FSH = follicle-stimulating hormone; LH = luteinizing hormone; ALP = alkaline phosphatase.

Melanosis coli (pigmentation of colonic mucosa) results from laxative abuse (Oster *et al.* 1980).

## Management

Most people are managed long-term as outpatients.

1. **Engagement** is crucial, and the initial interview requires time and great skill. The patient's family are usually involved early on.

2. **Psycho-education** advises on nutrition and health.

3. **Treat comorbid psychiatric illness** Depression, OCD, and substance misuse are all fairly common.

4. **Nutritional management and weight restoration** A realistic weekly weight gain target needs to be negotiated (usually 0.5–1kg/week). A target weight and eating plan are also established.

5. **Psychotherapies**
   - *Motivational interviewing* is an important approach when trying to engage ambivalent patients who lack insight into their disorder—or hold positive views of their illness (see p.98).
   - *Family therapy*—rather than simply focusing on the patient, this involves the whole family. Patients with a short history of early onset anorexia (onset before 19 years) show greatest response.
   - *Interpersonal therapy* aims at improving social functioning and interpersonal skills. This is better for patients with later onset or longer duration of illness.
   - *Cognitive behavioural therapy*—addresses control, low self-esteem, and perfectionism.

6. **Medical treatment** is especially important if there are physical complications, rapid weight loss, or BMI <13.5.

7. **Inpatient treatment** (preferably in a specialist eating disorders unit) may be necessary if:
   - BMI <13 or extremely rapid weight loss
   - serious physical complications
   - high suicide risk.

Day hospitals and partial hospitalization may be preferable to full-time admission. The Mental Health Act is occasionally needed to enable compulsory refeeding.

➡ Family members may share the patient's perfectionist traits, making the carer's role extremely stressful.

➡ Do not get into a battle of wills with people with anorexia nervosa—you will lose!

## Bulimia nervosa

### Clinical presentation

1. **Binge eating** Repeated bouts of overeating characterize BN. Patients experience irresistible cravings for food and *lose control,* eating enormous amounts, often of food usually regarded as 'forbidden' (sweet, high calorie, high fat), e.g. 15 doughnuts and a tub of ice-cream. Thousands of calories may be consumed and there is often a sense of desperate urgency and compulsion. Binges are frequently triggered by distress.

2. **Purging** Binges cause feelings of shame and guilt, and result in desperate measures to undo the 'damage', e.g. vomiting, use of laxatives or diuretics. Between binges, there may be episodes of fasting and excessive exercise to control weight.

3. **Body image distortion** Patients feel fat, are preoccupied with their shape and weight, and often hate their body.

4. **BMI >17.5** In contrast with AN, patients with BN are of normal or slightly increased weight and periods are usually present.

Patients are very secretive about their binging or purging behaviour. Since weight is usually normal, physical symptoms are mostly those secondary to vomiting and purging, e.g. arrhythmias (hypokalaemia) or convulsions (hyponatraemia).

### Investigations

These are similar to anorexia, paying particular attention to electrolytes and the ECG.

### Management

Most BN patients are managed in the community.

1. **Treat medical complications**.

2. **SSRIs** (fluoxetine) can reduce binging and purging through enhancing impulse control.

3. **Treat comorbid psychiatric illness** Depression, self-harm, and substance misuse occur frequently.

4. **CBT** is helpful in controlling symptoms. Longer-term psychotherapies may be needed to address underlying and comorbid problems.

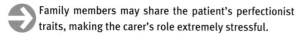 Prognosis

After 10 years, 50% of patients with AN have no eating disorder and 10% have died (suicide accounts for a third of deaths). The remaining 40% have ongoing problems and crossover to BN is common. Poor prognostic indicators include very low weight, bulimic features, later onset, or longer illness duration.

The prognosis for BN is better. Seventy per cent have recovered completely and only 1% have died at 10 years. A poorer prognosis is found in those with severe binging or purging, low body weight, and comorbid depression (Sullivan 2002).

! Urgent medical treatment is needed in high-risk patients with nutritional decompensation. Markers of this include:

- BMI <13
- weight loss >1kg/week
- purpuric rash
- cold peripheries
- core body temperature <34.5°C
- hypotension (systolic <80mmHg, diastolic <50mmHg)
- bradycardia (<40bpm) with prolonged QT interval on ECG

- inability to stand from squatting without using arms for leverage (squat test)
- electrolyte imbalance: $K^+ < 2.5$, $Na^+ < 130$ or $PO_4 < 0.5$.

Establishing adequate food intake in such patients can also be hazardous: *refeeding syndrome* is a recognized cause of mortality in the early stages of treatment. This is characterized by electrolyte imbalance (principally low serum phosphate, potassium, and magnesium) caused by their sudden intracellular movement due to the switch from fat to carbohydrate metabolism and associated increased secretion of insulin (Hearing 2004).

# REALITY

## General approach: tips, tricks, and cautionary tales

Many of these ideas apply to people who are under- *or* overweight.

### 1. Food and weight *aren't* the problem

You wouldn't tell a patient choking on a peanut to *breathe more*—you'd deal with the peanut! Telling someone with an eating disorder to *eat more* or *less* misses the point: food and weight are superficial signs of deeper problems. Recognize that they are probably struggling with big issues, including low self-esteem. Offering your support in understanding and working with their problems is a big deal: if these can be done, the rest should eventually fall into place.

### 2. Respect the patient's concerns

If someone is worried that their eating is a problem, then it *is* a problem (even with a normal BMI). People often worry that you will think them a 'fraud' or not 'sick enough' or 'thin enough' to need help. Overweight patients fear being dismissed as simply *fat*, *greedy*, *lazy*, or *weak-willed*. Respect their courage in asking for help —and take them seriously before the situation worsens.

### 3. Optimistic realism

Weight problems can feel overwhelming. Believe that your patient is capable of change, but be realistic, or you will set them up for failure and shame. Let your patient know that, as much as you would both love a *quick fix*, sustainable change takes longer. It is hard work and *very likely* that they will struggle at times, come to a standstill, or even go into reverse. It will help them to know beforehand that this is common and you won't be disappointed when they struggle.

### 4. Mind your language

People with weight problems are often exquisitely sensitive to comments, particularly perceived criticism: 'You look well/better' can be misinterpreted as *you are fat*. Describing weights or BMIs as *good* or *bad* can feel judgemental or a reflection on them being a *good* or *bad* patient. Similarly, beware of giving conditional praise (e.g. congratulating weight gain/loss). Rather, pay attention to the *process*: 'It looks as if you've worked hard/it was a challenge this week'.

It may sound obvious, but don't tell people with anorexia how *lucky* they are to be so slim. As well as being completely insensitive, it may reinforce their need to stay thin. Likewise, commenting on your own weight or weight problems is unhelpful and unprofessional.

People are often sensitive to control and will be very worried that you are trying to 'make them' lose or gain weight (AN and BN especially fear being made fat). They will engage more willingly if you are interested in *them* rather than focusing exclusively on their weight.

### 5. Jokes

Weight jokes are hurtful and inappropriate. Remember that weight is an obvious target for teasing from all sides: family, friends, even the general public. Although you'll forget the joke, your patient won't—even if they laughed politely with you at the time.

### 6. Put down the whip

People with eating disorders are usually rather hard on themselves. It *won't* motivate them to 'get better' if they receive additional punishment from you when they fail to improve. Punishment includes:

- frightening lectures about The Dangers of their weight
- insults or patronising comments
- frustrated sighs.

These tactics increase stress and make people revert back to old coping tactics. For example, having been berated for gaining weight, an overweight patient may leave, feeling that they have failed you—and binge to comfort themselves. You should feel partly responsible if they gain more weight or never return to see you again! Instead, recognize that they had a difficult week and try to understand why.

People *do* need to know about the dangers of extreme weight and weight loss methods—but give information in small and relevant chunks. Rather than scaring patients with health risks, use health benefits to reinforce their successes, e.g. 'Well done! You have lowered your risk of heart disease'.

## 7. Family matters

Families may feel stressed and helpless when dealing with eating disorders. They may be overly protective or directive, or break rules 1–6, accommodating or reinforcing eating disorder behaviours. Sharing ideas you find helpful in working with eating disorder patients can encourage families to rethink their own behaviours.

Your role is to facilitate discussions about problems in the family and keep everyone working together, *not* to take sides if arguments arise.

## 8. Treat people, not epidemiology

Most people with anorexia *are* young, white and female, but don't let this blind you to your older, ethnic minority, and male patients. Tune your clinical radar to symptoms and problems, not epidemiology.

## 9. A 'normal' BMI does not mean that your patient is well

People with eating disorders are suffering psychologically, whatever their BMI, and achieving a 'target weight' is not a 'cure' for this. BMIs are a useful marker of nutritional health, but can give a false sense of security unless viewed within your patient's overall context. For example, someone with a normal BMI may have life-threatening electrolyte abnormalities.

## The interview

### Anorexia or bulimia nervosa
*Eating and anorexic behaviour*

- How do you feel about your current weight?
- Are you trying to lose weight at the moment?

- How are you doing that? (calorie control, vomit, exercise, laxatives . . . ) Frequency? Triggers?
- What's your *ideal* weight?
- Can you take me through an average day?
- What are the *rules* of your weight loss plan?
- Do you worry that you'll lose control if you relax your rules a little?
- How do you feel about your body?
- What do your friends/family think about your weight?
- Do you ever lose control or binge? How often? What do you eat? How do you feel during and after?
- How do you manage the social side of eating? (eating with others, eating out)

*Physical problems*

- How's your physical health at the moment?
- Sometimes people on diets notice physical changes other than weight loss . . .
  - **periods** (*regularity and last one*), libido, dizziness, weakness, cold sensitivity, digestive problems.

*Screening for important psychosocial symptoms*

- What effect has this had on other areas of your life?
  - education/career/relationships with friends and family/ social life/spiritual life.

Rather than focusing on the details of the diet, look at the problems it causes and the overall pattern and *meaning* of eating.

---

**BOX 15.2** SCOFF screen

- Do you make yourself **S**ick because you feel uncomfortably full?
- Do you worry you've lost **C**ontrol over how much you eat?
- Have you recently lost more than **O**ne stone in a three-month period?
- Do you believe yourself to be **F**at when others say you are too thin?
- Would you say that **F**ood dominates your life?

One point for every 'yes': a score of 2 indicates a likely diagnosis of anorexia nervosa or bulimia

Morgan *et al.* 1999

---

Eating disorders are often a long war fought together by you, your patient, and their family. Don't expect to win every battle, or for problems to be solved quickly. If your patient vaguely trusts you after the first interview, you've started well.

# Eating disorder history (15 minutes)

## Candidate's instructions

You are a final-year medical student holding your own clinic in a GP surgery. Samantha O'Donoghue is a 17-year-old student. Her mother discovered her vomiting and brought her in. The practice nurse reports:

- height = 171cm
- weight = 51.0kg
- BMI = 17.4

Take a history of the eating disorder, sufficient to present Samantha to a senior colleague.

## Patient's brief

### Key characteristics

- I'm thin, annoyed, and wearing loose clothes. I fidget and chew gum.
- I won't divulge weight-loss methods unless directly asked.
- I grow sullen if I feel I'm being *told off* or pressurized to eat more.

I was sick! So? I finally take control of my life and everyone freaks out! I was bullied all through school for being fat: the other girls made fun of me and used to steal my lunch to 'help me lose weight'. I was a comfort-eater, eating whenever I was upset. Mum and Dad got divorced when I was sixteen after mum had an affair with Kevin (my step-dad now). I reached 80kg and couldn't go to my leavers' ball because I looked disgusting. When I got to college, eighteen months ago, I decided it was time to change. I joined a slimming club and got down to my target weight of 65kg in six months. Everyone said I looked great! I felt confident *at last*: no more bullying. I wanted to lose more weight but the slimming club wouldn't help, so I created my own diet and started running. I now weigh 51kg but I'll be happy when I'm 48kg.

I eat 500 calories a day: black coffee for breakfast; a *huge* salad at lunch; pasta and a piece of fruit for dinner. I cook for my family every evening but don't eat it. I chew my food and secretly spit it into a tissue. I let myself have a weekly chocolate bar but I throw up afterwards. That's how Mum caught me . . . I tried laxatives once but got awful stomach cramps; it was easier just to eat carefully. I don't use diet pills, diuretics, or anything else. I weigh and measure myself daily. I think about food and feel hungry all the time, but it'll be worth it when I'm thin enough to go to the summer ball.

I hate my body, especially naked. It's annoying when people say I'm skinny. They don't know what they're talking about: the cellulite, my fat belly and thighs . . . Euugh! I'm fit, though—I run three miles a day, never mind how tired I feel. My periods stopped a year ago but that often happens to athletes. My online friends understand me and they agree—everyone's worrying for no reason. I've a bright future; I'm predicted all A grades and I'm going to Edinburgh University to study law.

### Other history

- I'm constipated (bowels open weekly, small volumes) and my hands and feet are always cold. I get dizzy if I stand up too fast.
- I used to cut myself to cope with stress, but I only do it very rarely now.
- My sister was bulimic but recovered. She's *enormous* now.
- I was really close to my mum but things change . . .
- I don't drink or use drugs. I smoke 10 cigarettes a day.
- I'm not depressed or suicidal. I enjoy cooking, though I'm tired a lot.

### Questions

You won't tell Mum *everything*, will you?

### Worries

You want to make me fat.

# NEXT STEPS

## An underweight woman with fertility problems

You are a junior doctor working in a specialist out-patient clinic offering fertility treatment. Sean and Sarah Fox, both lawyers, have been unable to conceive for 2 years. Sarah is 33 and clearly underweight. When you speak with her alone she admits that her last period was 3 years ago, but protests that she 'eats normally'. You ask if she has ever seen a psychiatrist, but she curtly says she hasn't, 'because there *isn't* a problem'.

1. What further information do you need?
2. How could you encourage Sarah to accept that this is a problem?
3. Two weeks later she is weighed at her GP surgery and has gained 4kg. What are your thoughts on this?

### Issues

- Diagnosis
- Risk assessment
- Early management in a patient with apparently poor insight
- Confidentiality and relationship with husband

### Further information

You need to take a focused psychiatric history and perform a mental state and physical examination. As well as amenorrhoea, you must find evidence to support a diagnosis of AN: record an accurate BMI; ask about deliberate weight loss and distorted body image. You should look for comorbid problems such as suicidal ideation, depression, and substance misuse (including medications to aid weight loss).

The physical examination should pay particular attention to signs associated with high mortality, e.g. temperature, BP, pulse, and squat test (see p.179). Blood tests (p.179) and an ECG should be arranged immediately. You should be able to assess Sarah's risk; this will dictate the urgency of your referral. If the risk is low, you should inform her GP of your concerns by letter, to enable onward psychiatric referral. If you are worried that her risk is high (or you are *uncertain* of the level of risk), you should urgently contact a psychiatrist to discuss her case, asking her to wait in the clinic while you do so. Sarah may require an emergency psychiatric assessment, and—in extreme circumstances—admission to hospital for safe correction of nutritional decompensation.

### Enhancing motivation and understanding

It is important to assess Sarah's understanding of her condition and willingness to address problems. In a short appointment, you are unlikely to 'cure' her of a three-year history of AN, but you can help her to realize that there *is* a connection between her low weight and inability to conceive, which may be important in motivating her to gain weight in the longer term. If you listen to her worries and are sympathetic to her situation, you will increase her chances of engaging with her GP.

Other causes for infertility may need consideration, but anorexia nervosa is likely to be the problem and will need treatment before other causes can be addressed. Gain Sarah's permission to explain the situation to Sean; even if Sarah wants to hide the full extent of her eating problems, it would be reasonable to explain that you feel her weight is too low to conceive currently. This may be an opportunity to involve Sean in Sarah's treatment.

### 3. 4kg weight gain

This seems a lot and may be an erroneous result. Small variations in weight *matter* in this patient group, so always use the same scales and ensure that they are calibrated and accurate. Weighing should take place in normal indoor clothes (without shoes, coats, etc.). Pockets should be emptied of heavy objects beforehand, since patients sometimes fill them to simulate weight gain. Another 'trick' that can give the impression of weight gain is *water loading*, where patients drink excessively beforehand: look out for the wriggly patient who is desperate for the toilet at weighing time!

It is essential to look for all the symptoms of AN—not just a low BMI. Cancer, hyperthyroidism, AIDS, etc. could all lower a BMI to the point where conception was unlikely, although these patients would usually agree that they were too thin and wouldn't be worried about gaining weight.

**Film list**

*Malos Hábitos* (*Bad Habits*) (2007)

*The Best Little Girl in the World* (1981)

**Books**

Hornbacher, M. (1998) *Wasted*. London: Flamingo, 1999. One of the best autobiographical accounts of anorexia, including frank depiction of a number of classical and more inventive deceptive measures employed to maintain an image of recovery.

Lee, C. (2004) *To Die For: The True Story of a Broken Childhood*. London: Arrow Books, 2005. Biographical account of eating disorders written by the aunt of a sufferer, including diary sections.

Mantell, H. (1995) *An Experiment In Love*. London: Harper Perennial, 2004. Fictional look at how eating disorders can become manifest in pressured group situations, exploring contol issues relating to eating problems as well as social constructions of femininity and their relationship to thinness.

**Quotes**

Don't dig your grave with your own knife and fork.

**English proverb**

They are sick that surfeit with too much, as they that starve with nothing.

**William Shakespeare,** *Merchant of Venice*

You're only popular with anorexia

So I turn myself inside out

In hope someone will see

**Tori Amos,** *Jackie's Strength*

## Note

1. *Anorexic* by Eavan Boland. From *Selected Poems* published by Carcanet Press Ltd (1989).

## References/Further reading

Birmingham, C. and Beumont, P. (2004) *Anorexia Nervosa: A Practical Guide to Medical Management.* Cambridge University Press.

Hearing, S. (2004) Refeeding syndrome. *British Medical Journal*, **328**, 908–9.

Morgan, J.F., Reid, F., and Lacey, J.H. (1999) The SCOFF questionnaire: assessment of a new screening tool for eating disorders. *British Medical Journal*, **319**, 1467–8.

Oster, J.R., Materson, B.J., and Rogers, A.I. (1980) Laxative abuse syndrome. *American Journal of Gastroenterology*, **74**, 451–8.

Samuel, D.G. (2008) Personal view: the tale of an anorexic male medical student. *British Medical Journal*, **336**, 892.

Sharp, C.W. and Freeman, C.P.L. (1993) The medical complications of anorexia nervosa. *British Journal of Psychiatry*, **162**, 452–62.

Striegel-Moore, R.H., Schreiber, G.B., Lo, A., *et al.* (2000) Eating disorder symptoms in a cohort of 11 to 16-year-old black and white girls: the NHLBI growth and health study. *International Journal of Eating Disorders*, **27**, 49–66.

Sullivan, P.F. (2002) Course and prognosis of anorexia and bulimia nervosa. In *Eating Disorders and Obesity* (ed. C. Fairburn and K.D. Brownell). New York: Guilford Press.

Treasure, J. (1997) *Anorexia Nervosa: A Survival Guide for Sufferers and Those Caring for Someone with an Eating Disorder.* Hove: Psychology Press (this is a self-help book for people with an eating disorder and those who care for them).

Treasure, J., Schmidt, U., and Van Furth, E. (2003) *Handbook of Eating Disorders*. Chichester: John Wiley.

Wade, T.D., Gillespie, N., and Martin, N.G. (2007) A comparison of early family life events amongst monozygotic twin women with lifetime anorexia nervosa, bulimia nervosa, or major depression. *International Journal of Eating Disorders*, **40**, 679–86.

 Go to www.oxfordtextbooks/orc/stringer for an array of additional references, including indicative mark sheets for OSCEs, self-assessment questions, guidance, and exercises.

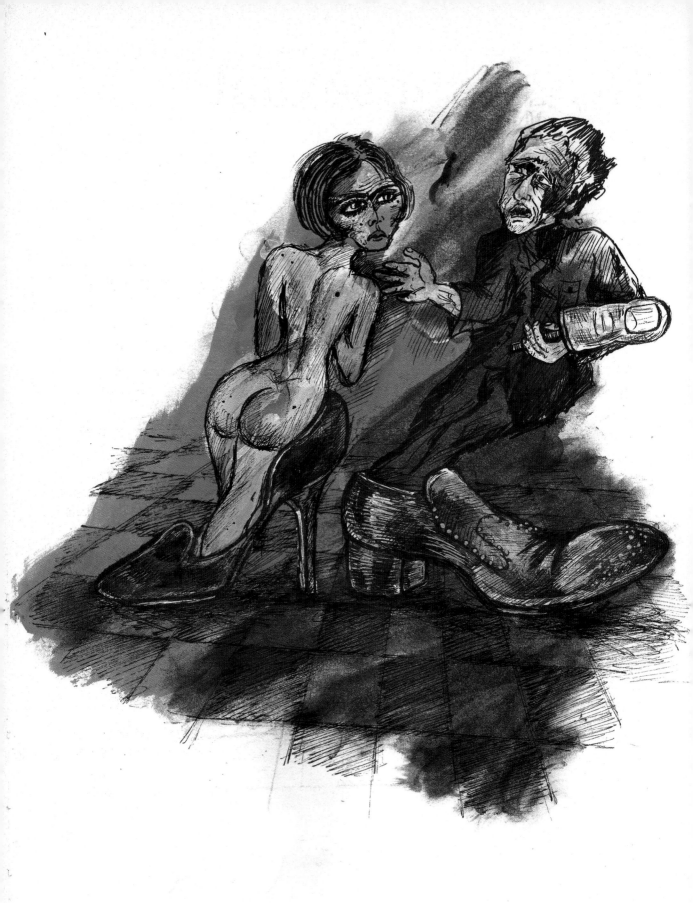

# 16 Psychosexual disorders

*Martin Baggaley*

## True or False? Test your existing knowledge—answers in the chapter and online

1. In sensate focus therapy, sexual intercourse is initially banned entirely.

2. Hypersexuality is more common in men than women.

3. Beta blockers are helpful in the treatment of erectile dysfunction.

4. Doctors are a recognised cause of erectile dysfunction.

5. SSRIs may improve premature ejaculation.

6. Vaginismus can affect women who have never been sexually active.

7. Paraphilias are treated with exposure therapy.

8. All transsexual patients must undergo psychiatric assessment before receiving gender reassignment surgery.

9. You should explain to patients that discussions about sex are afforded complete confidentiality.

10. A 48 year old woman becomes distressed during a smear test and discloses that she was raped. It is your clinical responsibility to inform the police if she refuses to do so.

## Contents

# PRINCIPLES

The world is not to be divided into sheep and goats. Not all things are black nor all things white. It is a fundamental of taxonomy that nature rarely deals with discrete categories. Only the human mind invents categories and tries to force facts into separated pigeon-holes. The living world is a continuum in each and every one of its aspects. The sooner we learn this concerning human sexual behaviour, the sooner we shall reach a sound understanding of the realities of sex.

*Sexuality in the Human Male*—A.C. Kinsey *et al.*[1]

## Introduction

Sexual problems adversely affect relationships and can cause, as well as result from, psychological disorders. It takes courage to raise sexual issues with a stranger, whether as a patient or a doctor, so it is important to demonstrate an understanding of sexual problems and be good at assessing them.

## Sexual dysfunctions

Sexual dysfunctions involve problems with libido, arousal, orgasm, or pain (Table 16.1). Problems are either *primary* (normal function never obtained) or *secondary* (loss of function). Epidemiology is unclear, but men present most commonly with erectile dysfunction (Box 16.1), and women with low libido.

### Sexual drive problems

#### Low libido

This is more common in women. Primary problems are normally idiopathic, but can be associated with childhood sexual abuse. New onset may relate to physical illness, depression, medication, relationship problems, or childbirth. *All* contact may be avoided for fear of it progressing to sex, which may leave partners feeling rejected.

Once the underlying causes have been addressed, treatment is psychological. Open communication is encouraged, with sex education if appropriate. *Sensate focus therapy* is used (Box 16.2). *Time-tabling sex* can help partners with very different libidos find a compromise.

#### Hypersexuality

Excessively high libido usually affects men and can damage their relationships. Exclude mania, substance misuse, and organic brain disorders (e.g. frontal lobe syndrome); then use CBT-based treatments.

### Arousal problems

#### Erectile dysfunction

In erectile dysfunction (ED), erections are insufficiently hard to allow penetration; the main causes are shown in

**TABLE 16.1** Common sexual dysfunctions

| Problem | Male | Female |
|---|---|---|
| Sexual drive | Low libido Hypersexuality | Low libido |
| Arousal | Erectile dysfunction | Failure of genital response |
| Orgasm | Premature ejaculation Delayed ejaculation | Anorgasmia |
| Pain | Dyspareunia | Dyspareunia Vaginismus |

---

**BOX 16.1** Causes of erectile dysfunction

**Organic**

- Diabetes
- Arteriosclerosis
- Neurological (e.g. autonomic neuropathy)
- Pituitary failure
- Medication, e.g.
  - antidepressants, antipsychotics
  - antihypertensives, beta-blockers, diuretics
- Substance misuse

**Psychological**

- Depression
- Performance anxiety

**BOX 16.2** The stages of sensate focus therapy

1. Intercourse is banned.

2. Non-genital caressing: focus on pleasure and relaxation.

3. Genital touching to achieve arousal and subsequently orgasm.

4. In time, intercourse occurs naturally (clitoral stimulation helps women reach orgasm).

**TABLE 16.2** Clues *suggesting* a physical/psychological cause of erectile dysfunction

|  | Physical | Psychological |
|---|---|---|
| Age | Older | Younger |
| Onset | Gradual | Sudden |
| *Any* erections? | No | Yes, e.g. early morning erections, masturbation |
| Risk factors | Yes, e.g. smoking, obesity, hypertension, alcohol | Alcohol |
| Illness | Physical, e.g. history of heart attack | Psychiatric, e.g. depression |

Box 16.1. In *performance anxiety*, there are fears of sexual 'failure', sometimes caused by a previous failure (e.g. while tired). Anxiety inhibits erections, triggering a vicious circle: worry causes erectile dysfunction, which causes more worry.

 Doctors often cause ED through the side effects of the medications they prescribe.

### Investigations

1. Physical examination including genitals (usually normal, but reassures patients).

2. Blood tests:
   - testosterone and sex hormones (low testosterone/hyperprolactinaemia)
   - glucose (diabetes), LFTs/γGT (alcohol misuse).

### Management

1. **Modifiable risk factors**:
   - Stop smoking, exercise, reduce weight and alcohol.
   - Treat diabetes, hypertension, etc.
   - Review medication (e.g. change fluoxetine to mirtazapine).

2. **Psychological approaches** as described above.

3. **Physical treatments** can overcome physical problems:
   - Phosphodiesterase-5 inhibitors, e.g. sildenafil (Viagra).
   - Intracavernosal prostaglandin self-injections prior to intercourse. This can be painful!
   - Vacuum pumps. A plastic dome and pump placed over the penis create a vacuum, producing an erection. This is maintained by slipping a tight ring around the base of the penis.

>> *See Reality for an erectile dysfunction OSCE (p.191).*

### Failure of genital response

Lack of lubrication causes pain on vaginal penetration. Causes may be psychological or secondary to physical problems, such as infection or menopausal atrophic vaginitis. Treatments include psychological approaches, lubricating gels, or hormone replacement therapy.

## Orgasm problems

### Anorgasmia

Although some women can achieve orgasm solely through vaginal penetration, many need direct clitoral stimulation. If women and their partners are unaware of this fact, sex education may resolve anorgasmia. Treatment then encourages self-exploration, masturbation, and sensate focus therapy (Box 16.1), although, sadly, some women never achieve orgasm.

### Premature ejaculation

This is very common in younger men, with ejaculation occurring before or just after penetration, and usually improves with practice. Squeezing the glans penis postpones orgasm (the stop–start technique), and serotoninergic antidepressants can also help (e.g. SSRIs).

### Delayed ejaculation

This term describes a delayed or absent male orgasm. Causes can be physical (e.g. SSRIs) or psychological (e.g. fear of conception). Treatment includes psychotherapy, advice on varying sexual techniques, and medication review.

## Painful disorders

### Dyspareunia

Dyspareunia is painful intercourse. Physical causes include:

- women—infection, episiotomy, endometriosis, tumour, vaginal dryness
- men—urethritis, protastatitis.

Psychological dyspareunia may reflect failure of arousal but is also associated with past abuse or relationship problems. Psychological treatments are used.

### Vaginismus

This is a painful, involuntary spasm of the vaginal muscles when penetration is attempted. Treatment involves education, relaxation, and self-exploration; insertion of 'trainers' (cylindrical plastic objects) of increasing sizes can accustom the patient to penetration.

## Paraphilias

Paraphilias are disorders of sexual preference, although the definition of 'normal' varies between cultures and over time. They occur almost exclusively in men and only need treatment if they cause harm or distress.

- **Fetishism**: sexual arousal and gratification rely on an object rather than a person, e.g. shoes, rubber, leather.
- **Paedophilia**: sexual arousal in response to children.
- **Sadism**: inflicting pain causes arousal.
- **Masochism**: humiliation or suffering cause arousal.

The unwanted arousal may be extinguished by *covert sensitization*. This pairs the arousal with aversive images (e.g. the patient imagines his manager discovering him in his wife's underwear). Patients should avoid activities that reinforce the paraphilia, e.g. fantasizing, looking at related pornography. Anti-androgens may be used in severe or dangerous situations (e.g. paedophiles who feel overwhelmed by sexual urges) but rely on the patient's motivation and cooperation.

Homosexuality is *not* a disorder! However, it is worth being aware that cultural change can be slow to take effect, and people may be reticent about discussing homosexuality.

## Disorders of gender identity

Transsexual people believe that their gender does not correspond to their body, and want to live and be accepted as a member of the opposite sex. It may begin in childhood and is much more common in biological males. Treatment options include hormone therapy and gender reassignment surgery, following careful joint assessment by psychiatrists and surgeons. The patient must demonstrate their ability to live successfully in their desired gender before surgery can be considered.

## Prognosis

Many disorders respond well to therapy, although low libido is very difficult to treat and paraphilias tend to show little improvement.

Where possible, check for knowledge of safe sex and offer sex education as needed. Even very sexually experienced patients may not be fully aware of the risks posed by their sexual activities.

# REALITY

## General approach: tips, tricks, and cautionary tales

Preferably see patients and partners together and alone.

### 1. Confidentiality

Explain confidentiality early on—it lets your patient understand that you respect their privacy and courage in talking. Remember that they may feel shy or ashamed; it's possible that they have *never* spoken to *anyone* about sex before.

If your patient tells you anything in confidence which suggests that their sexual activities are non-consensual or abusive, you *cannot* keep this information confidential.

### 2. Don't assume sexuality

Never assume that your patient is straight, gay, *or* bisexual—getting it wrong will make you both uncomfortable. Until you are sure of their partner's gender, use gender-neutral language:

- he/she = *they*
- boyfriend/girlfriend = *partner*.

A direct question might be:

- (I ask all my patients this.) Are you interested in men, women, or both?

Remember that your patient's current relationship may not reflect their sexual history.

Sexual health *isn't* necessarily the most pressing concern for most gay people. Don't spend all your time on STI screening.

## 3. Look unshockable

People engage in many kinds of sexual activities—which *can* be shocking. Try not to show it by fidgeting, changing the subject, or laughing. Sit still and make eye contact, and don't let your embarrassment prevent you from asking important questions.

## 4. Don't moralize

Regardless of your views on sex or sexuality, your duty is to care for your patient. This does not include approving *or* disapproving of their behaviour. Don't lecture people on how 'bad' you think they are, perhaps for homosexuality or sex before marriage.

## 5. Jargon

People have different words for sex acts and parts of the body. *You* should start with everyday terms (penis, vagina, 'having sex', oral sex); using your own slang terms could confuse or offend your patient. Encourage your patient to talk freely and ask them to explain words you don't recognize—then use these if appropriate.

## 6. Expose yourself!

Many doctors *do* feel shy or embarrassed when talking about sex. It's natural to begin with—but *you* need to overcome it. Exposure therapy is the key.

- Learn more about sex, e.g. read novels, watch movies.
- Discuss sex with a trusted friend or partner before you practise on a shy patient.
- Include sexual histories in general history-taking when relevant (detailed sexual questioning without reason is intrusive and inappropriate).
- Gain further experience in genitourinary clinics.
- Make an effort to meet gay, lesbian, bisexual, and transgendered people. Avoidance only increases your feelings of shyness or embarrassment.

Don't assume that elderly people simply *sleep* in bed! Many are sexually active, although vaginal dryness, erectile dysfunction, or lack of a partner may become a problem.

## 1. Psychosexual history (10 minutes)

### Candidate's instructions

You are a final-year medical student holding your own clinic at a GP surgery. Albert Arvine is a 48-year-old librarian who has attended to discuss a 'private matter.'

Please take a history of the presenting complaint.

### Patient's brief

*Key characteristics*

- I'm concerned about confidentiality.
- I'm hesitant and shy, but talk increasingly freely when taken seriously.
- I tend to gloss over details but respond well to direct questions.

My partner, Annabel, booked this appointment. She doesn't know what more she can do to help . . .

I should start at the beginning . . . I married Natalie at 25. She was my first partner and our sex life was really good to begin with. We had a son, Jim, who's now 20. Our sex life died off during a rocky patch in our marriage, 10 years ago. Natalie lost interest in sex, and I eventually gave up asking —I didn't like being rejected every night. Two years ago she admitted that she was having an affair. She was quite cruel about it, telling me how he satisfied her in ways I never had . . . I've been very lonely and depressed since she left me.

I met Annabel six months ago, and it was love at first sight. It's exciting to feel wanted again and Annabel made me feel like a love-struck teenager! We waited three months, to make sure it was what we wanted, and I planned a romantic weekend in Paris. Everything was going really well until . . . I just couldn't . . . keep my erection. I felt dreadful. She was very good about it, but we tried again and the same thing happened. Every time, since then. We make do with oral sex, but I never . . . um . . . orgasm. She keeps asking me if I find her attractive—and I *do*! She knows there were no problems like this in my marriage and worries that I still have feelings for Natalie—which I *don't*. I feel like a failure. I've been making excuses to avoid sex lately and I think I've hurt Annabel's feelings . . . she's now saying *she's* too tired for sex. It feels like my marriage all over again.

I don't feel depressed anymore, but if I lose Annabel, I think I'll probably get very low again—antidepressants or not.

*If specifically asked*:

- I don't get morning (or other) erections. I haven't masturbated in about a year. While I was depressed, it just wasn't something I wanted to do and until I met Annabel, I didn't realize it was a problem. Before I was depressed, I could always maintain an erection and ejaculate.
- During sex, I *never* get hard enough to penetrate Annabel. I bring her to orgasm with oral sex.
- *Nothing* Annabel does gives me a full erection.
- During sex I worry: 'I'm going to mess this up . . .'

*Other History*

- I don't drink, smoke, or take drugs.
- My eczema's bad because I'm stressed. I use steroid creams.
- I take fluoxetine 20mg for depression. This is my third bout, but I feel better now. I started my prescription a year ago and always take my tablets.
- I have no idea if anyone in my family had sexual or psychiatric problems. We didn't really talk about those things.

*Questions*

Is something seriously wrong with me?

*Worries*

If I can't satisfy Annabel, maybe she'll leave me for someone who can.

# NEXT STEPS

## Psychosexual problem in primary care

You are a junior doctor working in general practice. Frances Coney, a 48-year-old divorced woman, has come in for an overdue but routine smear test. She seems quiet and nervous today, and when you attempt to introduce the speculum she cries out in pain and is clearly distressed. You stop the procedure and sit with her; she tearfully explains that she has been having great difficulty because of pain ever since she was raped several years ago. Sex is painful and this is now becoming a problem for her and her partner, Tyler.

1. Describe how you will manage the problem further today.
2. What is the most likely diagnosis? Explain this to Frances.

### Issues

- Assessment and immediate management
- Diagnosis and explanation
- Further management

### Assessment and immediate management

Spend time building rapport and helping Frances feel calmer. If you are male, be aware that she may prefer to discuss this with a female colleague. Frances may also prefer to book another appointment, bringing Tyler for moral support. Gently take a sexual and relationship history, letting her set the pace and being sensitive to areas that she feels uncomfortable discussing. Check the temporal relationship between the rape and onset of pain; the problem may have been pre-existing.

Explore the issue of the rape—*if* she feels able to discuss it. Find out whether she reported it and if she gained support at the time. Psychological consequences include PTSD, depression, anxiety disorders, and substance misuse, and you should ask about symptoms of these. Frances may have been placed at risk of STIs through the rape, which could be a cause of concern to her and Tyler. Victims of rape often feel ashamed—and this, combined with her physical pain, may have stopped her from undertaking a sexual health check. STIs may be a source of further worry, and can contribute to pain during penetration.

### Diagnosis and explanation

The most likely diagnosis, in the absence of a lesion or infection, is vaginismus: 'The vaginal muscles quickly go into a very painful spasm; this can be triggered by smear tests, using tampons or having sex. For some women, this *just happens* for no obvious reason, while others find it begins after something painful or frightening, like a sexual assault. You are *not* deliberately tensing up—it happens automatically—but it *is* something that can be treated and cured.'

## Further support and management

If you are confident of the diagnosis of vaginismus, you can discuss management options. Self-help can be highly effective. Frances should be encouraged to explore her body through touching, at first on the outside and then, when comfortable, inserting a finger into her vagina. She can gradually build up from there (e.g. using vaginal trainers), involving Tyler in the treatment at any stage.

The rape itself may need your support. Frances may *still* wish to report the rape to the police, particularly if she knew her attacker. She may benefit from rape support groups, or from psychological input. Remember to treat comorbid psychiatric problems, e.g. chronic PTSD (see p.158). If Frances wishes to undergo STI testing, you might offer to write a covering letter, making staff at the clinic aware of her situation.

> Frances will still need to have her smear test completed at a later date. Delayed presentation is common for many intimate or embarrassing problems—empathy here may be life-saving!

### Film list
*Brokeback Mountain* (2005)—homosexuality.
*The Secretary* (2002)—fetishism and self-harm.
*Boys Don't Cry* (1999)—transexualism.

### Books
Boyle, T.C. (1999) *Riven Rock*. London: Penguin. Novel exploring hypersexuality at the turn of the century.

Ensler, E. (2001) *The Vagina Monologues*. London: Virago. Groundbreaking book, aimed at reducing myths and misapprehensions about the vagina.

Fowles, J. (1998) *The Collector*. London: Vintage. Obsession, asexuality, and the devastating effects of the repression of natural sexuality are explored in this novel.

### Quotes
In itself, homosexuality is as limiting as heterosexuality: the ideal should be to be capable of loving a woman or a man; either, a human being, without feeling fear, restraint, or obligation.
**Simone de Beauvoir**

Science is a lot like sex. Sometimes something useful comes of it, but that's not the reason we're doing it.
**Richard Feynman**

It comes down to how we love—not where we draw the line.
**Randall Williams**

## Note

1. Kinsey, A.C. *et al.* (1948/1998) *Sexuality in the Human Male*. Philadelphia, PA: W.B. Saunders; Bloomington, IN: University of Indiana Press.

## Further reading

Bancroft, J. (1983) *Human Sexuality and its Problems*. Edinburgh: Churchill Livingstone.

Kalamis, C. and Brennan, S. (2007) *Women Without Sex: The Truth About Female Sexual Problems* (3rd edn). London: Self-Help Direct.

Leiblum, S.R. and Rosen, R.C. (ed.) (2000) *Principles and Practice of Sex Therapy* (2nd edn). New York: Guilford Press.

Zilbergeld, B. (1999) *The New Male Sexuality* (revised edn). New York: Bantam Doubleday Dell.

 Go to www.oxfordtextbooks/orc/stringer for an array of additional references, including indicative mark sheets for OSCEs, self-assessment questions, guidance, and exercises.

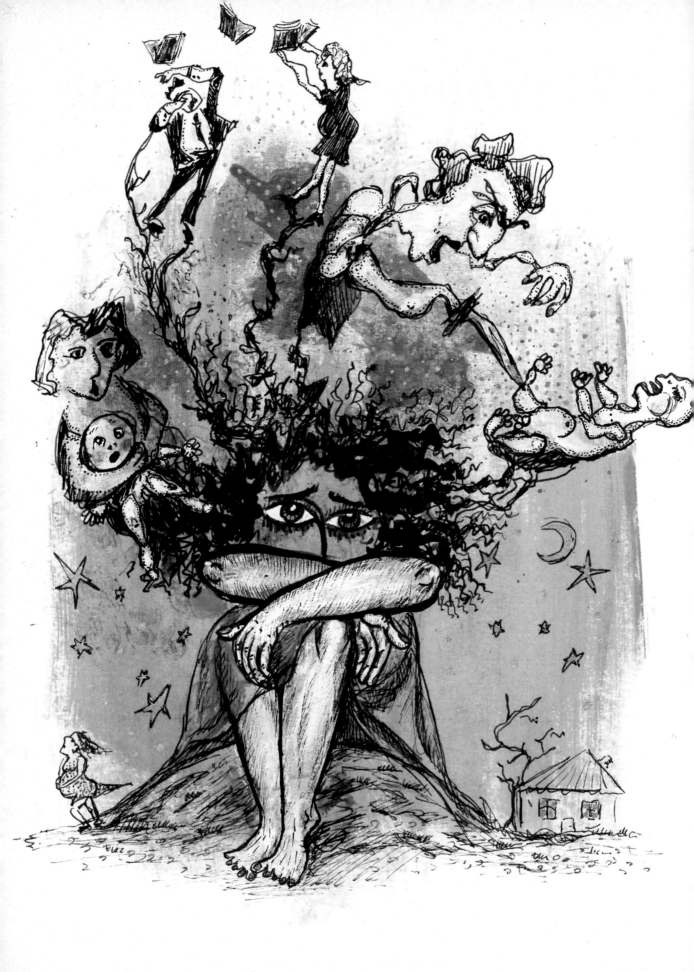

# 17 Problems following childbirth

*Sarah Cader*

## True or False? Test your existing knowledge—answers in the chapter and online

1. Pregnancy increases the risk of psychiatric illness.
2. Patients with bipolar affective disorder are at an 8-fold increased risk of relapse in the puerperal period.
3. Postnatal blues usually require only explanation and simple reassurance.
4. 1 in 20 women suffer postnatal depression in the year after childbirth.
5. Postnatal depression is usually treated in a Mother and Baby Unit.
6. Lithium is safe in breast-feeding mothers, as long as lithium levels are under 0.7mmol/L.
7. Electroconvulsive therapy is an effective treatment in postpartum psychosis.
8. Suicide is the number one cause of maternal death in the UK.
9. Struggling to cope with the care of a *single* infant is a sign of poor parenting skills.
10. The 24 year old mother of a 2 month old baby becomes tearful during a follow-up obstetrics outpatient appointment. The liaison psychiatrist must be involved before she can be discharged home.

## Contents

# PRINCIPLES

She, and hence I, have not slept for many hours. For perhaps the twentieth time in ten hours I feed her and put her down in her cradle. I am not asking for a solid stretch: I merely require a few minutes to myself gluing parts of my face back on and saying things allowed in front of the mirror to see if I've actually gone mad. At this point I don't just want her to go to sleep. She has to go to sleep otherwise I don't know what will happen. My position is at once reasonable, utterly desperate, and non-negotiable.

*A Life's Work: On Becoming a Mother*—Rachel Cusk[1]

## Introduction

Pregnancy is usually a time of mental well-being, when the risk of mental illness is not increased. However, the period *following* birth carries a higher risk of mental health problems. Although the 'baby blues' are easily managed, other post-partum problems are tricky and risky—don't be afraid to seek early specialist advise.

 The puerperium increases the risk of relapse in women with bipolar affective disorder (BPAD) eightfold.

## The blues

Postnatal blues are distressing but *normal*. They affect 50–75% of mothers a few days after the birth, and last only days. They feel weepy, irritable, and muddled; their moods seem 'all over the place' (labile) and they may have trouble sleeping. Explanation and reassurance are usually all that are required, although occasionally severe baby blues progress to postnatal depression.

## Postnatal depression

One in ten mothers suffers postnatal depression (PND) in the year after birth. The risk is increased by a personal or family history of PND or depression, younger maternal age, recent life events, marital discord, and poor social support. PND is very similar to normal depression (see p.32), although fatigue, irritability, or anxiety may be particularly marked. Depressive cognitions commonly relate to the baby, e.g. guilt or feeling a failure as a mother. Recurrent intrusive thoughts about harming the baby can occur as distressing obsessions or as part of a serious plan.

Management is as for depression generally, although antidepressants need to be used with care in breastfeed-

ing mothers (Box 17.1). Hospital admission should be considered if depression is severe with suicidal or infanticidal ideation. A mother and baby unit (MBU) placement is optimal under these circumstances, since it allows treatment without separation of mother and child. This enables bonding, staff support with childcare, and risk management.

Most women respond well to treatment within a month; some take longer and a few have difficulties for over a year. Unless there is a personal history of depression, any future risk is of PND and not depression *per se*. PND may affect the baby's attachment and have lasting effects on development and personality—early and effective treatment of PND is essential (Murray and Cooper 1997).

With a six-week-old baby it would be *abnormal* to have 'normal' energy, concentration and sleep! When assessing depression, focus on cognitive symptoms, e.g. guilt, hopelessness.

---

**BOX 17.1** Drugs during breastfeeding

Some psychotropic drugs are secreted in breast-milk, potentially affecting the baby, although this should not rule out medications if they are needed. Caution is advised with antidepressants, although low-dose amitriptyline (a tricyclic) is probably safe. Lithium should be avoided if possible and neuroleptics can cause lethargy, especially in high doses. Seek specialist advice.

---

## Puerperal psychosis

Psychosis follows one in 500–1000 births, usually occurring in the fortnight after childbirth. Those at highest risk have a personal or family history of puerperal psychosis or BPAD. Other risk factors include puerperal infection and obstetric complications (Blackmore *et al.* 2006). Onset is usually rapid, often beginning with insomnia, restlessness, and perplexity. Later, psychotic symptoms emerge, generally settling into one of three patterns:

- delirium (see p.117)
- affective (psychotic depression or mania, see pp.35, 41)
- schizophreniform (like schizophrenia, see p.75).

Symptoms can fluctuate dramatically and quickly—don't be misled by temporary symptom-free periods. Exclude an underlying delirium state or substance misuse (intoxication or withdrawal). Depending on the presentation, antipsychotics, antidepressants, or lithium may be needed, and benzodiazepines may be added to control agitation. In severe cases, electroconvulsive therapy may be life-saving. Admission is usually required for further management, preferably to an MBU. Most patients recover within 6–12 weeks and the overall risk of recurrence is about a third.

**!** Risk assessment is essential in all cases. Remember that suicide is the leading cause of maternal death in the UK (RCOG 2001). Always assess risk to the baby—through both neglect and violence. Look particularly for depressive delusions, e.g. that the baby is evil, dead, possessed, or abnormal. Some mothers may try to kill their baby because it is 'evil' or 'malformed'—or to save it from future 'doom'. Command hallucinations sometimes instruct mothers to harm their babies.

# REALITY

## General approach: tips, tricks, and cautionary tales

### 1. Give her a break

Arrange for a trusted member of staff or the family to look after the baby while you talk. An uninterrupted cup of tea while the baby is in safe hands is often a relief.

### 2. The Super Mum myth

New mothers often believe that ('good') mums naturally know everything and never need help. Therefore not being superhuman can make a woman wrongly feel she is a 'bad' mother. Explain that Super Mum doesn't exist—and 'good' mums struggle too. Praise her for admitting to worries or asking for help: it shows that she is in touch with her and her baby's needs.

### 3. Babies are hard work

Babies are deceptive—by looking small and cute, they convince us that they are easy to look after. Don't be fooled! Let your patient know that babies *are* exhausting and that it is *normal* to feel overwhelmed sometimes (especially when sleep-deprived). Hearing this can be hugely relieving and enables open discussion of problems. Are her partner, friends, and family aware of her stress and are they helping out?

### 4. Tough questions

Although delusions or thoughts of harming the baby are uncommon, you must ask about them. Look for unusual or guarded responses to open questions about the birth and the baby's development (e.g. feeding, sleeping, temperament). Then screen for delusions.

- How do you feel when you look at your baby?
- Do you ever worry that there might be something wrong with him/her?

Screen for thoughts of harm to self/baby:

- It can be very stressful looking after a baby. Do you ever feel like you can't cope?
- Are there times when he/she won't stop crying? How does that make you feel?
- How do you picture things in a month's time?
- Do you ever wish you hadn't had your baby?
- Do you have any worrying thoughts about your baby?

If she admits to being worried that she might harm her baby, don't panic! Stay calm, explore her thoughts, and undertake a full risk assessment.

### 5. Stay

Although the risk of a mum harming her baby is very low, don't leave her alone with her baby if she is psychotic, severely depressed, or agitated; stay with them until help or a second opinion arrives. Make your presence reassuring, rather than intimidating. Remember that perinatal psychiatrists do everything possible to keep even very unwell mothers safely with their babies, so don't try to separate them unless the risk is high.

**→** Mum's interaction with her baby will inform your risk assessment—is she warm, hostile, cold, etc.? Before judging this, ensure that you have looked after a baby by yourself for at least 24 hours . . .

# NEXT STEPS

## A tearful first time mother

You are a junior doctor seeing Carmel Pritchard, a 24-year-old woman, in obstetrics outpatients. Carmel's first child was born 2 months ago via forceps delivery. Carmel required an episiotomy and has since suffered problems with poor wound healing. During the appointment today Carmel is tearful and tells you that she is finding it very difficult to cope.

1. What are the important areas to cover with Carmel today?
2. What factors might make you seek an immediate psychiatric opinion?
3. What would be your further management?

### Issues
- Psychiatric assessment and diagnosis
- Physical health care
- Risk assessment
- Management

### Assessment

You do not have enough time to take a full psychiatric history, so concentrate on the presenting complaint ('not coping'), past history, and any information that will affect your risk assessment. Carmel will first need time to talk and not be hurried into a series of questions. Be empathic —she has had a difficult time and is not alone in finding the first months with a baby particularly difficult.

You need to decide whether she is clinically depressed and, if so, how severely. Assess for psychotic symptoms and any abnormal thoughts about her baby. Ask about her social situation, support within the home, and relationships with friends, family, and professionals. Her past psychiatric history, previous treatments for depression, and current drug and alcohol use are all important. During the assessment, look for signs of affection between mother and baby, e.g. whether Carmel seem interested in her child, how she reacts if the baby cries. Don't forget to assess her physical problems fully, since these will exacerbate her low mood.

### Immediate referral

Seek immediate psychiatric opinion if you have any serious concerns regarding the safety of Carmel, her baby, or other people (e.g. severe depression, psychotic symptoms, thoughts of suicide or infanticide). Psychiatric admission may be necessary—preferably to an MBU.

### Further management

Whether or not you refer to psychiatry, it is essential that you liaise closely with Carmel's GP. Remember that a follow-up letter to the GP may take a week or more to be sent out and reviewed, by which time Carmel and her baby may be in a more desperate state. Call the GP *now* to discuss your options over the telephone. It is also worth discussing problems with her closest supporters (e.g. partner, mother). It will usually be possible to support her at home with GP, health visitor, and mental health input. Social services may be able to help with additional childcare arrangements, and should be involved if there are risks to the baby.

Ensure that Carmel has adequate analgesia if she is in pain from her episiotomy wound; give shorter prescriptions with explicit primary care follow-up if there is any identified risk of suicide.

Because Carmel is more likely to neglect her own health during a depressive episode, the follow-up for her birth complications may need to be quite assertive, e.g. ensuring that reminder letters are sent and involving community midwives for a little longer than would be usual practice.

The Edinburgh Postnatal Depression Scale (Cox *et al.* 1987) is a five-minute screening test that helps health visitors to identify depressed mothers during routine home visits.

**Books**

Cusk, R. (2001) *A Life's Work: On Becoming a Mother*. London: Fourth Estate. Autobiographical struggle of motherhood (without perinatal problems).

Gale, P. (2007) *Notes From An Exhibition*. London: Harper Perennial, 2008. This novel follows the life and death of a mother with BPAD.

**Quotes**

. . . there had come merely an intense interiority, a sense of her world narrowing down to a focus no larger than her baby's dimpled head.
**Patrick Gale—*Notes From An Exhibition***

## Note

1. Cusk, R. (2001) *A Life's Work: On Becoming a Mother.* London: Fourth Estate, p.79.

## References/Further reading

Blackmore, E.R., Jones, I., Doshi, M., *et al.* (2006) Obstetric variables associated with bipolar affective puerperal psychosis. *British Journal of Psychiatry*, **188**, 32–3.

Bowlby, J. (1977) The making and breaking of affectional bonds. I: Aetiology and psychopathology in the light of attachment theory. *British Journal of Psychiatry*, **130**, 201–10.

Brockington, I. (1996) *Motherhood and Mental Health.* Oxford University Press.

Cox, J.L., Holden, J.M., and Sagovsky, R. (1987) Detection of postnatal depression: development of the 10-item Edinburgh Postnatal Depression Scale. *British Journal of Psychiatry*, **150**, 782–6.

Murray, L. and Cooper, P. (1997) Effects of postnatal depression on infant development. *Archives of Diseases in Childhood*, **77**, 99–101.

RCOG (Royal College of Obstetricians and Gynaecologists) (2001) *Why Mothers Die 1997–1999: Fifth Report of the Confidential Enquiries into Maternal Deaths in the United Kingdom.* London: RCOG.

 Go to www.oxfordtextbooks/orc/stringer for an array of additional references, including indicative mark sheets for OSCEs, self-assessment questions, guidance, and exercises.

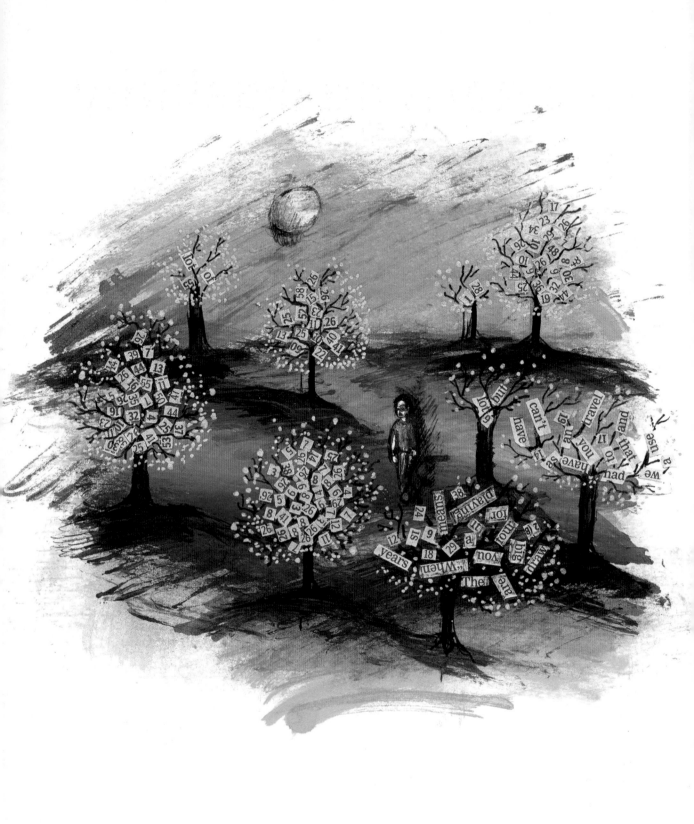

# 18 Learning disability

*Sarah Cader and Dimitrios Paschos*

## True or False? Test your existing knowledge—answers in the chapter and online

1. Learning disabilities are more common in males than females.

2. The number of people with a learning disability is rising.

3. The IQ level associated with a diagnosis of Severe Learning Disability is 35–49.

4. People with learning disabilities have higher rates of epilepsy.

5. There is an increased risk of schizophrenia in those with a mild learning disability.

6. Down syndrome is associated with congenital heart abnormalities.

7. Patients with Fragile X have expressive language deficits.

8. For optimal healthcare, people with learning disabilities should be encouraged to use specialist rather than mainstream services.

9. When talking to someone with a learning disability, you should use one idea per sentence to aid comprehension.

10. A 26 year old woman with Down syndrome begins to act in a sexualised manner at her residential home. A safeguarding vulnerable adults meeting can only be held with her consent.

## Contents

# PRINCIPLES

When I had to go to hospital the doctors would usually speak to my mum rather than speak to me. So I didn't bring her to the hospital anymore. Finally they started to recognize I'm the one, I need to understand, not my mum.

A young person with learning disability[1]

## Introduction

Learning disability is a developmental condition characterized by global impairment of intelligence and significant difficulties in socially adaptive functioning. The management of patients with these conditions can be challenging, owing to impairments in language and communication. Contact with doctors is frequent, since people with a learning disability are at increased risk of physical and mental illness.

## Epidemiology

Learning disability is slightly more common in males than females (3:2). Table 18.1 shows the prevalence, although many people with a *mild* learning disability are never formally diagnosed. It is estimated that the number of people with severe disabilities is rising, partly because of the increased survival of very premature babies.

## Aetiology

Specific causes of learning disability are listed in Table 18.2. Multifactorial causes are common and may represent environmental factors combined with *polygenic* inheritance.

## Clinical presentation

Learning disability usually presents in childhood, but may be missed if mild. Abilities can be *delayed*, *reduced*, or *absent* in:

- language
- schooling
- motor ability
- independent living
- employment
- social ability.

*Behavioural difficulties* may arise, secondary to a combination of communication problems, psychiatric or physical illness, epilepsy, or suboptimal support for individual needs. 'Behavioural phenotypes' are commonly recognized behaviours in particular syndromes, e.g. self-harm in Lesch-Nyhan syndrome.

**TABLE 18.1** Epidemiology of learning disability

| Learning disability | IQ level | Prevalence |
|---|---|---|
| Mild | 50–69 | 2.5% |
| Moderate | 35–49 | 0.4% |
| Severe | 20–34 | 0.1% combined |
| Profound | <20 | |

**TABLE 18.2** Some causes of learning disability

| Antenatal | Perinatal | Postnatal |
|---|---|---|
| Genetic (e.g. phenylketonuria) | Neonatal hypoxia | Social deprivation |
| During pregnancy | Birth trauma | Malnutrition |
|   Alcohol: fetal alcohol syndrome | Hypoglycaemia | Lead |
|   Drugs | Prematurity | Infections (e.g. meningitis) |
|   Medications | | Head injury |
|   Smoking | | |
|   Infection (e.g. rubella) | | |

Source: Bhate and Wilkinson 2006

## 1. Mild learning disability

- Language is usually reasonably good, although its development may be delayed.

- Problems may go undiagnosed, although individuals struggle through school or may be labelled with behavioural problems.

- With appropriate support, many people live and work independently.

## 2. Moderate learning disability

- Language and cognitive abilities are less developed.

- Reduced self-care abilities and limited motor skills may necessitate support.

- May need long-term accomodation with their family or in a staff-supported group home.

- Simple practical work should be achievable in supported settings.

## 3. Severe learning disability

- Marked impairment of motor function.

- Little/no speech during early childhood (some may develop during school years).

- Simple tasks can be performed with assistance.

- Likely to require their family home or 24-hour-staffed home.

## 4. Profound learning disability

- Severely limited language, communication, self-care, and mobility.

- Significant associated medical problems.

- Usually require higher levels of support.

People with a learning disability have increased physical mortality and morbidity, including higher rates of epilepsy. Problems are compounded by less frequent involvement in health screening and preventative interventions, e.g. although respiratory infections are a leading cause of death, levels of influenza vaccination are lower than that of the general population. Value judgements by healthcare professionals have been blamed for discriminatory practices, inadequate treatment, and disproportionate use of 'do not resuscitate' notices for people with more severe problems (Mencap 2004).

About 30–50% of people have additional mental health problems and associated autistic spectrum disorders (Smiley 2005). Mood and anxiety disorders are more common across the spectrum of learning disability and there is an increased risk of schizophrenia in those with a mild learning disability.

*Diagnostic overshadowing* describes the tendency to attribute *everything* to the learning disability itself. Changes in behaviour, mental state, or ability are dismissed, despite usually indicating physical or mental illness in people without a learning disability. For example, dismissing

**TABLE 18.3** Specific syndromes associated with learning difficulties

|  | Down syndrome | Fragile X | Fetal alcohol syndrome |
|---|---|---|---|
| Live birth rate | 1 in 700 | 1 in 4000 boys<br>1 in 8000 girls | 0.6 in 1000<br>(9 in 1000 *spectrum* disorders) |
| Cause | Trisomy 21 (most common)<br>Also translocations or mosaicism[a] of chromosome 21 | Mutation in FMR1 gene on X chromosome | Alcohol during pregnancy |
| Physical characteristics | Upward-slanting palpebral fissures<br>Epicanthic folds<br>Protruding tongue<br>Single palmar crease<br>Hypotonia | Elongated face<br>Prominent ears<br>High-arched palate<br>Large testes<br>Hyperextensible joints | Wide palpebral fissure<br>Smooth philtrum<br>Thin top lip |
| Associated problems | Congenital heart abnormalities<br>Thyroid problems<br>Epilepsy<br>Depression<br>Early-onset Alzheimer's disease<br>Leukaemia | Autistic type behaviour<br>Anxiety<br>Depression<br>Hyperactivity<br>Expressive language deficits | Behavioural difficulties<br>Fetal growth retardation<br>Neurological abnormalities |
| Comments | Most common genetic cause of learning disability<br>Risk increases in older mothers | Carriers have milder problems | Debate surrounds 'safe' drinking in pregnancy, although this problem can be entirely avoided by abstinence |

[a]Only a proportion of cells have the abnormality.

someone with a learning disability who cries and stops eating because: 'That's the way these people are sometimes'—when appendicitis is the problem.

➡️ **Never make assumptions about someone's quality of life. Most people with a learning disability report happy and fulfilling lives.**

## Differential diagnosis

1. **Autistic spectrum disorders**: people with Asperger's syndrome (autism with normal intelligence) may have significant social deficits, communication difficulties, and difficulties in living independently (see p.212).

2. **Epilepsy** may cause transient cognitive impairment. Very frequent uncontrolled seizures can mimic persistent cognitive impairment.

3. **Adult brain injury or progressive neurological conditions**: learning disabilities are neurodevelopmental disorders, occurring *while the brain is still developing*. If the patient presents late, it is important to decide whether or not impaired intellect was present *before* any adult illness.

4. **Psychiatric**: severe and enduring mental illness such as schizophrenia can lead to chronic cognitive impairment, reduced social functioning, and associated speech disorders—mimicking a learning disability. Exclude intellectual impairment prior to the onset of psychiatric symptoms.

5. **Educational disadvantage/neglect**: lacking the *opportunity* to learn must be distinguished from a learning disability.

## Investigations

1. IQ testing: is there global intellectual impairment?

2. Functional assessment of skills, strengths and weaknesses.

3. Detailed developmental history from parents, e.g. details of pregnancy and birth, language and motor skills development, schooling, emotional development, and relationships. School reports are helpful.

4. FBC, U&E, LFT, TFT, bone profile—to exclude reversible disturbances.

5. Additional blood tests for known causes of learning disability.

6. Investigations for associated physical illnesses, e.g. EEG for epilepsy.

7. Genetic testing if appropriate.

➡️ **Focus on your patient's *strengths* rather than their *weaknesses*. This will transform the way that you see your patient—and may reveal new management options.**

## Treatment issues

People with a learning disability should be supported to access and use mainstream services. More complex cases may involve specialist learning disability teams, which include psychologists, occupational therapists, nurses, psychiatrists, and speech and language therapists.

1. **Prevention**
   - Education, e.g. the risks of alcohol during pregnancy
   - Improved antenatal/perinatal care
   - Genetic counselling
   - Early detection and treatment of reversible causes, e.g. excluding dietary phenylalanine in babies with phenylketonuria.

2. **Treat physical comorbidity**

3. **Treat psychiatric comorbidity** The presentation of mental health problems in this population can be different because of cognitive, language, and communication difficulties. Diagnostic accuracy can be improved with the use of specialist guidelines, e.g. DC-LD (Royal College of Psychiatrists 2001). Although the usual treatment principles apply, patients may be particularly sensitive to medications, and so slower dose titration and careful monitoring are essential.

4. **Educational support** Early detection and a Statement of Special Educational Needs (in the UK) allow appropriate support, whether in mainstream or specialized schools, to maximize the child's potential.

5. **Psychological therapy** This may include counselling, group therapy, and modified CBT. Behavioural therapy can often help to improve unhelpful behaviour patterns. An *ABC Approach* is taken, identifying *Antecedents*, *Behaviour*, and *Consequences* of behaviour. This informs a management plan that is preferable to medicating behavioural problems, and may include:
   - avoiding antecedents
   - reinforcing positive behaviours
   - preventing reinforcement of negative behaviours (e.g. using distraction techniques)
   - helping people understand the consequence of their actions.

➡️ ***Change* in behaviour communicates any number of emotional or physical problems which cannot be verbalized, from toothache to heartache.**

6. **Other support** A comprehensive individualized support network is needed to provide specific help with daily living, housing, employment, and finances; as well as enabling integration into the local community. Carers' needs should always be assessed.

A learning disability is a lifelong condition, although the extent of effective support determines the degree of limitation. Life expectancy is reduced because of the comorbid physical illness and unmet health need (McGuigan *et al.* 1995).

People with a learning disability can be very vulnerable to neglect, abuse, and exploitation. Their problems may then be compounded by communication difficulties, and behavioural change may again be the only way of communicating distress. Be sensitive to this during assessments.

# REALITY[2]

## General approach: tips, tricks, and cautionary tales

### 1. Don't patronize

Adults with a learning disability must not be treated like children! Avoid:

- Using a patronising tone or language *below* their level of understanding.
- Referring to them as *girls* or *boys*.
- Addressing them by their first name or nicknaming without permission (e.g. changing Nicholas to 'Nicky').
- Assuming that things are too difficult for them to understand.
- Talking exclusively to their parent/carer, rather than to them.
- Assuming that they cannot make decisions ('*Does he take sugar?*').
- Ignoring their sexuality and sexual relationships because you think that these are *grown-up* issues.

### 2. Try

Always *try* to engage your patient first: greet them and gauge response. If there are communication problems, explain that you are going to ask their carer some questions to try to make it easier for the two of you to talk, and *then* talk to the carer. Find out how your patient usually communicates and ask the carer to demonstrate. Options include:

- facial expressions and gestures
- sign language (or adapted sign language, e.g. Makaton)
- communication boards (e.g. with symbols and pictures)
- speaking computers
- photographs
- objects of reference—objects with individualized symbolic meanings (e.g. a fork meaning *meals*, a model car meaning *travel*).

Sometimes carers can act as interpreters, especially when speech is unclear or specialized skills are needed to communicate. Remember, your patient's view may differ from that of their carer; don't assume carers know *everything* going on inside your patient's head.

### 3. Pitch

Follow your patient's lead for pitching level and pace. Speak clearly and simply, using short words and sentences with *one* idea per sentence. Avoid abstract language, as some people will apply literal meanings, causing confusion, e.g. '*The doctor will give you a ring later*'. Others may only pick up a few key words from a sentence. For example:

**You:** You'll be pleased to know that we have excluded cancer and you are not going to die.

**Liz:** Cancer? Die!

Checking for understanding is essential.

 Try rephrasing questions to check that you still get the same response.

### 4. Silence

Understanding a question, thinking of an answer, finding the right words, and getting the words out may all take longer than they would for you. *Wait* for a response; it's frustrating to be asked a question but not given time to answer. If there really is no response, try asking the same question in a simpler way before moving on. Be patient if speech is very slow or laboured—it's rude to finish people's sentences for them.

### 5. Sort out sensory problems

Deafness and visual impairment are more common; identify and address problems early on.

## 6. Be understanding

Always check that *you* have understood what your patient is trying to say, e.g. 'Your leg hurts? Is that right?' The harder they are to understand, the more frequently you must check. People will be patient with you if you explain that you are checking because you want to know what *they* think.

Sometimes—despite your best attempts—you won't understand what your patient is trying to say. Although you don't understand *them*, don't assume that they can't understand you. Be mindful that your patient may still be listening and want to hear what you have to say, even if they cannot respond. Keep them involved in the conversation.

Remember that people with a learning disability may want to please you and appear to understand when they don't. Repetition does not mean comprehension, so always get them to explain in their own words. For example:

> **You:** Do you feel depressed?
>
> **Liz:** Yes.
>
> **You:** How does it feel to be depressed?

## 7. More than words

Speech is only a small part of communicating. 'Total communication' is using *whatever works* to communicate with an individual who has limited language skills. This might involve gestures and facial expression when talking, to help get your message across, e.g.

- 'Do you feel *sad*?' (make a sad expression).
- 'Does your arm hurt?' (point to your arm, rub it and make a pained expression).

Drawing simple explanatory pictures may be useful, even if your artwork is bad.

📖 Your patient may be very anxious about meeting you or coming to hospital. Giving them some idea of what will happen and offering choices, where possible, can considerably reduce anxiety.

# NEXT STEPS

## Behavioural change in a woman with Down syndrome

You are a junior doctor working in general practice and receive a phone call from the manager of a residential group home for people with learning disabilities. He describes a 26-year-old woman, Nathalie Rowell, who is exhibiting rather worrying new patterns of behaviour.

Nathalie has Down syndrome and a mild learning disability. She has lived at the home for three years and has been doing very well, despite of a lot of changes in staff and residents. Over the past week Nathalie has been 'very emotional and behaving in a disinhibited, sexualized manner'. She wanted to go out to a nightclub late last night and was wearing heavily applied make-up and a skirt that she had cut herself, making it very short. Something is clearly not right, and the manager would like you to see Nathalie urgently. He is worried that she may have to leave the home because of the disruption and risk she is causing.

1. What is the differential diagnosis?
2. Describe your assessment.

### Issues

- Diagnosis
- Risk assessment
- Management
- Ensuring security of her placement
- Possibility of abuse.

### Differential diagnosis

- Manic episode
- Substance abuse
- Organic disorder, e.g. delirium, dementia, or post-ictal state
- Psychotic episode
- Behavioural change secondary to traumatic event, e.g. victim of sexual abuse
- Adjustment disorder, possibly secondary to environmental change
- No disorder

### Assessment

With this differential diagnosis in mind, the history and mental state examination will need to be detailed and cover a wide range of possibilities. Before seeing Nathalie, gather as much information as you can from her medical notes, social services, any psychiatric team involvement, and the staff in the home. You will also need to find out more about Nathalie's family; her parents may need to be involved in the assessment process and should be kept informed of any changes or referrals.

Nathalie should be seen urgently; ideally on her own for at least part of the interview (and with a chaperone, in view of her disinhibited behaviour). Take a history to elicit mood symptoms, particularly mania (e.g. subjective mood, energy levels, and enjoyment). Look for evidence of labile affect and psychotic symptoms. Assess her cognition, comparing her current ability with her usual ability. For example, does she recognize staff and know where her room is—or is she confused? Ask about her physical health and whether there has been any substance misuse. Sensitively explore her relationship history and how she has been getting on with staff members and other residents at the home. Is she frightened of anyone, or does she become tearful or excited when certain staff or residents are mentioned? Has a favourite companion left the home or found a new friendship circle? You must conduct a full physical examination, and consider appropriate investigations (e.g. urine dipstick for possible urinary tract infection).

You should assess the risk of self-harm, harm to others, and Nathalie's vulnerability in her current state. There appears to be a high risk to Nathalie, since her sexualized behaviour may make her a target for the sexual advances of others and she may not have the skills to negotiate safe boundaries. In addition to this vulnerability, her placement could break down if the situation does not improve quickly. Unless the cause of her behaviour is both immediately clear *and* easily managed, she should be urgently referred to a specialist community mental health team for people with a learning disability. If Nathalie discloses abuse (sexual or otherwise), urgent referral to social services will be needed to protect her from this point onwards.

Moving Nathalie from her residential home will almost certainly worsen her distress and, by separating her from friends and familiar places, may disable her longer term. Remind staff that Nathalie does not normally behave like this, and will probably return to her usual state once the underlying issue has been identified and resolved. No sudden transfers should be made—especially not against Nathalie's will. Her capacity must be assessed. Although there are many possible and serious causes of her behavioural change, the entire episode may be due to excitement at meeting a new partner!

## Film list
*I am Sam* (2001)
*The Other Sister* (1999)
*Forest Gump* (1994)
*What's Eating Gilbert Grape* (1993)
*Charly* (1968) —the film of *Flowers for Algernon*

## Books
Cook, D. (1980) *Walter*. Harmondsworth: Penguin. Novel exploring the effect and treatments of learning disability in the era of segregation and institutionalization.

Keyes, D. (1966) *Flowers for Algernon*. New York: Harcourt. Charlie Gordon is a janitor with an IQ of 68 until he volunteers for an experiment which will boost his IQ, but only temporarily . . . This examines the treatment of and attitudes to people with a learning disability as well as the effect on their lives.

Mardell, D. (2005) *Danny's Challenge: Learning to Love My Son*. London: Short Books. Autobiography describing the impact of having a child with unexpected Down syndrome.

## Quotes
I'm not a smart man . . . But I know what love is.
**Forest Gump**

We should take care not to make the intellect our god; it has, of course, powerful muscles, but no personality.
**Albert Einstein**

Sometimes I've got words in my mind, and I'm trying to explain it in the best possible way, but it doesn't always come out.
**A young person with a learning disability[1]**

## Notes

1. From *Mencap Guide: Communicating with People with a Learning Disability*. Available at: www.mencap.org.uk
2. Many thanks to Mencap for their support in preparing this section. For further information go to: www.mencap.org.uk

## References/Further reading

Bhate, S. and Wilkinson S. (2006) Aetiology of learning disability. *Psychiatry*, **5**, 298–301.

Bouras, N. and Holt, G. (ed.) (2007) *Psychiatric and Behavioural Disorders in Intellectual and Developmental Disabilities* (2nd edn). Cambridge University Press.

Cooper, S.A., Smiley, E., Morrison, J., *et al.* (2007) Mental ill-health in adults with intellectual disabilities: prevalence and associated factors. *British Journal of Psychiatry*, **190**, 27–35.

Harris, J.C. (2006) *Intellectual Disability, Understanding its Development, Causes, Classification, Education, and Treatment.* New York: Oxford University Press.

IASSID (International Association for the Scientific Study of Intellectual Disabilities) (2001) *Mental Health and Intellectual Disabilities. Addressing the Mental Health Needs of People with Intellectual Disabilities, Report to the WHO.* Geneva: WHO.

McGuigan, S.M., Hollins, S., and Attard, M. (1995) Age-specific standardized mortality rates in people with learning disability. *Journal of Intellectual Disability Research*, **39**, 527–31.

Mencap (2004) *Treat me Right! Experiences of Using Health Services.* London: Mencap Campaigns Department.

Odom, S., Horner, R., Snell, M., and Blacher, J. (ed.) (2007) *Handbook of Developmental Disabilities.* New York: Guilford Press.

Royal College of Nursing (2007) *Mental Health Nursing of Adults with Learning Disabilities.* London: Royal College of Nursing.

Royal College of Psychiatrists (2001) *DC-LD: Diagnostic Criteria for Psychiatric Disorders for Use with Adults with Learning Disabilities/Mental Retardation.* London: Gaskell.

Smiley, E. (2005) Epidemiology of mental health problems in adults with learning disability: an update. *Advances in Psychiatric Treatment*, **11**, 214–22.

 Go to www.oxfordtextbooks/orc/stringer for an array of additional references, including indicative mark sheets for OSCEs, self-assessment questions, guidance, and exercises.

# 19 Child and adolescent psychiatry

*Gregory Lydall and Philip Collins*

## True or False? Test your existing knowledge—answers in the chapter and online

1. Most babies babble by the age of 2 months.

2. Poor parenting style is a recognized cause of autistic spectrum disorders.

3. 75% of children with autism have significant learning disabilities.

4. The first-line treatment for childhood depression is psychodynamic psychotherapy.

5. Girls are twice as likely to suffer from an anxiety disorder as boys.

6. Encopresis is defined as inappropriate defaecation after the age of 3.

7. The Conner's rating scale is used in the assessment of children with suspected conduct disorder.

8. The main risk of using stimulant medications in the treatment of ADHD is the risk of dependency.

9. Using basic street slang usually helps with rapport when talking to teenagers.

10. Shortly before discharge home from the paediatric ward, a 12 year old boy claims that his mother has been hitting him. He can be sent home to her care as long as a referral has been made to social services.

## Contents

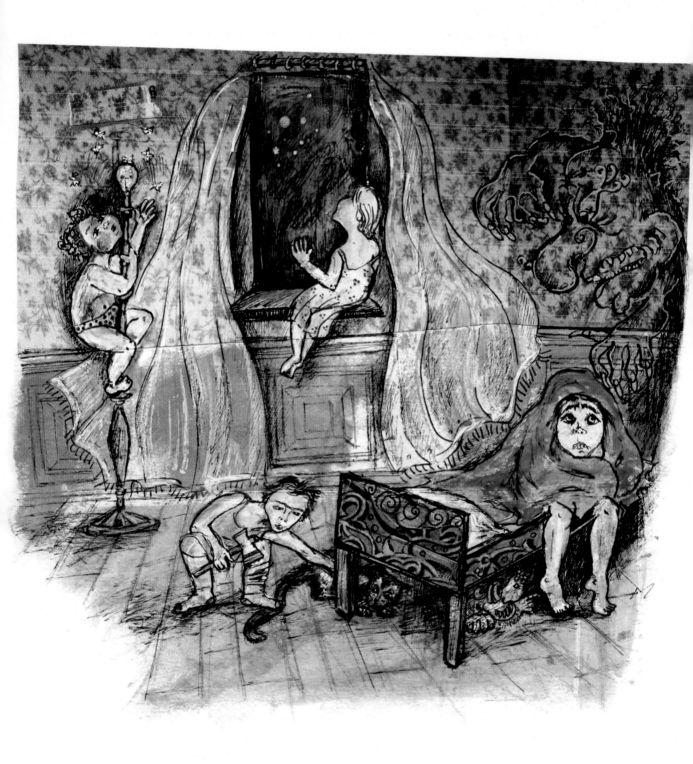

# PRINCIPLES

I have quite a few worries. I have made a list of them in my notebook—it's a notebook for worst worries—because people say things aren't so bad if you make a list. And then you can tick things off when they are solved. So far I haven't ticked anything off.

*Clarice Bean, Don't Look Now*—L. Child[1]

## Introduction

Children are not immune to mental illness. Sadly, up to 15% are affected by psychiatric problems at any one time—with potentially devastating effects on their social development and education. Therefore early recognition and intervention are crucial, although children rarely present themselves to doctors, even when extremely distressed. Parents or teachers usually raise concerns, and problems that cannot be dealt with by GPs or school support may be referred to Child and Adolescent Mental Health Services (CAMHS). CAMHS teams vary in size, but usually include a psychologist, specialist nurse, psychiatrist, and social worker.

Interactions between the child, their family, and their environment contribute to the overall risk of childhood mental health problems.

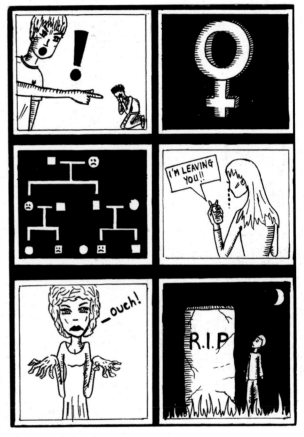

FIGURE 19.1 General risk factors for childhood mental health problems

### BOX 19.1 To optimize your reading

Child and adolescent psychiatry deals with *any* mental illness in this age group. Problems such as depression, anxiety, and self-harm are covered only briefly here, but are comprehensively discussed in their own chapters; read *with* this one for best effect! Similarly, we refer you to the dedicated chapter on eating disorders.

TABLE 19.1 Risk factors for childhood mental health problems

| Child | Family | Environment |
|---|---|---|
| Male | Family breakdown/conflict | Inner city |
| Sensory impairment | Separation/death and loss | Overcrowding |
| Physical illness | Abuse/neglect | Migration |
| Developmental delay | Inconsistent discipline | Homelessness |
| 'Difficult' temperament, | Hostility | Trauma |
| e.g. impulsive, intense | Large families (>4 children) | Poor social support |
| negative emotions | Parental | Peer criminality |
| Genetic factors | Psychiatric illness | |
| | Physical illness | |
| | Substance misuse | |
| | Personality disorder | |
| | Criminality | |

!  Child abuse may be subtle and does not always present with obvious behavioural problems or unexplained bruises. Stay alert for neglect. A neglected child could also go unnoticed by health professionals who treat them. Remember that child protection is *everyone's job*; discuss any concerns that you have with your senior colleagues immediately[3].

## Normal development

Failure to meet normal developmental milestones may simply be a 'late developer', but could signal underlying problems, which if corrected in time, can avert enduring disability (e.g. speech delay due to deafness). If there are concerns about delay, further assessment can be arranged.

**TABLE 19.2** Milestones

| Milestone | Average age | Limit age |
|---|---|---|
| Eye contact/follows face | 1–4 weeks | 3 months |
| Smiles responsively | 4–6 weeks | 8 weeks |
| Reaches for objects | 4 months | 6 months |
| Good head control when sitting | 4 months | 6 months |
| Turns to a voice | 7 months | 9 months |
| Tuneful babble | 5–6 months | 10 months |
| Sits unsupported | 7–8 months | 10 months |
| Pincer grip | 9–10 months | 15 months |
| Walks independently | 11–13 months | 18 months |
| Builds two cubes | 13–15 months | 19 months |
| First word | 8–18 months | 2 years |

Adapted from Sheridan 1997.

## Developmental disorders

Although learning disabilities are developmental problems, these are discussed in Chapter 18.

### Autism

Autism affects one in 1000 children, with as many again having autistic spectrum disorders (i.e. not meeting the full diagnostic criteria, but similar to autism). The male-to-female ratio is 4:1. There is no single cause, although obstetric complications, perinatal infection (e.g. maternal rubella), and genetic disorders such as tuberose sclerosis, Down syndrome, and fragile X are all risk factors.

 Neither parenting style *nor* measles–mumps–rubella (MMR) vaccination cause autism.

#### Clinical presentation

There are problems with the following domains:

1. **Reciprocal social interaction** Autistic children are not interested in people; they appear aloof, tend to play alone, and lack the ability to 'read' emotional states in others. Attachments are impoverished, without mutuality or warmth; these children do not turn to parents for comfort. Eye contact may be odd, either avoidant or 'looking through' you.

2. **Communication abnormalities** Expressive speech and comprehension are delayed or minimal. Ideas are taken literally (concrete thinking). Gestures are usually absent (e.g. pointing, waving goodbye). Later, speech may consist of monologues, interminable questions, or echolalia (repeating what has been said), but there is no exchange. Classically 'I' and 'me' are confused with 'you', 'he', and 'she' (pronominal reversal).

📖 When talking to autistic children, remember that eye contact is difficult for them. They may well be listening to you, even if they are staring intently at something else.

3. **Restricted behaviours and routine** Autism is characterized by repetitive, stereotyped behaviours and restricted interests—rather than imaginative play. Even small changes in routine (e.g. the wrong spoon) can result in intense tantrums.

Additionally, 75% of children have significant learning disabilities and 25% suffer from seizures. Overactive behaviour is common.

→ One patient's special interest was prawn shells. He spent hours categorizing his huge, smelly collection.

#### Differential diagnosis

1. **Deafness** causes poor language acquisition.
2. **Asperger's syndrome** (Box 19.2).
3. **Specific language disorder**: delayed speech but normal IQ and social ability.
4. **Learning disability**: IQ problems but relatively intact social skills.
5. **Rare disorders**, e.g. childhood schizophrenia, Rett's syndrome.
6. **Neglect** can lead to language delay and poor socialization—reversible unless severe.

#### Investigations

1. Hearing tests.
2. Speech and language assessment.
3. Neuropsychological testing—assess IQ and confirm diagnosis.

#### Management

1. **Support and advice for families**, e.g. the National Autistic Society.
2. **Behaviour therapy** (p.204)—reinforce positive behaviours.

3. **Speech and language therapy.**
4. **Special education.**
5. **Treat comorbid problems** (e.g. epilepsy).
6. **Antipsychotics or mood stabilizers** are *occasionally* used for extreme aggression or hyperactivity.

### Prognosis

Only 1–2% of adults gain full independence, with most needing lifelong support and care. Good prognostic indicators are an IQ over 70 and acquisition of some useful language.

---

**BOX 19.2** Asperger's syndrome

.........................................................

- An autistic spectrum disorder.
- Male:female = 8:1.
- Poor social skills and restricted interests.
- *Normal* language and IQ.
- Tendency to literal interpretation of language and difficulty in reading social cues.
- Management: advice, support, routine, social skills training.
- Prognosis is much better than for autism.

---

 A patient with Asperger's syndrome, obsessed with train timetables, became a very successful train conductor.

## Emotional disorders

### Depression

One to two per cent of children and 8% of adolescents are affected. The sex ratio is equal before puberty, but girls outnumber boys thereafter (Anderson *et al.* 1987). The presentation is similar to that in adults, although children are more likely to complain of somatic problems (e.g. headaches, tummy-aches). Irritability and deteriorating school performance may be reported by teachers. First-line treatment is cognitive behavioural therapy (CBT). Antidepressants are only prescribed by specialists in severe cases. The prognosis is generally good, but severe episodes are likely to recur.

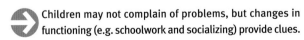 Children may not complain of problems, but changes in functioning (e.g. schoolwork and socializing) provide clues.

You may miss essential problems unless you offer young patients time to speak with you without their parents. Take a colleague to chaperone.

### Anxiety disorders

Anxiety disorders affect boys and girls equally and the presentation is similar to that in adulthood. Psychological therapies are the mainstay of treatment.

### Separation anxiety disorder

Children present as clingy, becoming distressed on separation from their parents, often fearing that it will be permanent. Tactful exploration of the family history may reveal a threatened or unmourned loss, with which the family can be helped while managing the child's anxiety by increased periods of separation with reunion.

### School refusal

Unlike truancy, this is *unconcealed* absence from school. It is common at times of transition, e.g. a new school or a new sibling. Bullying, fear of failure, or an unsympathetic teacher may be implicated. It may occur in families with 'precious' children (death of a sibling, difficulty conceiving) or vulnerable parents (life-threatening illness, agoraphobia). The child typically has tummy-ache just before school, but never at weekends or holidays.

First help the parents tackle the problem, enlisting the school's support to deal with anxiety about performance, bullying, etc. A rapid return to full attendance carries the best prognosis. Failure to achieve this signals deeper problems—depression or separation anxiety (in parent or child).

## Enuresis

Poor bladder control affects up to 10% of 5-year-olds and 1% of adolescents. There is often a family history of similar problems. Enuresis can be *primary* (toilet training was never mastered) or *secondary* (dryness was achieved for at least a year but has been lost). Nocturnal enuresis (bed-wetting) is more common in boys; diurnal enuresis affects girls more frequently.

Primary enuresis is usually due to delayed maturation of the bladder's nervous innervation or more generalized developmental delay, although stress and excessively relaxed or strict toilet training can also play a role. Secondary causes are usually stress related, e.g. starting at a new school.

### Management

1. **Refer** organic causes of enuresis to paediatrics, e.g. epilepsy, urinary tract infection, constipation, diabetes.
2. **Reassure** the family and the child that the problem is common and is no one's fault. Address stressors and review the toilet training received so far.
3. **Restrict fluids** before bed.
4. **Star charts** celebrate each dry night (positive reinforcement).
5. **Bell and pad**: this 'underpants alarm' clips onto pyjamas and wakes the child if moisture is detected, teaching normal voiding.

6. Medication, e.g. imipramine (tricyclic antidepressant) or desmopressin (synthetic antidiuretic hormone).

## Encopresis

Encopresis is inappropriate defecation after age 4, when bowel control is expected. Again, boys are more commonly affected and the problem can be primary or secondary.

Most cases relate to constipation ('overflow incontinence'). Constipation may be due to:

- dehydration
- painful defecation (e.g. anal fissure)
- fear of punishment
- toilet fears (e.g. monsters in the toilet)
- Hirschsprung's disease (rarely, bowel obstruction due to an aganglionic section of colon).

When constipation is not an issue, reasons for incontinence include diarrhoea, learning disabilities, and occasionally hostility (e.g. angrily defecating in Mum's shoe). Some children simply feel defeated by the transition from the potty to the toilet, and punitive toilet training may have compounded this. Stress can trigger secondary incontinence.

### Management

1. **Laxatives** and stool softeners for constipation; treat other physical causes.
2. **Reassure**, address stress, and review toilet training.
3. **Star charts.**

Sixty to ninety per cent become continent within a year.

## Elective mutism

An electively mute child *can* speak, but doesn't in certain situations, e.g. at school. This affects four in 1000 children (girls slightly more often than boys), often beginning around the time of starting school. The child is commonly very talkative at home, but painfully shy and completely silent elsewhere. Treatment involves reassurance, reducing stress, and sometimes behavioural management (Labbe and Williamson 1984).

## Behavioural disorders

## Attention deficit–hyperactivity disorder (ADHD)

Hyperkinetic disorder or ADHD affects 2% of UK children and is three times more common in boys. The cause is unknown, although genetics plays an important role; dopamine and noradrenaline deficiencies and frontal lobe abnormalities are implicated.

### Clinical presentation

Problems should present by the age of six, and must be persistent and pervasive across different situations. A child who is calm at school but over-excited at home would not be diagnosed.

### Hyperactivity

Children are boisterous with excessive energy. They seem constantly on the move: running, jumping, climbing, unable to sit still for any length of time without fidgeting, squirming, or wandering about. They are usually noisy and garrulous.

### Inattention

Children are distractible and unable to concentrate, flitting chaotically between activities and leaving tasks unfinished.

### Associated features

These children are impulsive and reckless, rarely stopping to consider the consequences of their actions. This can result in risky behaviour, e.g. poor road safety. They tend to be clumsy and accident prone, and may be disobedient, although often through impulsivity rather than deliberate naughtiness. Additionally, they are socially disinhibited, paying little attention to normal social conventions; they interrupt others and find it hard to wait their turn. Learning disability and conduct disorder are associated.

### Differential diagnosis

1. **Depression/anxiety**—both can cause agitation.
2. **Mania** (extremely rare in childhood).
3. **Conduct disorder.**

### Investigations

1. Questionnaires, e.g. Conner's Rating Scales (Conners 1970), completed by the child, parents, and teacher to rate ADHD-related behaviours.
2. Classroom observation of the child by the clinician may help.
3. Educational psychology assessments.

Teachers are excellent sources of information, partly because they understand the range of 'normal' behaviours for a particular age.

### Management

1. **Family**: education on ADHD; advice on parenting and boundaries.
2. **Behavioural management.**
3. **Support for teachers**: appropriate schooling placement.
4. **Family therapy.**

5. **Stimulant medication** (e.g. methylphenidate, dexamphetamine). This increases monoamine pathway activity, improving concentration and allowing learning and maturation. Adverse effects include appetite suppression and insomnia. 'Drug holidays' (weekends and school holidays) limit growth retardation to 1cm finally. Stimulant medications are *not* addictive in ADHD.

 Many parents report benefits from dietary changes, e.g. increasing oily fish/excluding certain foods. No firm evidence exists for this but *anything* that helps is a bonus for exhausted parents!

### Prognosis

Children with ADHD may suffer low self-esteem, peer rejection, educational under-achievement, and harsh parenting. Although symptoms often improve in adolescence, up to 50% of adults have ongoing problems (up to 30% retain the diagnosis) (Gittelman *et al.* 1985). Untreated ADHD is a risk factor for later dissocial personality disorder, criminality, and substance abuse.

## Conduct disorder (CD)

CD affects 10% of 10-year-olds and is four times more common in boys. It runs in families, although no genes have been identified. Risk factors include urban upbringing, deprivation, parental criminality, harsh and inconsistent parenting, maternal depression, and a family history of substance misuse. Antisocial behaviour is often learned from parental or societal models, and may be rewarded (e.g. by increased attention) and thus reinforced.

### Clinical presentation

Behaviour is persistently antisocial, not merely 'rebellious', e.g. bullying, stealing, fighting, fire-setting, truancy, and cruelty to animals or people. In *socialized* CD the child has a peer group (often sharing in the antisocial behaviour). Children with *unsocialized* CD are rejected by other children, which often makes them more isolated and hostile.

### Differential diagnosis

1. **Oppositional defiant disorder**: a milder form of CD, occurring in children under 10, with provocative, angry, and disobedient behaviour towards adults. No extreme antisocial behaviour is present.

2. **ADHD**

3. **Depression**: some children present with antisocial behaviour.

### Management

1. **Family education**: the family members need to understand CD and recognize that they may reinforce problems.

2. **Parent management training**: teaches parents to reward good behaviour and deal constructively with negative behaviours.

3. **Family therapy**: the family meets with a skilled therapist to discuss current problems. They are helped to cooperate in problem solving.

4. **Educational support.**

5. **Anger management** for the child.

6. **Treat comorbid problems**, e.g. ADHD.

### Prognosis

Up to 50% develop substance misuse problems or dissocial personality disorder as adults (Robins and Price 1991).

Inpatient admission is reserved for children with complex or risky presentations.

## Miscellaneous disorders

### Tic disorders

Tics are repetitive, involuntary, and purposeless movements or vocal utterances. They are categorized as simple (e.g. blinking, throat-clearing) or complex (e.g. self-hitting, swearing). Transient simple tics affect 10% of children, and are three times more common in boys. There is often a family history of problems and obsessive–compulsive disorder is commonly comorbid. Stress or stimulant medications usually worsen tics. They recede when the sufferer is concentrating on something else. Tics can be voluntarily suppressed at the cost of internal tension, which is relieved by their expression. Reassurance and stress management are effective treatments, but clonidine (adrenergic agonist) or haloperidol (antipsychotic) are also useful.

In Gilles de la Tourette syndrome there are multiple motor tics with at least one vocal tic. It tends to worsen in adolescence and persist into adulthood.

# REALITY

## General approach: tips, tricks, and cautionary tales

### Children (especially under-eights)

#### 1. Start with the family

Young children usually feel overwhelmed if asked to explain why their parents have brought them in, so greet the whole family and ask the child if they are happy for you to start by asking their parents some questions. Explain that they can join in to add things, or if they disagree or don't understand. This also reinforces the message that they should not talk to strangers; respect a child's natural wariness of you and ensure that they realize you are talking to them with parental permission.

 Remember that older children may want to speak *before* their parents.

#### 2. Starting the conversation with a child

Begin with easy cheerful topics (e.g. a recent birthday, favourite activities). If the child is clutching a toy or book, ask them about it—they may feel confident about discussing it, since it is their specialist subject!

- Under five years—observe their play and play a little yourself, chatting as you do so.
- Over five years—it may help to ask them to do a drawing. Chat and use directed questioning to take more of a history (suggested by Goodman and Scott 2005).

Remember, showing interest is your most powerful communication tool!

#### 3. Shy/frightened children

 Young children may find you less intimidating if they know your first name; as a doctor you might introduce yourself less formally, e.g. 'Dr Laurence' rather than Dr Church.

The key to engaging shy or scared children is remembering that the harder you try, the harder they will hide from you. Try a graded exposure approach. Take your focus off them for a few minutes by talking to their parents about something *other* than the child. Placing an interesting toy or paper and pens near them (but not too close to you) and leaving them alone may help them relax. Shy children often eavesdrop as they play,

and may even creep closer as they feel safer. Try building their confidence by dropping their name into the conversation intermittently or asking them an easy closed question ('Do *you* like Mummy's new car?'). Next try asking about their toy or drawing. They may let you look at or talk about it before they make eye contact or talk about themselves. Speak softly and kindly.

There can always be a follow-up interview if needed. The main benefit of the first interview may be dispelling fears, e.g. that doctors give painful injections or send 'bad' children to hospital. If the child remembers you as 'the nice doctor', hopefully they will feel braver next time.

 Get into your chair (or closer to the child's level) as soon as you can. Even short adults appear like giants to children! Also, remember children often feel safer sitting on their parent's lap rather than in a chair.

#### 4. Excitable children

Children naturally have more energy than adults; with their additional excitement or anxiety about *seeing the doctor*, they may resemble little firecrackers. If you forget this, you will over-diagnose ADHD! Although tempting, don't increase their excitement by bouncing around, chasing or tickling them—or by shouting for order. Remember that *you* won't be taking them home in a worked-up state! Speak calmly and encourage them to settle with a (quiet) toy or task.

#### 5. Worries are big when you are little

Although they may differ from your main clinical concerns, listen very carefully to a child's problems or worries. Some worries may seem silly (e.g. about falling down the toilet) but to a child they are very serious.

#### 6. Normal versus abnormal

If you have never worked with children and have none of your own, the normal–abnormal line can feel very hard to judge (a little like the first liver you palpated: *Was that normal?*). You need comparisons against which you can gauge children, and this is mostly down to clinical experience. When in doubt, defer to experienced colleagues, teachers, and parents.

#### 7. Don't infantilize

Children are often very sensitive to being patronized or treated like babies, e.g. ruffling hair, pinching cheeks, describing them as *cute*, or calling them *champ*, *sport*, etc. If *you* wouldn't like it, don't do it to them.

## Teenagers

### 8. Don't try to be 'cool'[2]

Don't try speaking or acting *like a teenager* as a way of gaining rapport—it looks ridiculous and feels patronizing. You are more likely to gain rapport by treating young people as adults and being interested, understanding, and non-judgemental. These traits in an adult are actually quite 'cool'.[2]

### 9. Don't stereotype

Lots of people judge teenagers as lazy, violent, disrespectful, promiscuous, etc., based on appearance and the fact that they are *the youth of today*. We were all *the youth of today*, once! The person inside the image may well be gentle and articulate, with a passion for human rights politics, even if they *do* wear their trousers halfway down their buttocks.

### 10. Language

Be aware that teenagers may use words with a different meaning to you; they may also use language that they don't fully understand (especially when trying to gain your respect). It's always worth checking meaning to ensure that you understand each other. As with all patients, avoid medical jargon.

## Parents

### 11. Talking to Mum and Dad

Parents often feel apprehensive or guilty about their child's problems. Having a *no blame* attitude helps—and once parents relax, children often follow suit. Occasionally, parents are very clearly a part of the problem (e.g. abusive). It's important not to become punitive or angry, since this can have a detrimental effect: parents may disengage or take their anger out on the child.

➜ *Mentally* perform two MSEs: one for the child and one for their family. Your observations are an essential part of the assessment and offer insight into family dynamics, parenting skills, personalities, and sociability.

## Child and adolescent history (10 minutes)

### Candidate's instructions

You are a final-year medical student holding your own clinic in a general practice. Mr Michael McMahon has attended to discuss his five-year-old son, William.

Take a history sufficient to allow referral to a specialist if required.

### Patient's brief

*Key characteristics*

- I'm not a 'touchy feely' person and see Will as being like me.
- I don't want to believe that there's anything wrong with Will.
- I worry that I'm not a good enough dad and I've done something wrong.

Will's teacher thinks he's a bit 'different'—she said I should talk to you about him. His pregnancy was easy but he was born by Caesarean after the placenta burst. Charlotte (my girlfriend) died from blood loss... Will needed the Special Care Baby Unit, but was out the next day and he's been fine ever since. All his baby checks were normal and he walked at nine months—quite the athlete! His first word was *cup*, when he was 18 months. He's not chatty like his sister Lily, but he can speak if he wants to. *(If pushed)* He's never really got into sentences—mostly he just names things and I know what he means ... *cup* or *bread* or whatever. *(If asked)* I can't remember seeing him point or wave goodbye, but I guess he *must*. He doesn't nod or shake his head, but he can say *yes* and *no*, so doesn't need to.

He's always been very independent—a *man's man*. Right from when he was little, he just got on with things. He doesn't mind if he's left alone (unlike Lily, who still cries, even though she's seven)—he's no wimp! Even when he falls over he doesn't come running for help—just cries and then gets on with things. He's not cuddly, but then neither am I—there's nothing wrong with that. Lily's his biggest fan and very protective of him, even though, if the tables are turned, he doesn't really pay it back ... Yesterday she fell over and was wailing her head off but Will just walked straight past and paid no attention! I guess he's still too little to realize she was hurt. He likes his own company—plays by himself all day if you let him. He's not into hanging out with the other boys just yet—he's not really interested at the moment.

Will's very determined and single-minded. He'll play with his toy cars for hours on end, just lining them up or holding them in the air and spinning the wheels round. Maybe he'll be a mechanic when he grows up. It's funny, but he has a real thing for yellow plastic forks and likes to stroke the prongs along his arm, over and over. He's never been interested in soft toys or bedtime stories or anything—but you give him a yellow plastic fork and he'll be no trouble for hours! He has tantrums if he can't find it, so I always carry a spare! He doesn't like things that are bright red (even forks) and we keep red things away from him to prevent more tantrums. We both like routine: get up, breakfast, playschool, home, supper, bed. We stick to that so that no one gets confused and Will reminds me if I get it wrong (tantrum).

I was told autistic children don't make eye contact—but Will *does*: it's such a keen stare, it's like he's looking right through you . . .

### Other history

- He's had all his vaccinations and never gets anything worse than a cold.
- His hearing is excellent.
- No one in the family has any mental health problems.

### Questions

He can't be autistic, can he?

### Worries

- I'm to blame. Maybe if his mum was still alive, he'd be more cuddly . . .
- I shouldn't have let him have the MMR vaccination.

# NEXT STEPS

## Hyperactivity and non-accidental injury

You are a junior doctor in paediatrics. Dwayne Rutherford (12 years old) has been admitted three times in the past six months with asthma attacks. He is very popular on the ward and has formed close relationships with the staff. During his last admission he asked your colleague if they could keep a secret and told them that he had been smoking cigarettes—triggering the asthma attack. Dwayne promised never to smoke again and your colleague agreed not to tell his parents.

Dwayne has a diagnosis of ADHD and is prescribed methylphenidate by the CAMHS team. You are aware that he has been through a tough time, with his parents divorcing two years ago. He has been in trouble at school lately, and you think that his mother may be having difficulties managing his behaviour.

On this admission he was noted to have bruises on his back. He had explained that they resulted from playground fights, but now, on the day of his discharge, he has approached you asking if *you* can keep a secret. You say that you can, and he tells you that the bruises were from his mother hitting him, which has been happening quite a lot recently.

1. How will you respond to his disclosure?
2. What longer-term interventions could help the family?
3. How could Dwayne's ADHD affect his asthma? What could be done?

### Issues

- Risk
- Disclosure of information told to you in confidence
- Management

### Response

You will need to let Dwayne know that he has done the right thing in talking to you, and is not in any trouble. You should listen carefully, showing that you do believe him and recording what he tells you without *pushing* him to disclose information. You will explain how you plan to help him, and that you have a duty to act to ensure his safety. Dwayne may consent for you to pass on his information, but if he still refuses after your best efforts to explore any reluctance, you should proceed, since he is at considerable risk of harm. You will urgently refer Dwayne to the children's duty social worker—both by telephone and by immediately completing a referral form. You will also inform your consultant, the nurse in charge, and the child protection lead for the team.

As a rule, you should communicate openly and honestly with Dwayne's parents unless you think that this might place Dwayne (or someone else) at increased risk of significant harm.

The initial assessment will take place urgently with Dwayne remaining in hospital until the lead social worker recommends that he can be safely discharged. Dwayne will probably be able to return home with safeguards and a follow-up plan in place. If the social worker assesses Dwayne as a 'child in need', a meeting will be arranged involving social work, the police, and other relevant agencies (e.g. CAMHS, GP). Further enquiries, a child protection conference, and a child protection plan may be necessary, depending on the risks to Dwayne.[3]

## Interventions

Help for the family is needed, regardless of the outcome of the disclosure, since this incident signals that Dwayne and his family need support. Interventions include:

- **Dwayne**: emotional support from school or CAMHS, further assessment, and optimal ADHD treatment. His educational needs and performance at school should be addressed.

- **Mother**: practical/emotional support; parenting skills groups especially tailored to caring for children with ADHD. Does Mum have mental health needs of her own?

- **Family**: family therapy, preferably with both parents, at CAMHS.

## Effect of ADHD

Dwayne's ADHD may affect his ability to remember to take his asthma medication, because of difficulties concentrating on tasks and his impulsive behaviour. He will also be more likely to forget to carry his short-acting beta-2 agonist inhaler. You should check that he understands when he should take each inhaler and consider strategies to remind him to use them. Complicated prescribing regimes will result in missed doses, so once- or twice-daily treatments will help Dwayne manage his ADHD and asthma.

📖 **Never offer unlimited confidentiality!** Dwayne should have been told, 'I can keep most secrets, unless you tell me something that makes me worry that you or someone else might be hurt. If I'm really worried I'll have to tell other people so that we can keep you safe. OK?

### Film list
*Kidulthood/Pretty Persuasion* (CD)
*Thirteen* (2003) (self-harm and substance misuse in adolescence)
*Rain Man* (1988) (autism in adulthood)

### Books
Haddon, M. (2003) *The Curious Incident of the Dog in the Nighttime*. London: Vintage, 2004. Explores how people with autistic spectrum disorders perceive the world; the narrator has Asperger's syndrome.

Haden, T. (1988) *Just Another Kid*. London: Harper Element, 2006. A special needs teacher's tale of working with children with selective mutism, autism, learning disability, schizophrenia, and conduct disorder.

Ray, R. (1998) *A Certain Age*. London: Penguin. Self-harm in adolescence.

### Quotes
A characteristic of the normal child is he doesn't act that way very often.
**Anonymous**

Even when freshly washed and relieved of all obvious confections, children tend to be sticky.
**Fran Lebowitz**

Children's talent to endure stems from their ignorance of alternatives.
**Maya Angelou, *I Know Why the Caged Bird Sings***

Don't give up! I believe in you all! A person's a person, no matter how small!
**Horton, *Horton Hears a Who* (Dr Seuss)**

## Notes

1. Child, L. (2006) *Clarice Bean, Don't Look Now*. Copyright Orchard Books, London.
2. The author apologizes for the lame term 'cool'. She thought that it was what all the kids were using today.
3. For further information see HM Government publication *What to do if you're worried a child is being abused* (www.everychildmatters.gov.uk).

## References/Further reading

Anderson, J.C., Williams, S., McGee, R., and Silva, P.A. (1987) DSM-III disorders in preadolescent children: prevalence in a large sample from the general population. *Archives of General Psychiatry*, **44**, 69–76.

Conners, C. (1970) Symptom patterns in hyperkinetic, neurotic, and normal children. *Child Development*, **41**, 667–82.

Costello, E.J., Mustillo, S., Erkanli, A., *et al.* (2003) Prevalence and development of psychiatric disorders in childhood and adolescence. *Archives of General Psychiatry*, **60**, 837–44.

Gittelman, R., Manuzza, S., Shenker, R., and Bonagura, N. (1985) Hyperactive boys almost grown up. I: Psychiatric status. *Archives of General Psychiatry*, **42**, 937–47.

Goodman, R. and Scott, S. (2005) *Child Psychiatry* (2nd edn). Oxford: Blackwell.

Kanner, L. (1943) Autistic disturbances of affective contact. *Nervous Child*, **2**, 217–50. Reprinted in *Acta Paedopsychiatrica*, **35**, 100–36, 1968.

Labbe, E.E. and Williamson, D.A. (1984) Behavioral treatment of elective mutism: a review of the literature. *Clinical Psychology Review*, **4**, 273–92.

Robins, L.N. and Price, R.K. (1991) Adult disorders predicted by childhood conduct problems: results from the NIMH Epidemiologic Catchment Area project. *Psychiatry*, **54**, 116–32.

Rutter, M. (1999) Psychosocial adversity and child psychopathology. *British Journal of Psychiatry*, **174**, 480–93.

Rutter, M., Tizard, J., Yule, W., *et al.* (1976) Research report: Isle of Wight Studies, 1964–1974. *Psychological Medicine*, **6**, 313–32.

Scott, S. (2008) An update on interventions for conduct disorder. *Advances in Psychiatric Treatment*, **14**, 61–70.

Sheridan, M.D. (1997) In *From Birth to Five Years* (ed. M. Frost and A. Sharma). London: Routledge.

Taylor, E., Sandberg, S., Thorley, G., and Giles, S. (1991) *The Epidemiology of Childhood Hyperactivity*. Oxford University Press.

 Go to www.oxfordtextbooks/orc/stringer for an array of additional references, including indicative mark sheets for OSCEs, self-assessment questions, guidance, and exercises.

# 20 Personality disorders

*Laurence Church*

## True or False? Test your existing knowledge—answers in the chapter and online

1. Cluster A disorders include paranoid and histrionic personality disorders.

2. Multiple personality disorder is the diagnosis given to people showing traits from each of the three personality clusters.

3. Overall, personality disorders are equally common in men and women.

4. To fulfil ICD-10 diagnostic criteria, evidence of a personality disorder must be present from adolescence onwards.

5. A family history of alcohol dependency is a risk factor for the development of personality disorder.

6. *Reaction formation* is an ego defence mechanism where a person behaves in a way opposite to their unacknowledged and unacceptable desires or impulses.

7. Personality disorders, by definition, are untreatable conditions.

8. The severity of a personality disorders may fluctuate over the course of a patient's life time.

9. It is important to have very flexible boundaries when working with patients with personality disorders.

10. A diagnosis of dissocial personality disorder means that a person cannot be held responsible for their actions.

## Contents

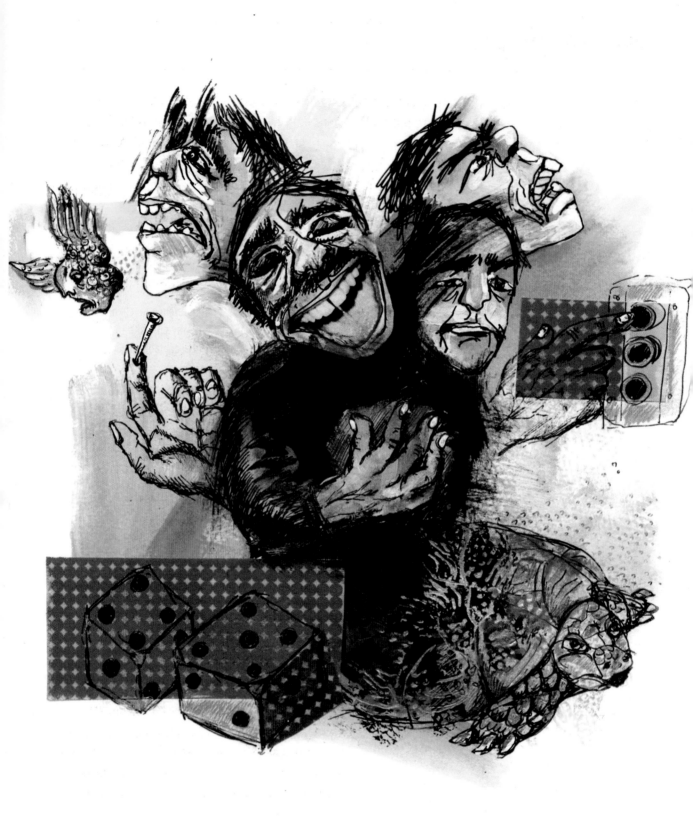

# PRINCIPLES

'Why do I think I'm here?' After five doctors, I have the first visit procedure down and can go through the routine on autopilot, laying out the relevant data points like setting the table for a five-course meal. Anorexia at age ten, bulimia at twelve, alcoholism and sexual promiscuity with the onset of puberty; lying, nightmares, and self-mutilation for as long as I can remember.

*The Good Patient*—Kristen Waterfield Duisberg[1]

## Introduction

**Personality** is derived from the Greek *persona* or *mask*. In ancient theatre, masks were used to identify characters.

Personality refers to a set of consistent thoughts, feelings, and behaviours shown across time in a variety of settings. People with a personality *disorder* experience difficulties in interpersonal relationships which, in a medical setting, may present as *difficulties in getting their needs met* or being labelled as *difficult patients*. Patients may evoke strong opposing reactions in staff, some of whom want to help and others to keep away. This group of patients has been stigmatized and regarded as 'untreatable' for years—but understanding and support are actually required.

Have you seen a patient who evoked strong reactions in staff? How did you feel about them?

## Personality traits and disorders

Personality is made up of characteristics, or *traits* (Box 20.1). There is no such thing as a 'bad' trait; all have strengths and weaknesses which manifest in different situations. For example, doctors may be perfectionists—a valuable trait for their patients. However, in an emergency, most patients would prefer a doctor who acted quickly to one who found a dictionary to check that their spelling was correct in the notes!

*3Ps* distinguish personality *disorder* from traits:

- Pervasive—occurs in all/most areas of life
- Persistent—evident in adolescence and continues through adulthood
- Pathological—causes distress to self or others; impairs function

ICD-10 requires the following criteria for a diagnosis of personality disorder (REPORT):

### BOX 20.1 The 'big five'—five-factor model

This describes five broad personality factors (OCEAN), consisting of groups of traits:

- **O**penness to experience: curiosity, imagination and appreciation of art, adventure and emotion
- **C**onscientiousness: ability to plan and be self-disciplined to achieve goals
- **E**xtraversion: predisposition to experience positive (social) events
- **A**greeableness: tendency to be cooperative, trusting, and kind
- **N**euroticism: predisposition to negative emotions, e.g. anxiety, anger, or depression

- **R**elationships affected
- **E**nduring
- **P**ervasive
- **O**nset in childhood/adolescence
- **R**esult in distress
- **T**rouble in occupational/social performance

This behaviour must not be attributable to brain damage or disease, or another psychiatric disorder.

The rare and controversial *multiple personality disorder* is classified within dissociative disorders (p.170).

Personality disorders commonly coexist, falling into three broad groups or *clusters*. According to ICD, these are:

- **Cluster A** ('odd or eccentric'): paranoid, schizoid.
- **Cluster B** ('dramatic, erratic, or emotional'): histrionic, emotionally unstable, and dissocial.
- **Cluster C** ('anxious and fearful'): anankastic, anxious (avoidant), and dependent.

Don't confuse *cluster A* with *type A personality*, a rather dated term describing impatient, aggressive, competitive people, thought to be at higher risk of heart disease.

## Epidemiology

The prevalence of personality disorder varies greatly according to the setting and the diagnostic criteria used (Table 20.1). Men have higher overall rates, particularly cluster A, dissocial or anankastic types; histrionic or emotionally unstable borderline personality disorders are more common in women.

**TABLE 20.1** The prevalence of personality disorders/clusters in different settings

| Setting | Prevalence of personality disorder | Predominant cluster |
| --- | --- | --- |
| Epidemiological community survey | 10% | — |
| Primary care | 20% | C |
| Psychiatric outpatients | 30% | B |
| Psychiatric inpatients | 40% | B |
| Prison | 50% | B |

## Aetiology

### Genetics

Genetics determine 50% of our personality and personality traits show a monozygotic:dizygotic twin concordance rate of 50%:30% (Loehlin and Nichols 1976). Personality disorder is associated with a family history of personality disorder, as well as a history of depression and alcohol dependency.

### Childhood temperament

Temperament describes an infant's pattern of activity, attention span, response to new situations, and intensity of emotional responses. The temperament of children as young as 3 can predict personality traits in adulthood (Caspi and Silva 1995). Children with 'difficult' temperaments have greater problems coping as adults, possibly because they find it harder to develop supportive relationships, and are more distressed by negative events. Early attachment difficulties are also associated with personality disorder.

### Childhood experience

Personality disorder is associated with insecure attachment and traumatic, neglectful, or chaotic upbringing. Many people experience traumatic childhoods, and it is not understood why most are resilient, whilst others develop a personality disorder or another mental illness (e.g. depression, eating disorders, or schizophrenia).

## Theories of personality disorder

### Cognitive and psychoanalytical theories

The quality of early relationships and the nature of the environment in which someone is raised influence their expectations about themselves and the world. For example, people feel lovable because they were first loved, feel fearful if others were unpredictable or frightening, and behave cruelly if first treated with cruelty.

Behaviour is viewed as being motivated by a combination of beliefs and desires, with cognitive theories favouring beliefs and psychoanalytic theories emphasizing desire. Both agree that our expectations tend to be fulfilled and perpetuated. For example, open, confident people more often receive a friendly response, confirming to them that others are friendly and encouraging them to continue being confident and open. Aggressive people tend to spark hostility in others, 'proving' their view that people are threatening and deserve a heavy-handed approach.

### Psychological defences

Defence mechanisms are unconscious strategies that are used to manage uncomfortable feelings. They are often adaptive, but sometimes they cause trouble. They become pathological when people are overly reliant on them, causing conflict with others or never addressing their underlying emotions. Some are listed below, with reference to the later personality disorder subtypes that illustrate them (pp.225–7).

- **Acting out** Impulses are expressed through actions, without conscious awareness of the underlying emotion (e.g. Phoebe's self-harm rather than sadness).
- **Splitting** Other people are thought of in polarized terms and either idealized or denigrated. This protects 'good' people from hostility by directing it at 'bad' people (e.g. Phoebe's views of her boyfriend).
- **Projection** Uncomfortable feelings are 'put onto' someone else and then experienced as belonging to them (e.g. Reuben rids himself of hostile feelings by projecting them onto his colleagues).
- **Fantasizing** Using imagination to escape from the painfulness of reality (e.g. Masson's daydreams prevent him from feeling lonely).
- **Reaction formation** behaving in a way that is opposite to unacknowledged and unacceptable desires. (e.g. Reece's excessive punctiliousness keeps worrying criminal impulses at bay).

## Neurotransmitter theories

There is evidence of lower serotonin levels in dissocial personality disorder (Virkkunen *et al.* 1987). Serotonin has been implicated in regulation of impulsivity and aggression. Other monoamines have received less attention, but may be involved in predicting certain patterns of behaviour, e.g. dopamine for novelty seeking and noradrenaline for persistence and dependency to rewards.

## Clinical presentation of personality disorders

As well as REPORT, *at least three* of the features listed below are required to diagnose a specific personality disorder.

## Paranoid personality disorder

| Features | Example |
|---|---|
| Sensitive<br>Unforgiving<br>Suspicious<br>Possessive and jealous of partners<br>Excessive self-importance<br>Conspiracy theories<br>Tenacious sense of rights | Reuben suspected that his colleagues at the Post Office were getting preferential treatment, despite his certainty that he was the best worker there. When he was offered overtime, it was 'only the shifts that no-one else wanted'. This confirmed his suspicion, and so he resigned, feeling insulted. Five years later he is still convinced that his boss was corrupt. |

**Differential diagnosis**: schizophrenia, persistent delusional disorder

## Schizoid personality disorder

| Features | Example |
|---|---|
| Anhedonic<br>Limited emotional range<br>Little sexual interest<br>Apparent indifference to praise/criticism<br>Lacks close relationships<br>One-player activities<br>Normal social conventions ignored<br>Excessive fantasy world | Masson was a night security guard, content with solitude and daydreaming his shift away. His manager passed on complaints from the day staff that he left a 'body odour smell' in the office, but he didn't try to wash. Although people thought he was odd, he really didn't care. He wasn't interested in having friends or a sexual partner, preferring his own company. He was neither happy nor sad about this; that was just life. |

**Differential diagnosis**: Asperger's syndrome, agoraphobia, social phobia, psychosis, depression

## Histrionic personality disorder

| Features | Example |
|---|---|
| Attention seeking<br>Concerned with own appearance<br>Theatrical<br>Open to suggestion<br>Racy and seductive<br>Shallow affect | Paige met her boyfriend for lunch. He suggested a bottle of wine, so she ordered champagne! Tottering on her pink stilettos, she fell into his lap as she got out of her chair. Everyone stared but Paige shrieked with laughter! She became bored and flirted with the waiter, but when he ignored her she left, announcing loudly, 'I'll *never* eat here again!' |

**Differential diagnosis**: hypomanic/manic episode, substance misuse

## Emotionally unstable personality disorder

**Features of both subtypes**

Affective instability

Explosive behaviour

Impulsive

Outbursts of anger

Unable to plan or consider consequences

**Borderline type (borderline personality disorder)**

| Features | Example |
|---|---|
| Self-image unclear<br><br>Chronic 'empty' feelings<br><br>Abandonment fears<br><br>Relationships are intense and unstable<br><br>Suicide attempts and self-harm | Phoebe had been on two dates with her *perfect* university lecturer—she already *knew* they'd get married! When he cancelled a date because of work, Phoebe felt so alone. A familiar numb feeling of emptiness returned, reminding her of when her ex-boyfriend left. Phoebe told him she was going to kill herself and it was his fault. She slammed down the phone and cut her wrists with scissors—she couldn't bear to be alone again. The bastard! |

**Differential diagnosis**: adjustment disorder, depression, psychosis (patients occasionally experience fleeting psychotic features)

**Impulsive type**

| Features | Example |
|---|---|
| Lacks impulse control<br><br>Outbursts or threats of violence<br><br>Sensitivity to being thwarted or criticized<br><br>Emotional instability<br><br>Inability to plan ahead<br><br>Thoughtless of consequences | Layla and her dad had a great day together. When he went out to collect her mum, she suddenly decided to cook a surprise roast dinner. There were no potatoes and not enough time, so dinner was only half ready when her parents returned with a takeaway. Her dad asked why she had bothered going to the trouble of cooking, and Layla's patience snapped. She swore at him and threw all the food away. Why did this always happen to her? |

**Differential diagnosis**: affective disorder, adjustment disorder, adult ADHD

## Dissocial personality disorder (antisocial personality disorder)

| Features | Example |
|---|---|
| Forms but cannot maintain relationships<br><br>Irresponsible<br><br>Guiltless<br><br>Heartless<br><br>Temper easily lost<br><br>Someone else's fault | Jake joined the local snooker club and was getting on well with the other members until he accused his opponent of cheating during a 'friendly' game. Jake quickly lost his temper, breaking the other man's nose with his cue and storming out. He was banned from the club, but felt that it was 'the other guy's fault' for cheating; he deserved his broken nose. |

**Differential diagnosis**: acute psychotic episode, manic episode

## Anankastic personality disorder

| Features | Example |
|---|---|
| Doubtful<br>Excessive detail<br>Tasks not completed<br>Adheres to rules<br>Inflexible<br>Likes own way<br>Excludes pleasure and relationships<br>Dominated by intrusive thoughts | Reece, the cricket club's treasurer, had developed his own detailed filing system. When the chairman delivered a big box of receipts, the day before the committee meeting, Reece was annoyed—this would take ages to sort out! The chairman tried to help, but kept ruining the system, and Reece sent him away, staying up all night to do the job *properly*. The next day, he couldn't stop wondering whether he had made mistakes. |
| **Differential diagnosis**: obsessive–compulsive disorder, autistic spectrum disorder | |

## Anxious (avoidant) personality disorder

| Features | Example |
|---|---|
| Avoids social contact<br>Fears rejection/criticism<br>Restricted lifestyle<br>Apprehensive<br>Inferiority<br>Doesn't get involved unless sure of acceptance | Luca had wanted to attend an evening class for ages, but was too anxious to go alone. When a friend finally took him, Luca kept silent. He knew he wasn't as clever as everyone else and worried they would dislike him. He also worried that his friend would stop going and he wouldn't have anyone to talk to. Better to stay at home than be rejected. |
| **Differential diagnosis**: social phobia, autistic spectrum disorder, schizophrenia, depression | |

## Dependent personality disorder

| Features | Example |
|---|---|
| Subordinate<br>Undemanding<br>Feels helpless when alone<br>Fears abandonment<br>Encourages others to make decisions<br>Reassurance needed | Hanne lived with her younger sister Rebecca. Hanne did the housework, but needed Rebecca's advice for even the simplest tasks: 'Rebecca is *so* clever and capable—she makes *all* the important decisions! How would I ever cope without her if she got married and left me alone?' |
| **Differential diagnosis**: reliance on others because of cognitive impairment, anxiety disorder | |

## Investigations

1. Second interview and collateral history: confirm whether *traits* amount to a personality *disorder*.
2. Psychology/psychotherapy assessment.

## Management

Personality disorders *are* treatable. A long-term approach is needed, encouraging the patient to *take responsibility* for their actions. Boundaries are essential and all staff require a clear understanding of the plan and their respective roles.

### Psychotherapy

A range of approaches are used in personality disorders, most drawing on ideas from cognitive behavioural therapy (CBT) and psychoanalysis to varying degrees. CBT models focus very practically on interactions between thoughts, feelings, and behaviours, *here and now*. Psychoanalytical models use the relationship between therapist and patient to understand the past and how this relates to current interpersonal difficulties. Therapies include:

- CBT
- dialectical behavioural therapy (DBT)
- cognitive analytical therapy (CAT)
- mentalization
- therapeutic communities
- psychodynamic and psychoanalytical psychotherapy.

## Medication

Medication is occasionally used to try to improve certain symptoms, facilitating psychosocial treatments. **Antipsychotics** may reduce impulsivity and aggression. **Antidepressants** may have general effects in reducing impulsivity and anxiety. **Mood stabilizers** have been used for labile affect but their effects are unimpressive.

## Treat comorbid problems

Comorbidity (e.g. substance misuse, affective and anxiety disorders) requires management.

## Prognosis

Personality disorders disrupt relationships, education, and employment; some are associated with child abuse and domestic violence. Although personality disorders are persistent, they may change in severity over time. For example, cluster B disorders become less common with increasing age, possibly due to maturation, 'burning out', and the high rates of mortality (suicide and accidents) in this group.

**!** The consensus is that people with a personality disorder are responsible for their actions. Nevertheless, clinicians still have a duty to consider risk modification. Self-harm and violence are most important, usually relating to dissocial and emotionally unstable personality disorders. Consider the emergency assessment of a patient with borderline personality disorder who has self-harmed and continues to threaten suicide. Their *long-term* risk is likely to be high (10% suicide rate) although admission to a psychiatric ward could dramatically reduce their *short-term* risk. However, in some cases, admission may be counter-productive, fostering dependence and disempowering the patient from adopting safer coping strategies. If violent behaviour features, further information is advisable, e.g. from police, probation services, etc. Discussion with senior colleagues is essential.

# REALITY

## General approach: tips, tricks, and cautionary tales

These tips relate particularly to people with borderline or antisocial traits, but may help with any patients who generate strong emotions.

### 1. Wonder 'why?'

If you met a patient scarred head to foot from burns, you would immediately realize that they had been through something awful—it would be obvious that your sympathies would go out to them. Unfortunately, the 'scar' of a challenging personality evokes much less sympathy, despite the possibility of horrific early trauma. Bear this in mind as you speak to them.

### 2. Draw the line

People with personality disorders may have difficulties 'knowing where to stop'. You need to set clear boundaries from the start. Don't recite a list of interview rules, but *expect* appropriate behaviour and deal with problems when they arise: explain *what* they are doing, *why* it is unacceptable, and what *will happen* if it continues (usually ending the interview).

### 3. Know your limits

Your role is to listen and learn from your patients—but you must go home at the end of the day and leave the ward for ever after your attachment ends. You don't have the resources to provide 24-hour support, so be clear about your availability and don't raise your patient's expectations that you will 'be there' for them whenever they need you. Care equally: spend your resources at a rate that allows long-term work with many patients, rather than a few intense days with one.

### 4. Don't believe the hype!

Patients may declare you their super-hero. Be alert to phrases like, 'You're going to be the *best* doctor, ever!' or 'You're not like all the others'. *Don't fall for it!* Those who idealize quickly will often denigrate you at the slightest imperfection, unable to see any middle ground. Expect: 'You're going to be the *worst* doctor ever . . . you're *just* like all the rest'. It feels as bad to be the villain as it felt great to be the superhero—the temptation is then either to reject the patient or to work harder to regain their praise. Don't. Treat them the same as your other patients and take *none* of it to heart. Realize how unstable and disappointing their world is, when people seem so changeable.

## 5. Little things

Rather than promising miracles, be reliable. If you say you'll visit at 2pm. for 20 minutes, do so—no more, no less. This demonstrates that people *can* be reliable, and that in your busy day, they were as important as everyone else.

## 6. How they feel about you ('transference')

People with personality disorders, *by definition*, think and behave in ways that make them difficult to get on with. Their reactions to others are often outdated responses to people and situations that occurred in the past—and may be triggered by seemingly insignificant conversations or actions. They may show any number of emotional responses to your well-meaning bedside manner, e.g. anger, desperation, fear. This can feel confusing and unfair, but acknowledge their feelings and try to think together about what triggered the reaction.

➡ Does the patient have a history of eerily similar relationships, always following the same pattern? This may indicate that some unresolved childhood problem is being played out over and over.

## 7. How you feel about them ('countertransference')

You *will* feel different emotions towards your patients. An awareness of these feelings allows you to decide whether it is appropriate to show them or act on them. A clingy, dependent patient might make you feel that you want to rescue them *or* run away. A common response is to shut off completely from the patient, preventing *anything* good coming from the interaction. Remain neutral and see what happens next, rather than responding automatically. Understand the emotions as a first-hand experience of the way your patient's friends and family feel—remembering that knee-jerk responses won't get you any further than it got them.

## 8. Accept the patient's behaviour as the solution to their problems

Self-harm, shouting, fighting, drug-taking, or casual sex may not be *your* way of dealing with problems, but for your patient, these were the best solutions they had *at the time*. Think about what the behaviour communicates, e.g. drug-taking may be an attempt to sedate painful memories, and casual sex may indicate a need for closeness —to *anyone*.

## 9. Judgements

It is easy to believe that difficult personality-disordered people are 'undeserving' of our care. If likeability defined the role of the patient, we would all be treating very nice but completely healthy people! Be polite and respond professionally to their needs.

➡ If you are having similar sorts of feelings about *all* your patients irrespective of their differing issues, the likelihood is that *you* are the one with the personality problem!

>> *See Safety (p.17) and Mania reality: (p.50) for further tips on boundaries; there is more on transference and countertransference in Suicide Reality (p.64).*

# NEXT STEPS

## An angry husband in primary care

You are a junior doctor working in general practice. Last week you saw Mrs Samantha Charlton, who has been the victim of domestic violence for several years. She finally took your advice and went to a women's refuge. You know the location of this refuge, but her husband, Gavin, does not. You notice that Gavin is due to see you later today. Although he has always been polite and charming towards all the surgery staff, you are aware that he has previous convictions for assault and is a heavy drinker.

You are concerned that he may attend in a very angry mood and demand to know Samantha's whereabouts.

1. What precautions will you take before you see Gavin?
2. Highlight the main points of your risk assessment.

### Issues
- Safety of yourself and others in the surgery
- Maintaining a therapeutic relationship with Gavin, if possible
- Samantha's ongoing safety
- Risk assessment
- Screening for evidence of mental illness
- Management

### Precautions

Speak with the staff on reception and other members of staff at the practice that afternoon, as they are also at risk from Gavin. They need to know a little bit about the situation and possible foreseeable problems. Reception should let you know as soon as he arrives—keeping him waiting is not going to help matters! If he appears intoxicated with drink or drugs, he should be asked to rebook his appointment, maybe for a morning slot to reduce his substance misuse opportunities. Police should be called if he refuses to leave in this situation.

Arrange to see Gavin in a private room, close to the busiest part of the building, e.g. a room off reception is better than one at the far end of an empty corridor. Ensure that it has a panic alarm or, at the very least, a telephone to contact reception for assistance. If you have one, wear a personal alarm and check that it works *beforehand*. Remove clutter from the room, since unnecessary objects may obstruct your exit or be used as missiles or weapons. Arrange the seats in advance (see Safety, p.17). Finally, ensure that the receptionists know where you are seeing Gavin and ask them to check on you frequently.

## Risk assessment

Make sure you have a clear idea of Gavin's agenda before launching into your risk assessment. He may be presenting for purely physical concerns and need treatment. If Gavin has come to find out where Samantha is, be clear regarding your duty of confidentiality—you cannot tell him but you are also his doctor and therefore want to deal with *his* problems.

You must assess the risk that Gavin poses to himself and others (e.g. you, Samantha, other staff and patients in the surgery, Samantha's family, any children). This requires that you take a brief psychiatric history and MSE, focusing on any evidence of mood disturbance, psychosis, morbid jealousy, or threats to harm himself or others. You should ask about current drug and alcohol use and whether he has any plans to act violently or ever carries weapons. Gather information about any previous violence or self-harm and discuss details of violent offences if possible, e.g. why he thinks they happened and whether he feels any remorse.

You may need to speak with the police if you identify a high risk to an identified person (e.g. Samantha) and consider psychiatric referral if there is evidence of mental illness.

➡ Gavin has a diagnosis of dissocial personality disorder and alcohol dependency. He shows consistent patterns of violent behaviour that are impulsive, irresponsible, and lack any sense of remorse or empathy. When intoxicated he can be extremely volatile, and his threshold to act violently is even lower. However, intoxicated or not, he is still answerable for his actions and must take full responsibility for them. In order to legally defend criminal behaviour the mental illness must impair cognition and volition *substantially*. This is not so in Gavin's case.

### Film list

*Girl, Interrrupted* (1999)—borderline and dissocial personality traits

*Lock, Stock and Two Smoking Barrels* (1998)—dissocial personality disorder (Big Chris)

NB: Monica from the American sitcom *Friends* has anankastic personality disorder

### Books

Boyle, J. (1977) *A Sense of Freedom*. London: Pan Books. Autobiography examining dissocial personality disorder within its social context.

Duisberg, K.W. (2003) *The Good Patient*. New York: St Martin's Press. Fiction following a patient with borderline personality disorder as she travels from self-harm through psychotherapy, finally emerging with an understanding of herself and relationships. Demonstrates the potential for improvement, if not cure.

Wurtzel, E. (1994) *Prozac Nation*. London: Quartet Books, 1996. Despite Wurtzel's formal diagnosis of depression, she demonstrates clear borderline traits.

### Quotes

I knew that I had come face to face with someone whose mere personality was so fascinating that, if I allowed it to do so, it would absorb my whole nature, my whole soul, my very art itself.
**Oscar Wilde**

Everyone is a moon, and has a dark side which he never shows to anybody.
**Mark Twain**

Before you judge me, try hard to love me,
Look within your heart then ask, Have you seen my childhood?
**Michael Jackson, *Childhood* (song)**

## Note

1. Kristen Waterfield Duisberg (2003) *The Good Patient*. New York: St Martin's Press.

## References/Further reading

Balint, M. (1957) *The Doctor, His Patient and the Illness*. London: Tavistock Press.

Bateman A.W. and Fonagy, P. (2004) *Psychotherapy for Borderline Personality Disorder: Mentalization Based Treatment*. Oxford University Press.

Campling, P. and Haigh, R. (1999) *Therapeutic Communities: Past, Present and Future*. London: Jessica Kingsley.

Caspi, A. and Silva, P.A. (1995) Temperamental qualities at age 3 predict personality traits in young adulthood. *Child Development*, **66**, 486–98.

Dolan, B., Warren, F., and Norton, K. (1997) Change in borderline symptoms one year after therapeutic community treatment for severe personality disorder. *British Journal of Psychiatry*, **171**, 274–9.

Linehan, M.M. (1993) *Cognitive Behavioural Treatment of Borderline Personality Disorder*. New York: Guilford Press.

Loehlin, J.C. and Nichols, R.C. (1976) *Heredity, Environment, and Personality: A Study of 850 Sets of Twins*. Austin, TX: University of Texas Press.

Main, T. (1987) *The Ailment and Other Psychoanalytic Essays*. London: Free Association Books.

Ryle, A. and Kerr, I.B. (2002) *Introducing Cognitive Analytic Therapy: Principles and Practice*. Chichester: John Wiley.

Virkkunen, M., Nuutila, A., Goodwin, F.W., *et al.* (1987) Cerebrospinal fluid monoamine metabolite levels in male arsonists. *Archives of General Psychiatry*, **44**, 247.

 Go to www.oxfordtextbooks/orc/stringer for an array of additional references, including indicative mark sheets for OSCEs, self-assessment questions, guidance, and exercises.

# INDEX